By the same author (books in French):

– *Sugar and Nutrition*
– *The Enslaved Patient*
– *The Paths To Individual Sovereignty*
– *GMO, Meat-bone Flour And Other Nasties*
– *Forbidden Discoveries, The Beljanski Case*
– *Being Happy, The Theater of Life*
– *Let's Not Be Fooled!*
– *The Beginning of a Change is Coming!*

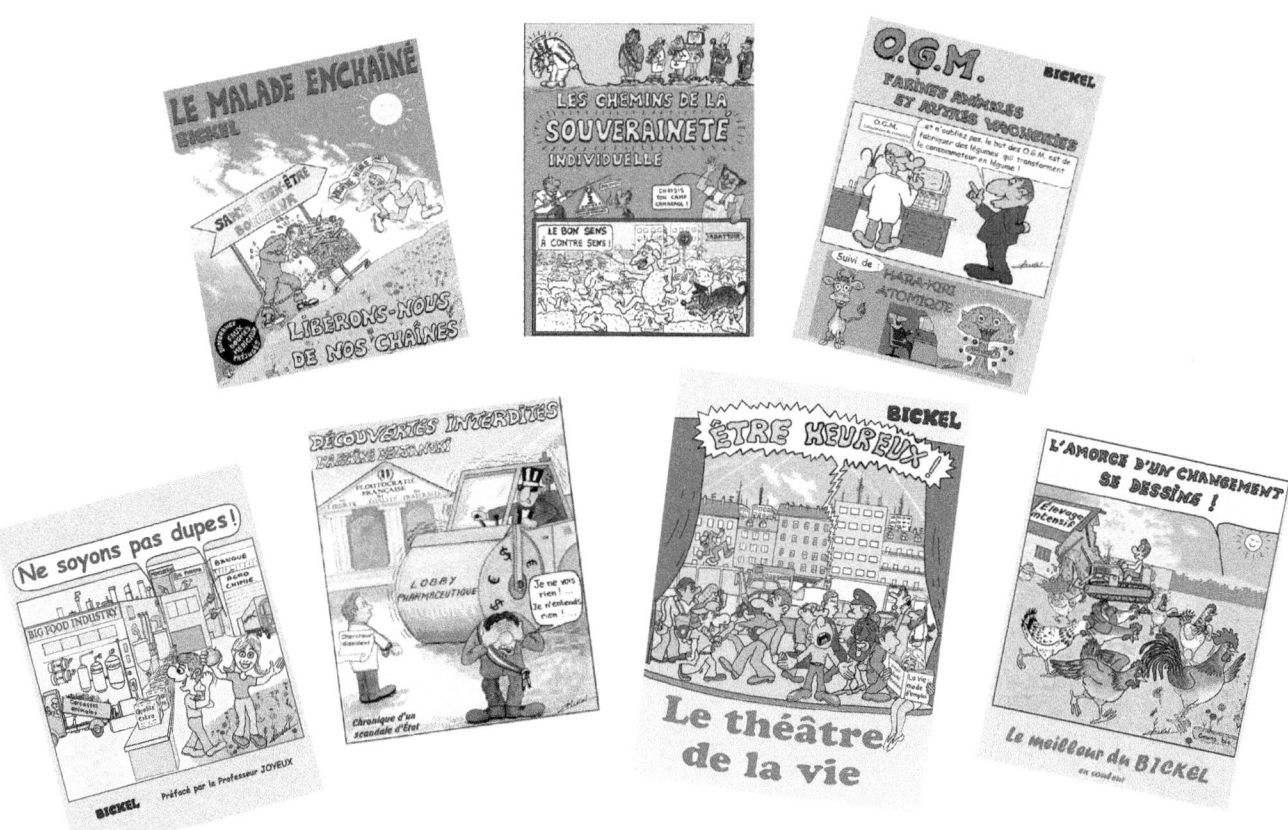

Talma Studios
231, rue Saint-Honoré
75001 Paris – France
www.talmastudios.com
info@talmastudios.com

© Bickel (www.bickel.fr)
All rights reserved

ISBN: 979-10-96132-54-6
EAN: 9791096132546

VACCINATION: THE GREAT ILLUSION

Drawings, texts and layout by Bickel

2nd Edition (2020)

Translated by Antoine Metaxian

Reviewed by Catherine Frompovich,
Ingri Cassel and Dewey Ross Duffel

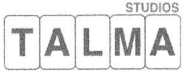

Commentary

Common sense and a sense of humor are the same thing, moving at different speeds. A sense of humor is just common sense, dancing.

William James (1842-1910)
American philosopher &
physician

René Bickel's *Vaccination: The Great Illusion* illustrates just how farcical the pharmaceutical industry's spin about vaccines actually is. If we can apply Dr. James' quotation as allegory, Bickel's superbly illustrated book about the history of vaccines and vaccinations 'dances' and even 'rocks'. Cartoonist René Bickel's ingenious use of humorous illustrations makes translating Big Pharma's stories about vaccines surprisingly funny, if not just plain common sense. I am very pleased to have been asked to be the consultant for the English translation of this French artist's exceptional depiction, via art and humor, of one of the more seriously-flawed medical and supposed preventive healthcare measures of modem times, in my opinion as a consumer health researcher and author.

Catherine J. Frompovich
www.catherinefrompovich.com

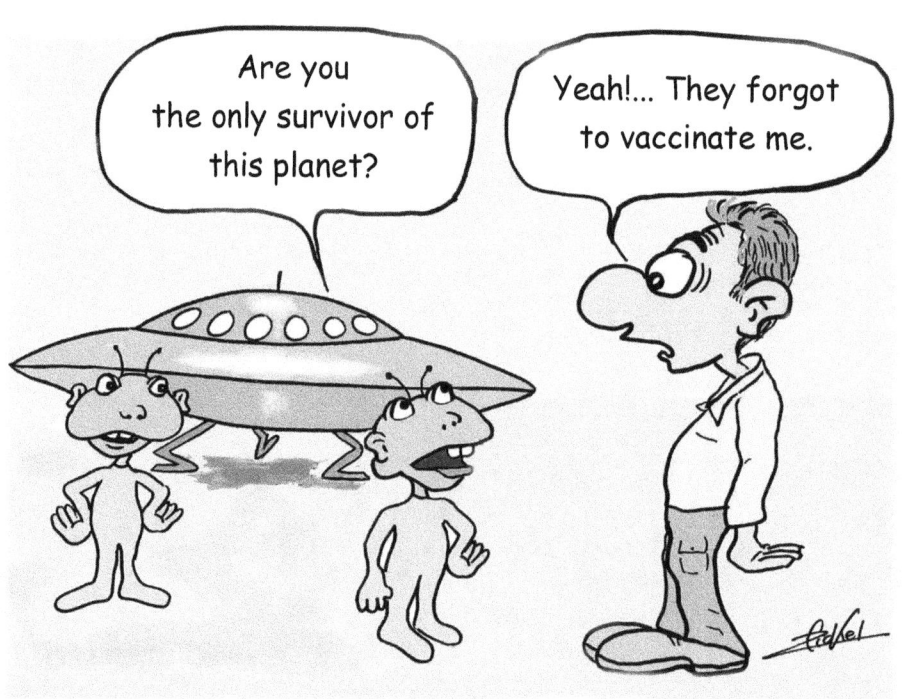

Foreword

As a physician who practiced medicine for fifty years, I saw many cases where patients undoubtedly experienced adverse reactions to vaccines/vaccinations that other physicians did not recognize as such. Early on in my practice I saw the unfortunate damage that vaccines and vaccinations were causing children, so I devoted my energies to medical research about vaccines. What I uncovered revealed disastrous information that vaccine makers were not publicizing in their studies. As a result of personal experiences with both patients and science, I made the conscious decision to become a physician advocate for vaccine safety, patient and parents' rights to information regarding vaccines.

I was one of the "early birds" to publish papers about vaccine damage and as such have written numerous papers and books about vaccines in my time. Even though my work was from a medical scientific viewpoint, I can appreciate and recommend the efforts that cartoonist René Bickel puts forth in this book that graphically details in humor the history of vaccines and vaccinations along with the perils that medicine and the pharmaceutical industry keep under wraps.

I applaud Mr. Bickel for his efforts in trying to bring some semblance of reality to a very serious health problem: vaccines, their ineffectiveness, and most of all, their adverse side effects.

I hope readers enjoy his cartoons as much as I did.

Harold E Buttram, MD
Board Certified,
Environmental Medicine (USA)

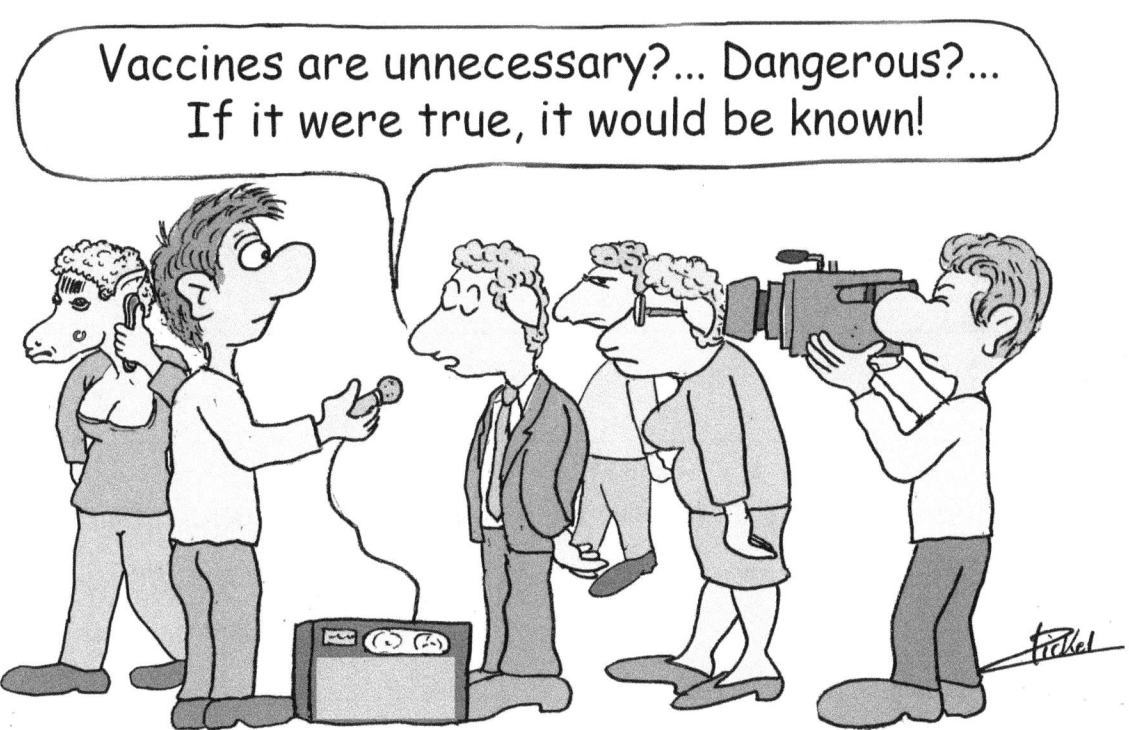

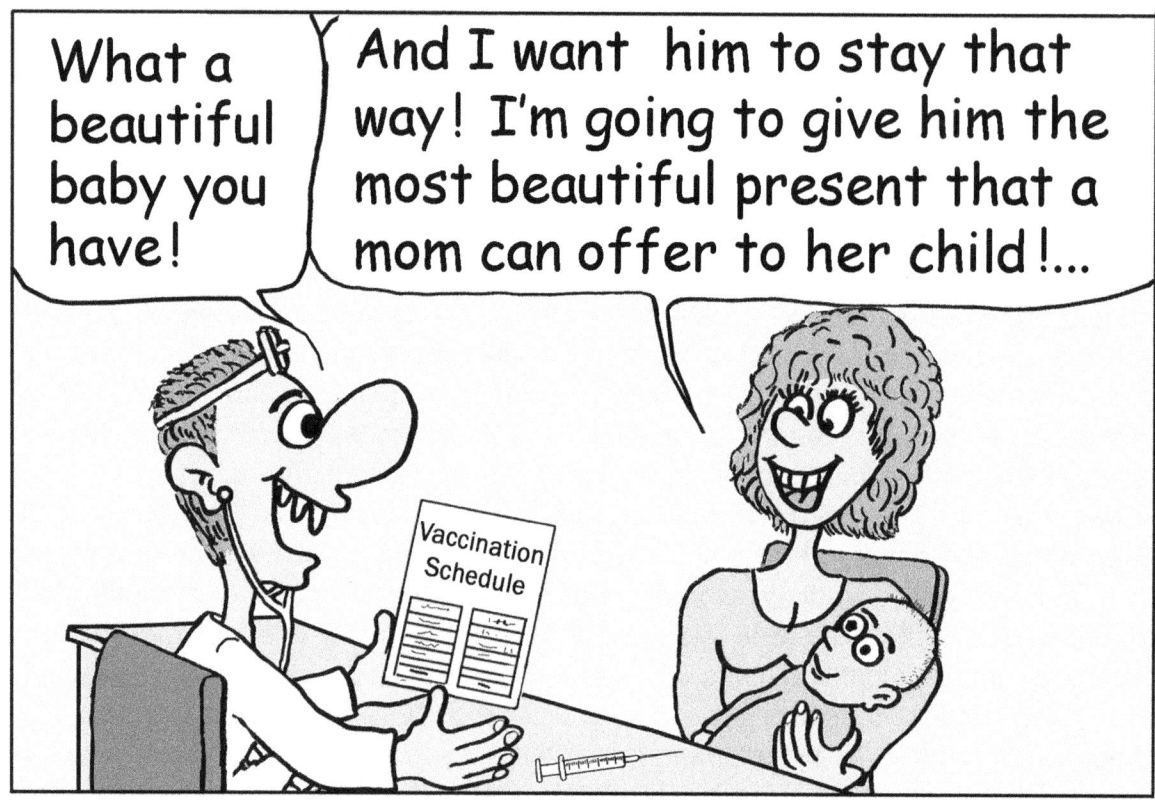

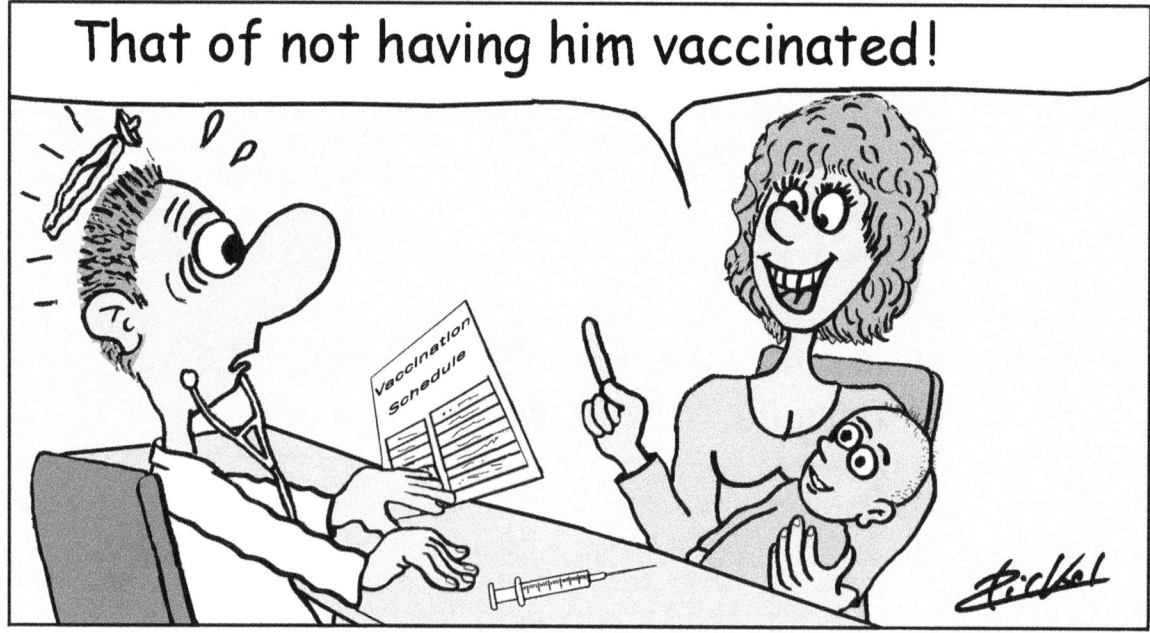

> Vaccines are the backbone of the entire Pharmaceutical Industry. The vaccinated children become clients for life.
>
> Dr. Sherri TENPENNY

In the newspapers and encyclopedias, in schools and universities, everywhere error rides high and basks in the consciousness of having the majority on its side.

GOETHE

Presentation

Hi! My name is Healthrix. My girlfriend is Libertix. We present this book to provide crucial information for your health and life.

This book belongs in everyone's hands.

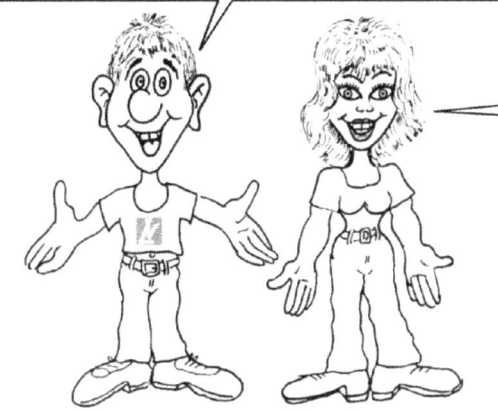

All the information in this book can be verified scientifically and historically.

A bibliography is provided to support this work.

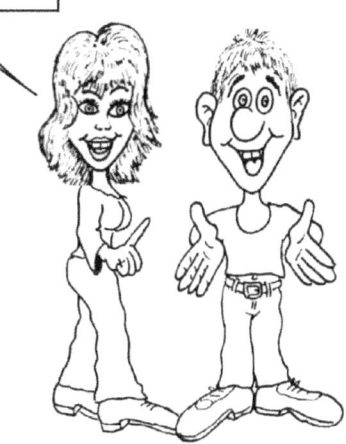

Those who manufacture vaccines do not want parents and healthcare consumers to know the facts because that would ruin their money-making business.

Vaccines: The Great Illusion

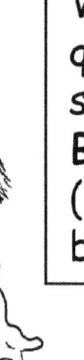
"We have been taught and lied to that vaccines prevent disease and save lives."

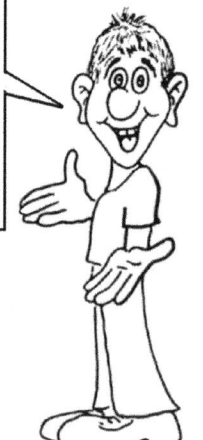
"When you study vaccinations, many questions arise which, for many of us, seem impossible to believe.
But what if the opposite were true?
(in other words, vaccines do not prevent but contribute to disease.)"

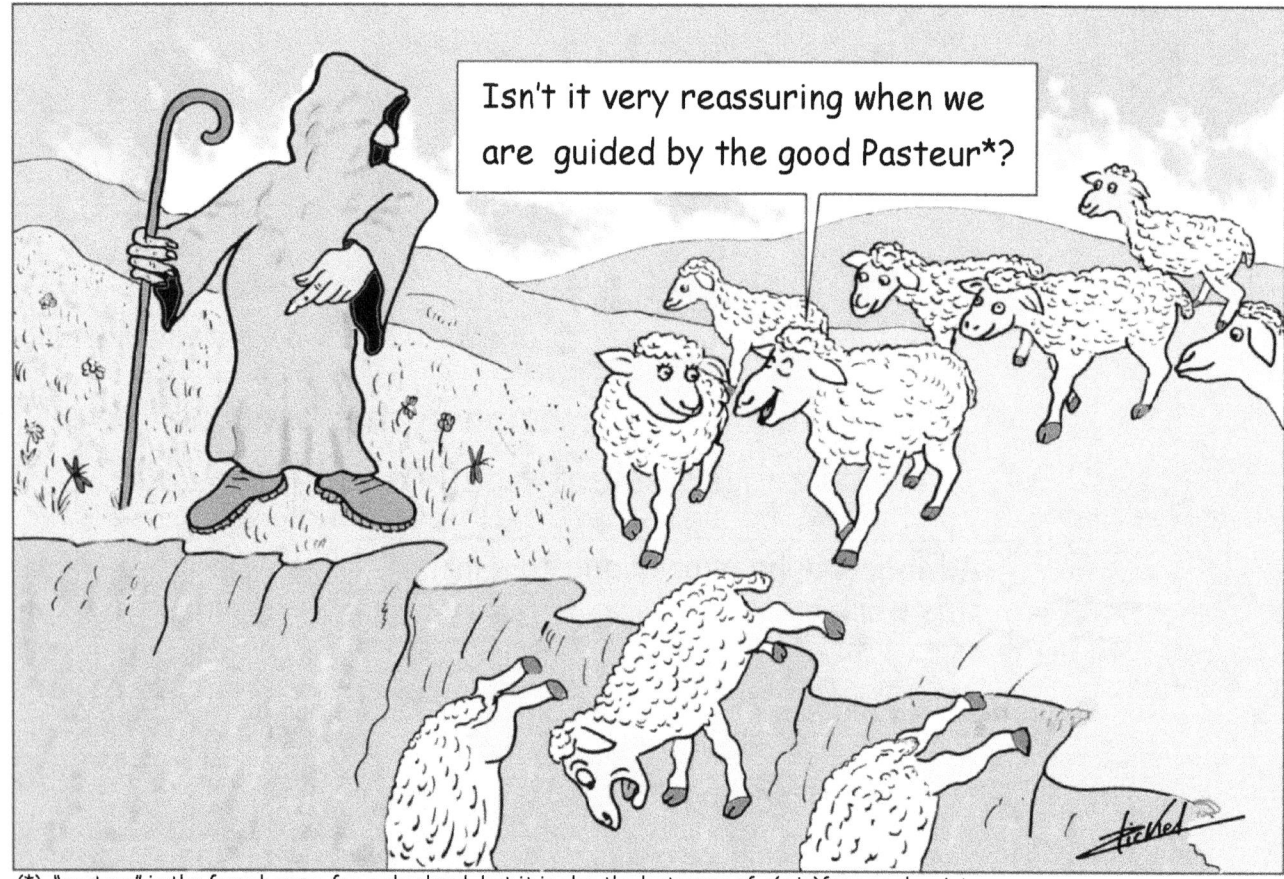
"Isn't it very reassuring when we are guided by the good Pasteur*?"

(*) "pasteur" is the french name for a shepherd, but it is also the last name of a(n in)famous chemist...

> *Communities tend to be guided less than individuals by conscience and a sense of responsibility. How much misery does this fact cause mankind! It is the source of wars and every kind of oppression, which fill the earth with pain, sighs and bitterness.*
> Albert EINSTEIN

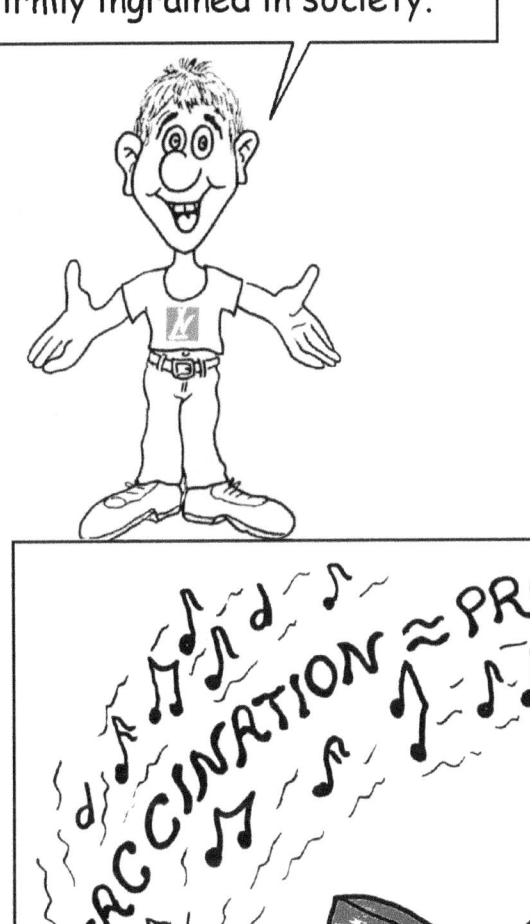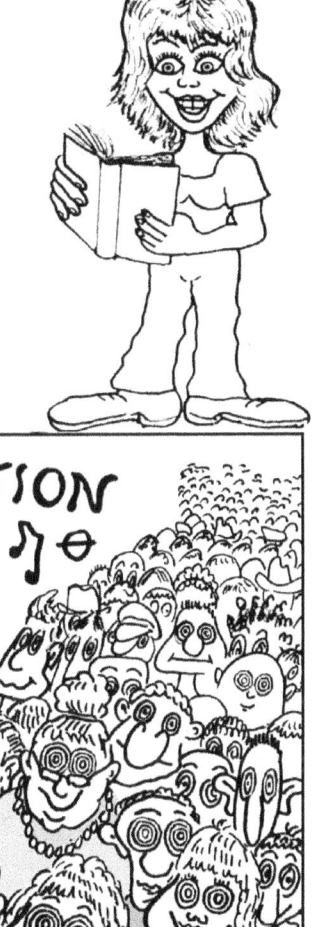

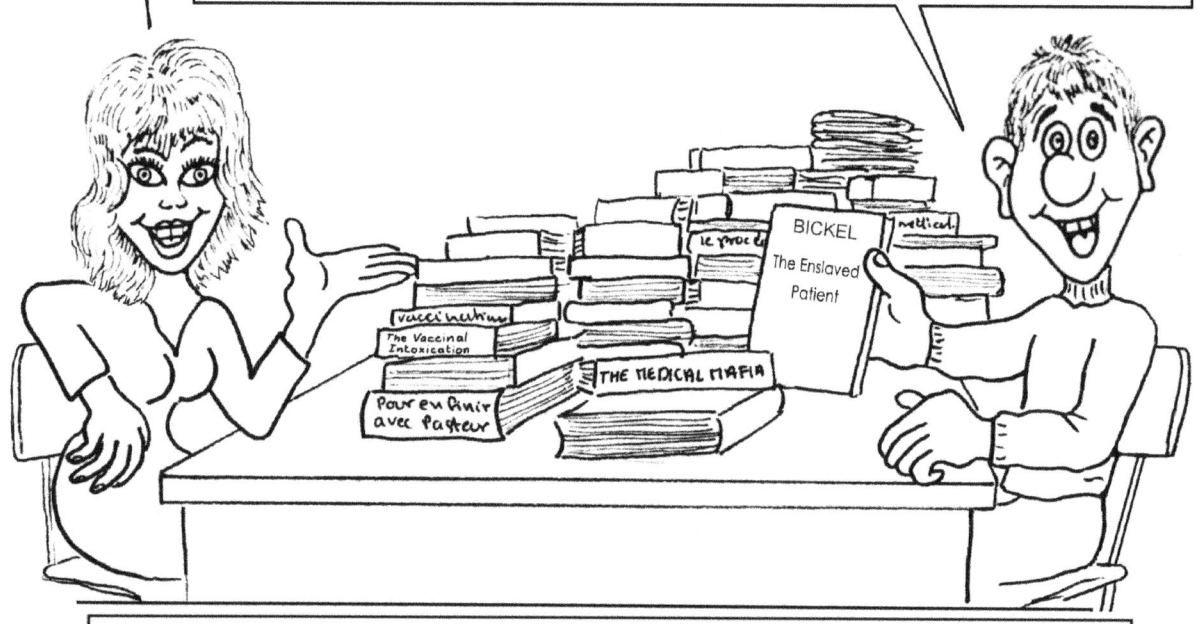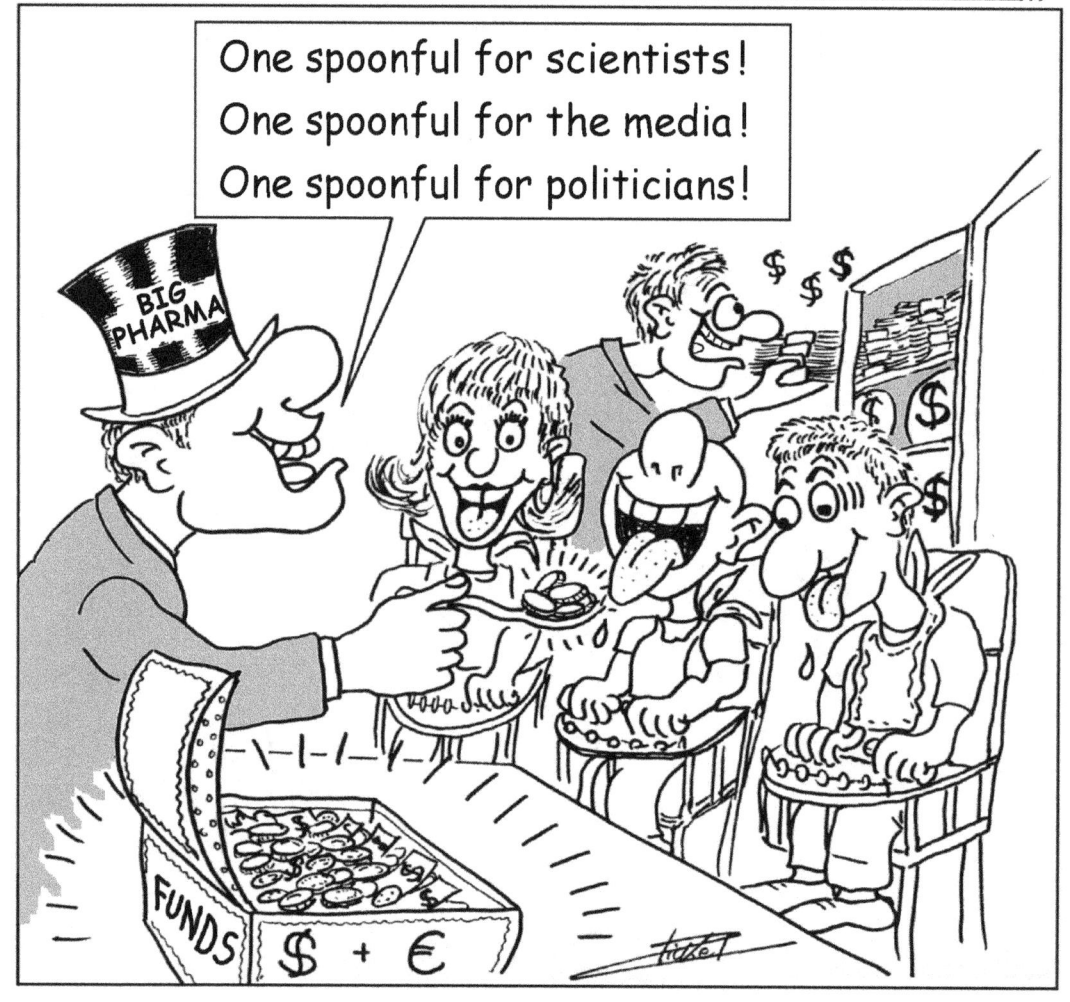

Vaccines: The Great Illusion

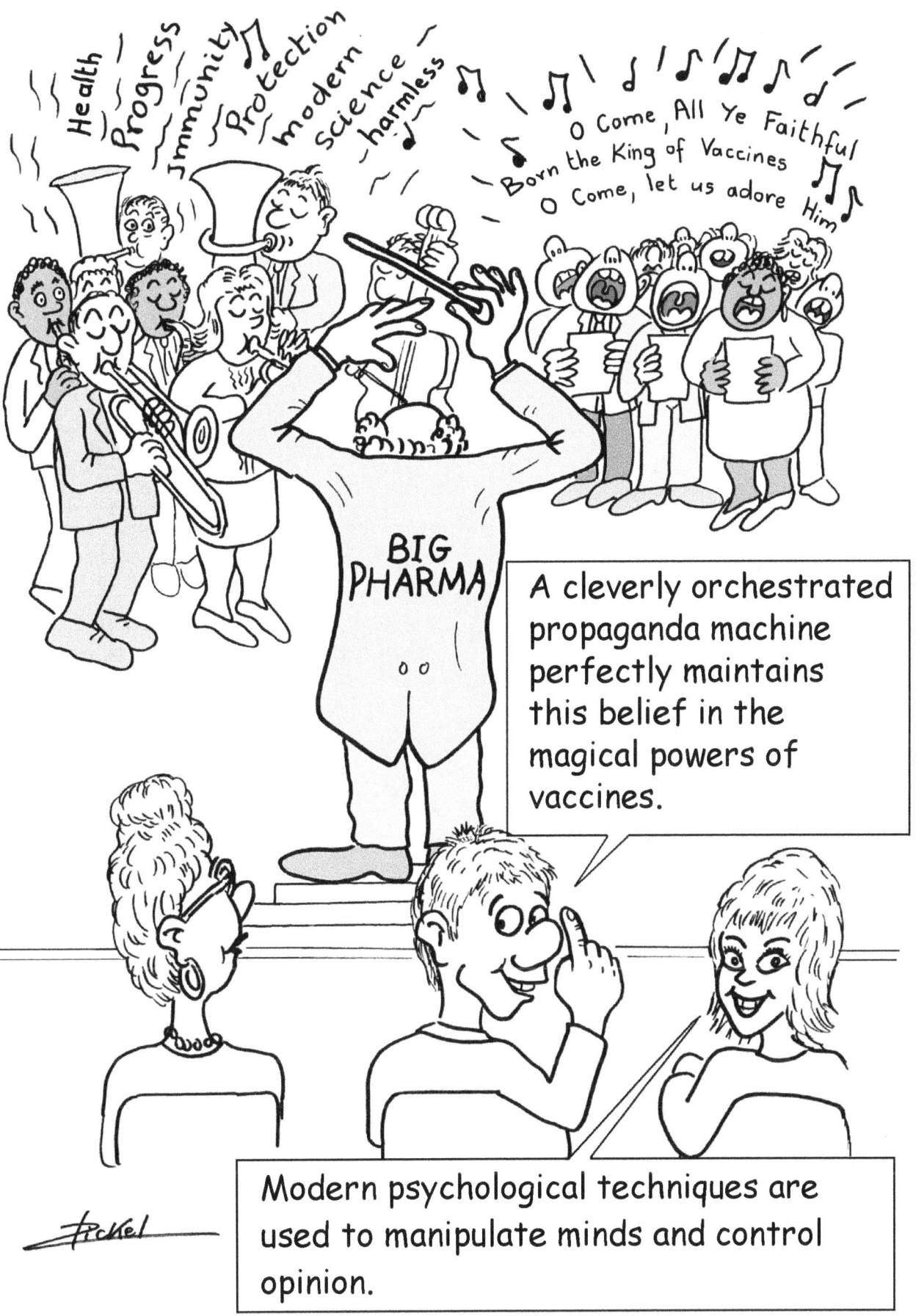

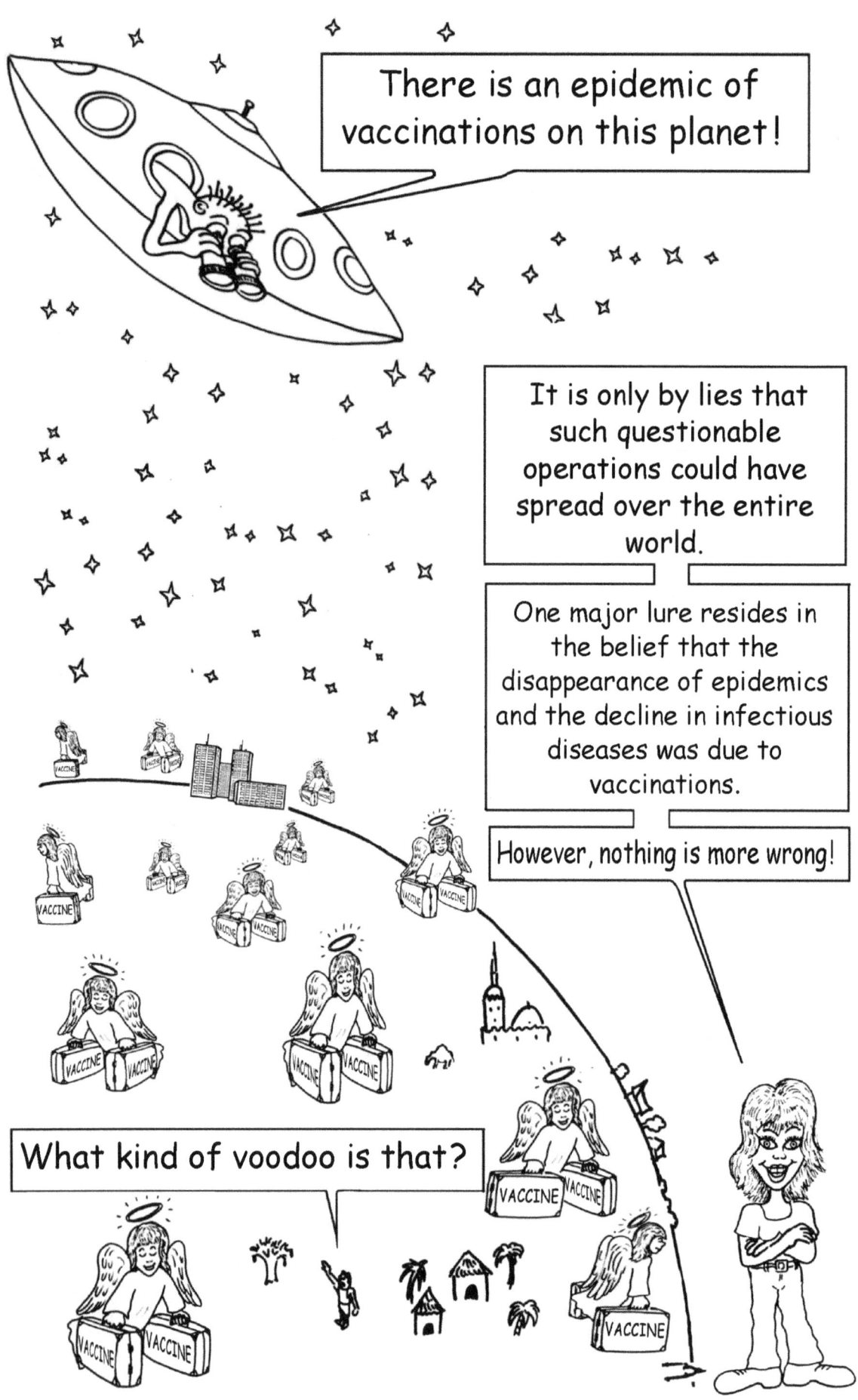

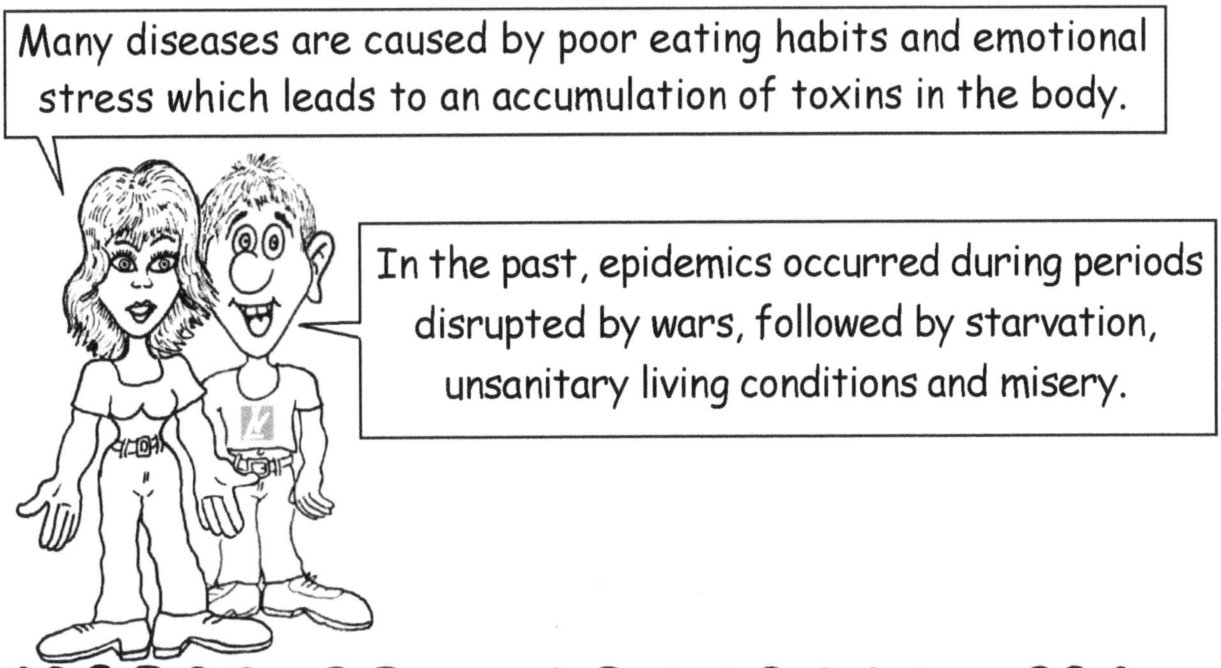

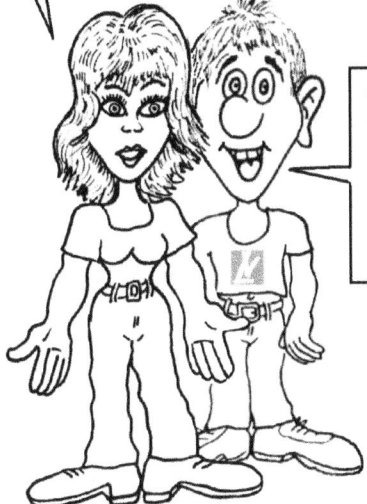

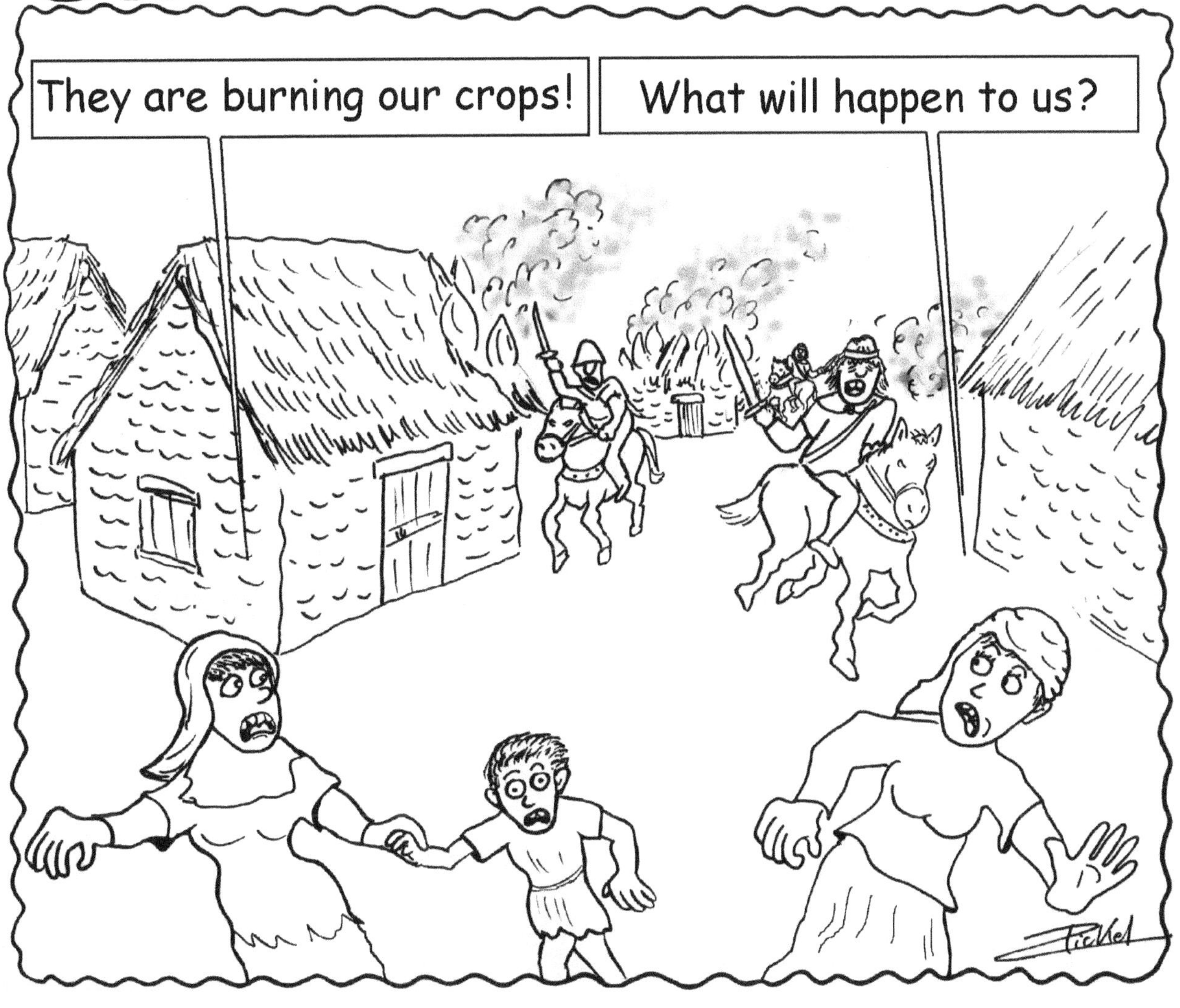

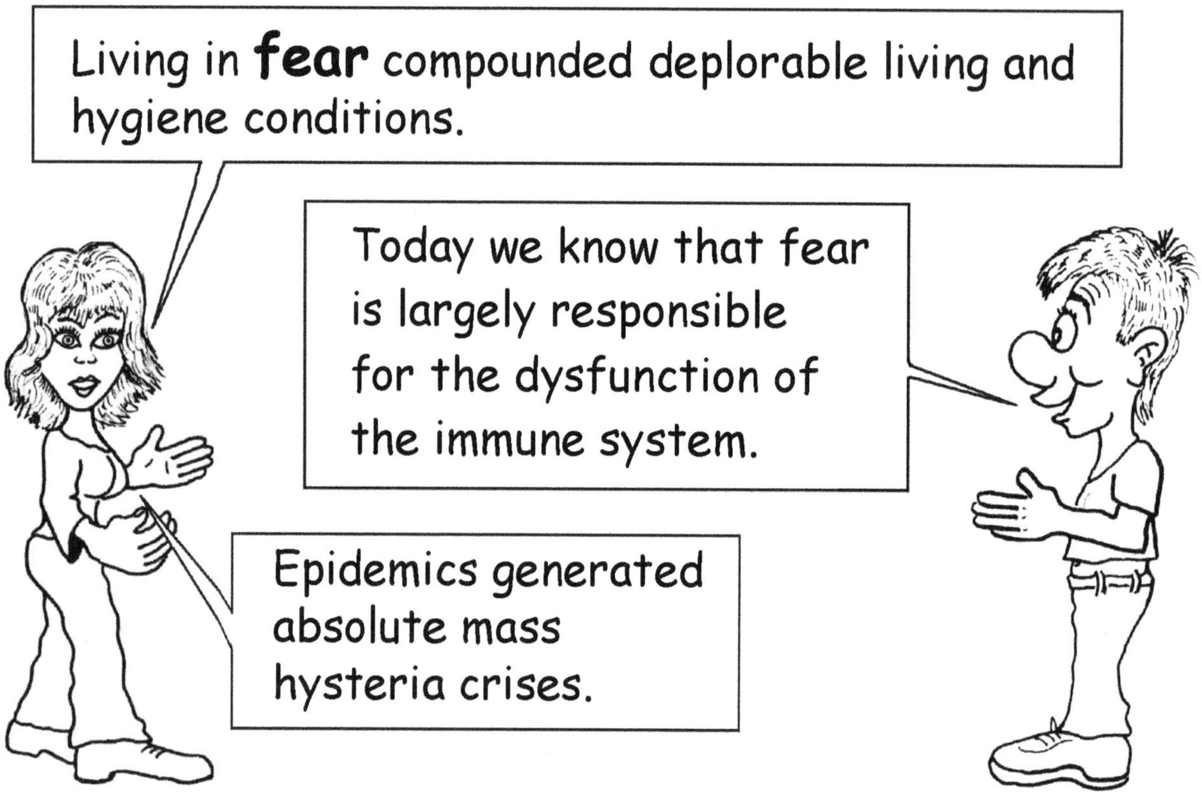

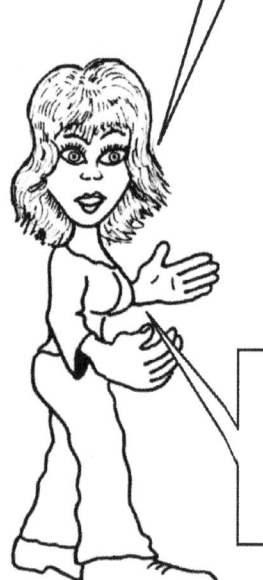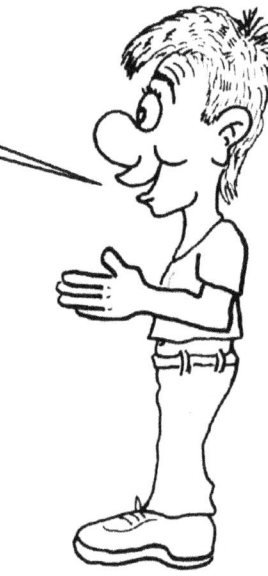

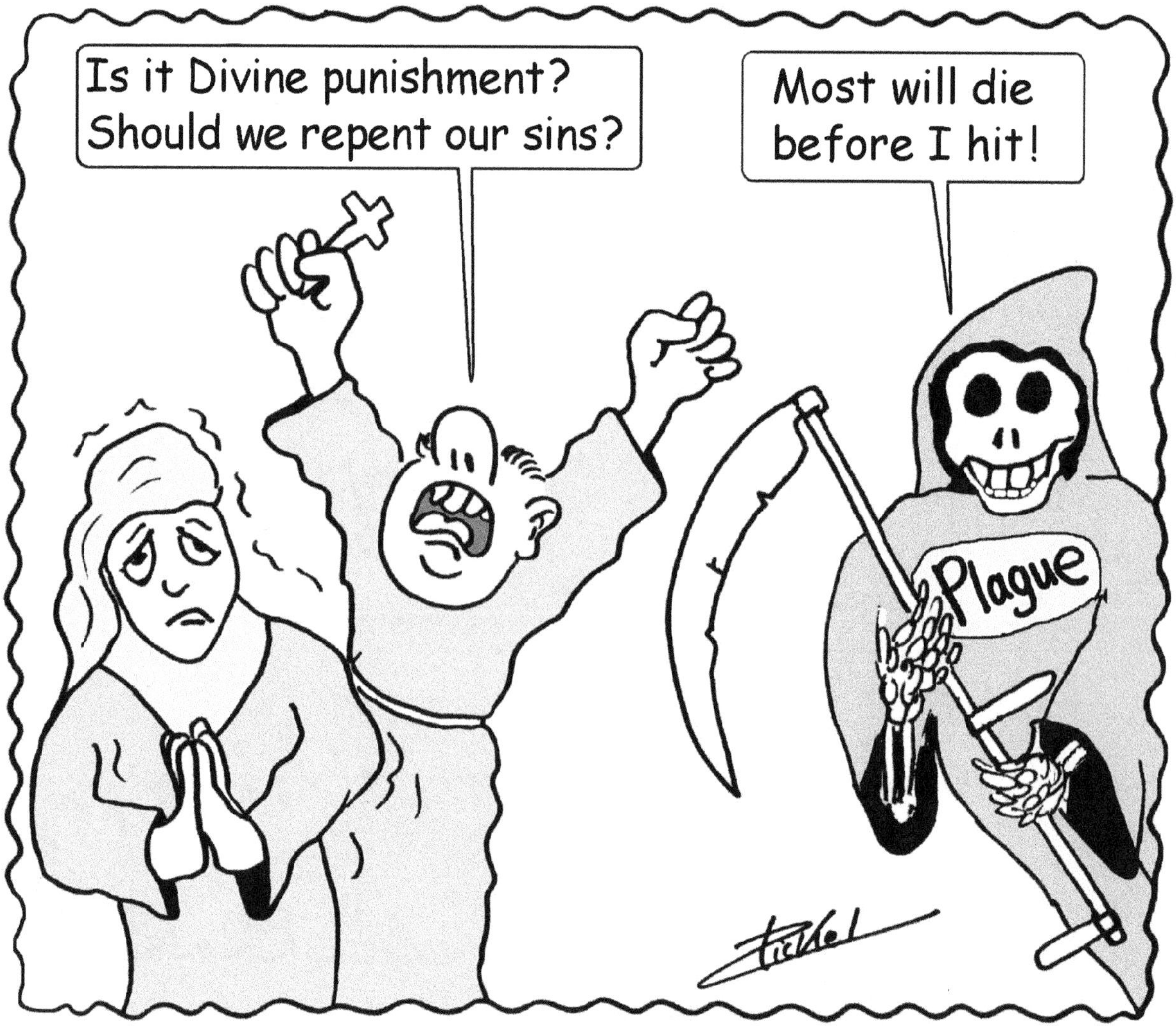

Slaves at the beginning of the industrial era

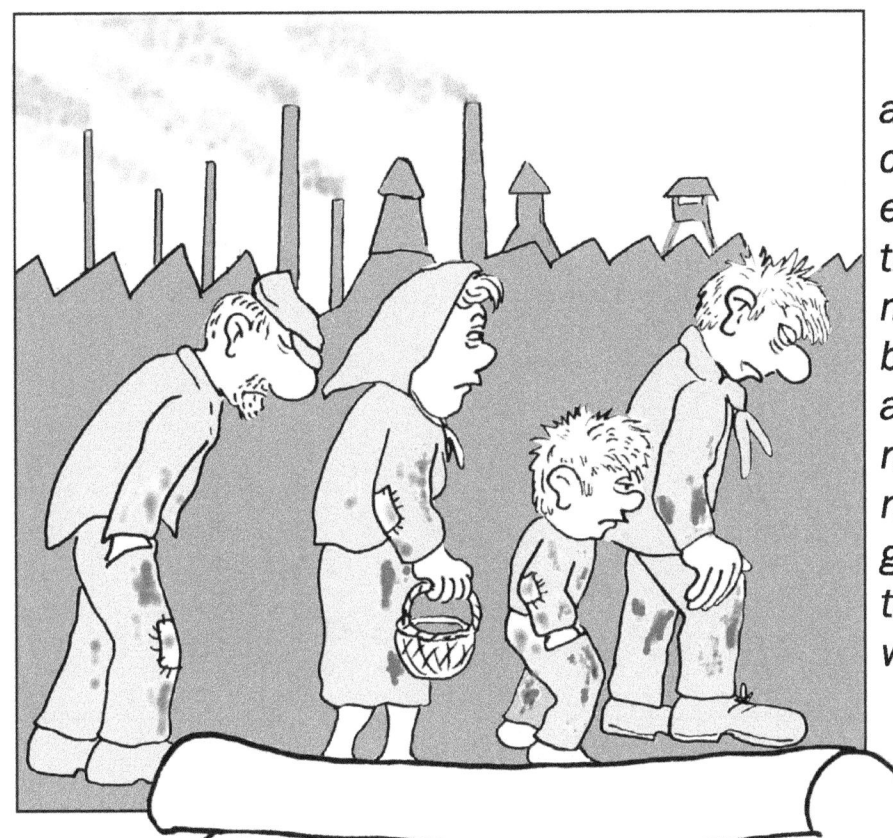

You should see them arrive every morning in the city and leaving every evening. There is among them a multitude of pale, meager women, walking barefoot in the mud ... and an even larger number of young children no less dirty, nor less gaunt, dressed in rags totally stained with the oil of works.

Doctor Villermé (1840)

We are told about the ethics of life; we have no right to commit suicide; suicide is a cowardice ...
Yet, every day we partially commit suicide.
- I am committing suicide when I consent to remain inside premises in which the sun cannot penetrate ever.
- I am committing suicide when I spend hours on a work that I know is useless.
- I am committing suicide when I do not satisfy my stomach with the quantity and quality of foods that I need.
- I am committing suicide every time that I agree to obey men and laws that oppress me.

Libertad (1907)

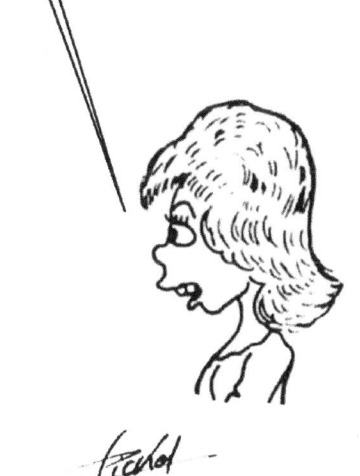

The working class living conditions were inhumane. Daily they worked between 12 and 16 hours, sometimes from childhood.

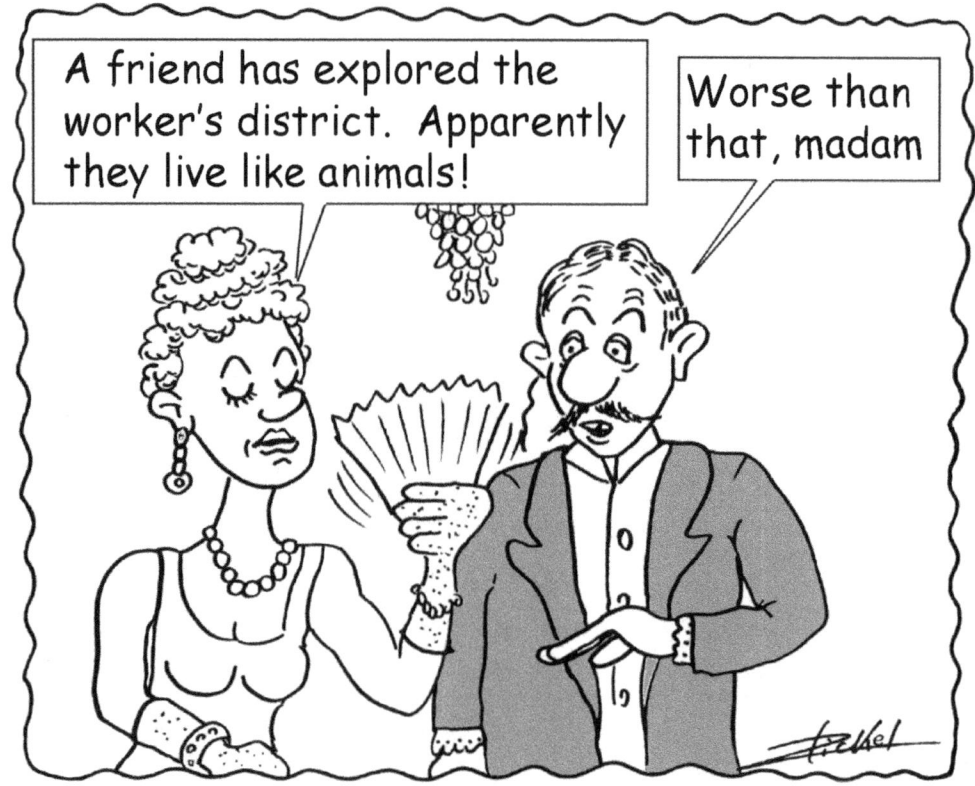

Due to a lack of means, families were cramped together in unhealthy slums, without clean tap water, without latrines and lived in rooms where the sun never penetrated.

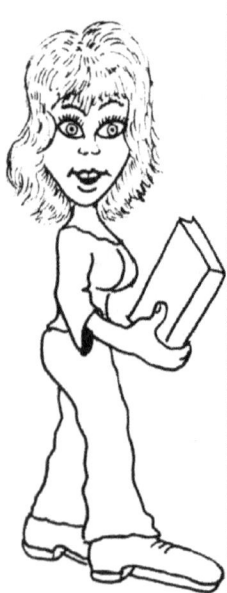

"To live, for them, means not to die."

This tragic sentence is that of Doctor Guépin, describing in 1835 the life in Nantes of a homeworking weaver:

"If you want to know how he is housed, for example go to the street of the manures, which is almost exclusively occupied by this class; enter, bowing your head, into one of these cesspools, opened on the street and located below its level.
One must have walked down these aisles where the air is damp and cold as in a cellar; one must have felt his foot slipping on the dirty ground and feared falling into this mud, in order to get an idea of the terrible sensation that is felt upon entering the home of those wretched workers.
Enter, if the foul smell that you breathe does not make you step back.
Be careful, because the uneven floor is neither paved nor tiled, or if it is, the tiles are covered with such a thick layer of grime that one cannot see them at all.
And you see these three or four beds, poorly supported and leaning, because the twine which attaches them to their cankered frames has not resisted well itself. A bench, a blanket made of tattered fringes, seldom washed because there is only one. This is the place where, often without fire in winter, without sunlight in the daytime, in the brightness of a candle of resin in the evening, men work during fourteen hours for a salary of 15 to 20 sous."
The workers in the factories, many of who were women and children, were equally unfortunate.

Living in a state of slavery and submission weakens immunity.

Alcohol caused enormous devastation among the lamblike workers.

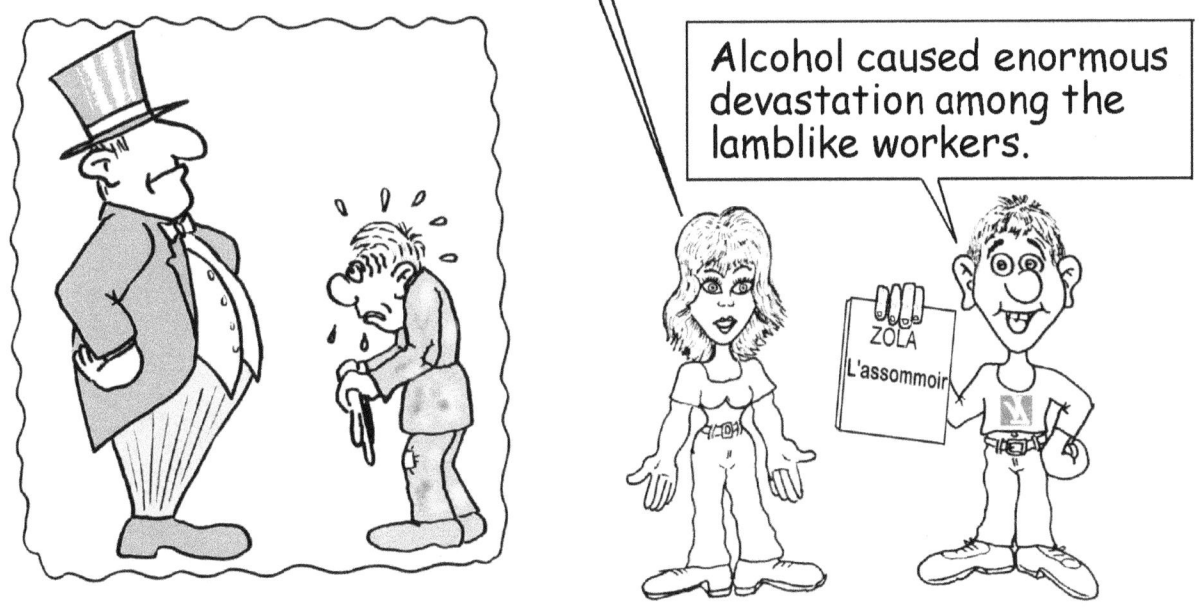

Adding to this was a diet lacking (or deficient in) vital nutrients such as vitamin C [1] and protein. Hence, all conditions were present to cause high mortality by infectious diseases or premature aging.

Nowadays, we can find fresh produce in all seasons, even though they may be sprayed with pesticides.

Workers' meager budgets drove them to buy only bread and potatoes. Fruits and vegetables were considered less nutritious.

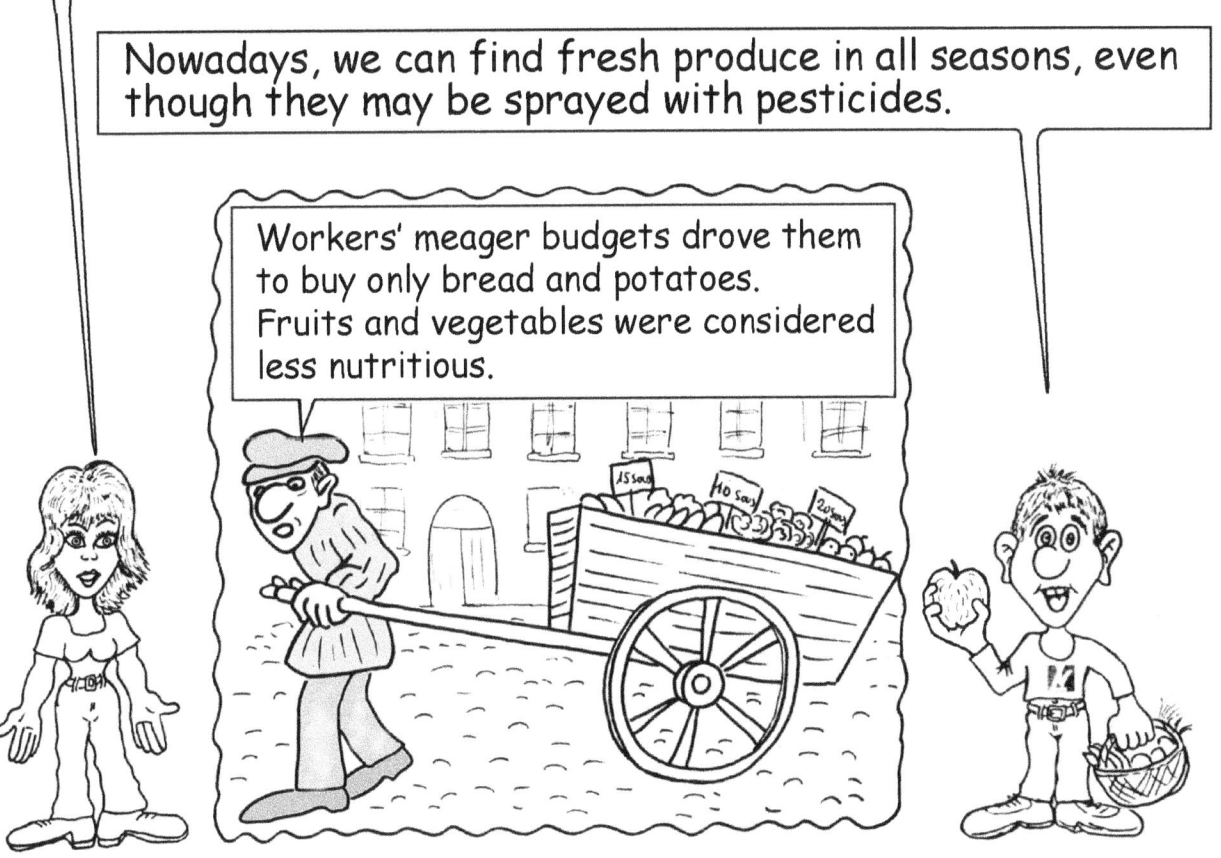

[1] Vitamin C plays a crucial role in the metabolism of the body.

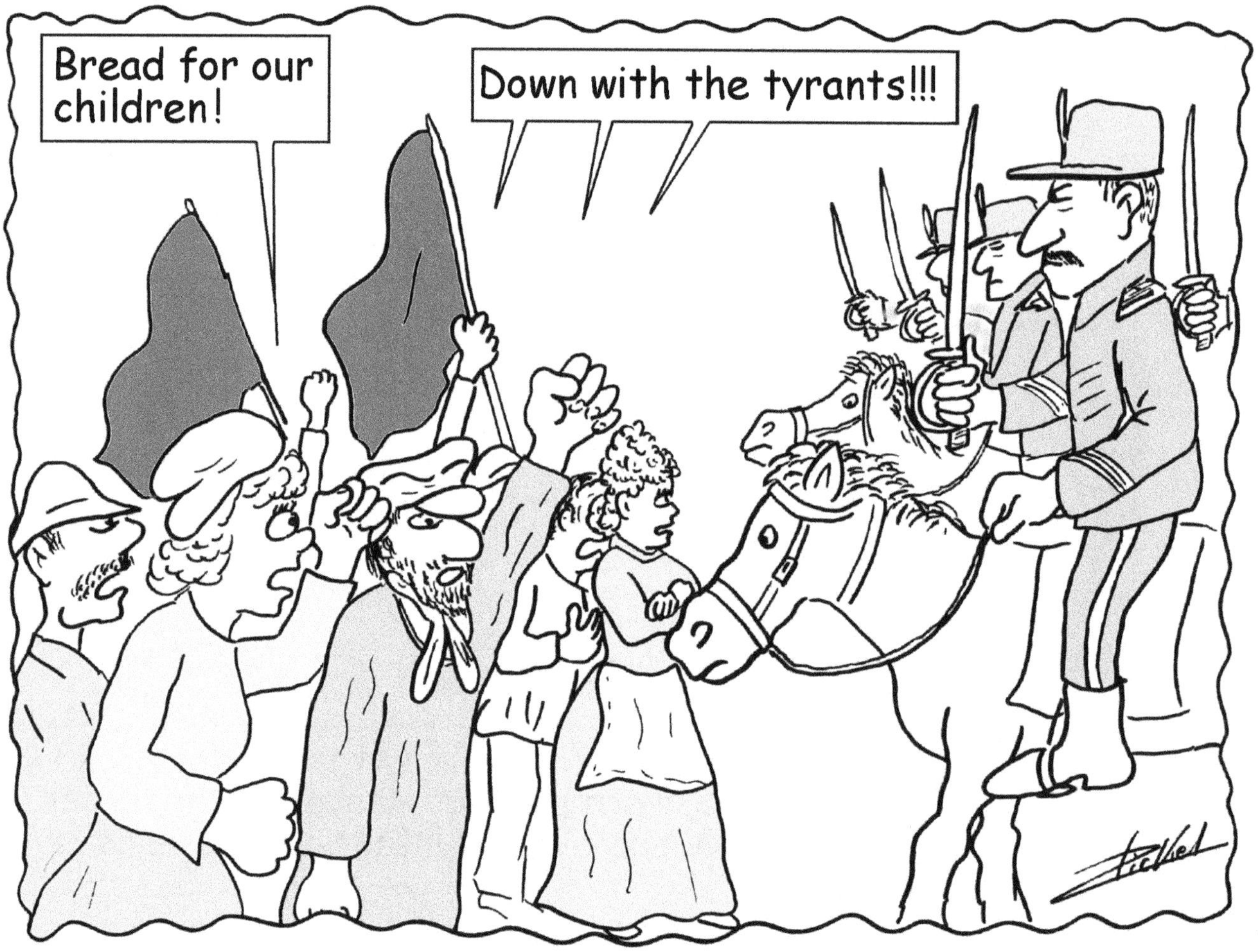

> **Bread for our children!**
>
> **Down with the tyrants!!!**

Confronted with ruthless bosses often bribing political authorities, workers rebelled in spite of violent repressions.
Thanks to many men and women who were abused and suffered greatly, conditions essential for health have improved gradually. Civic and social changes made significant improvements in health, spuriously attributed to medicine, and vaccines in particular.

> The vaccines, which gradually appeared at that time, did not play a beneficial role in health: quite the contrary.

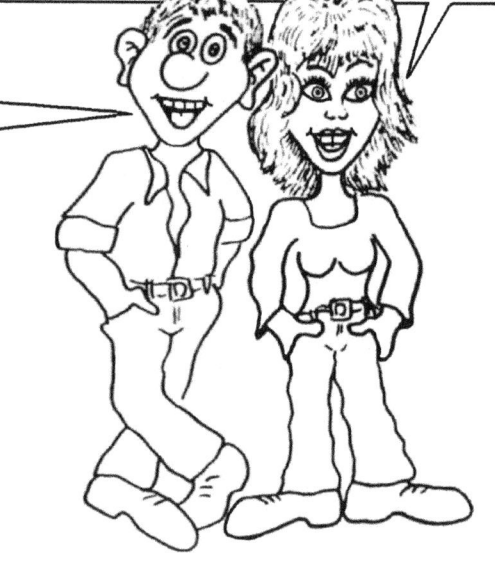

Vaccines: The Great Illusion

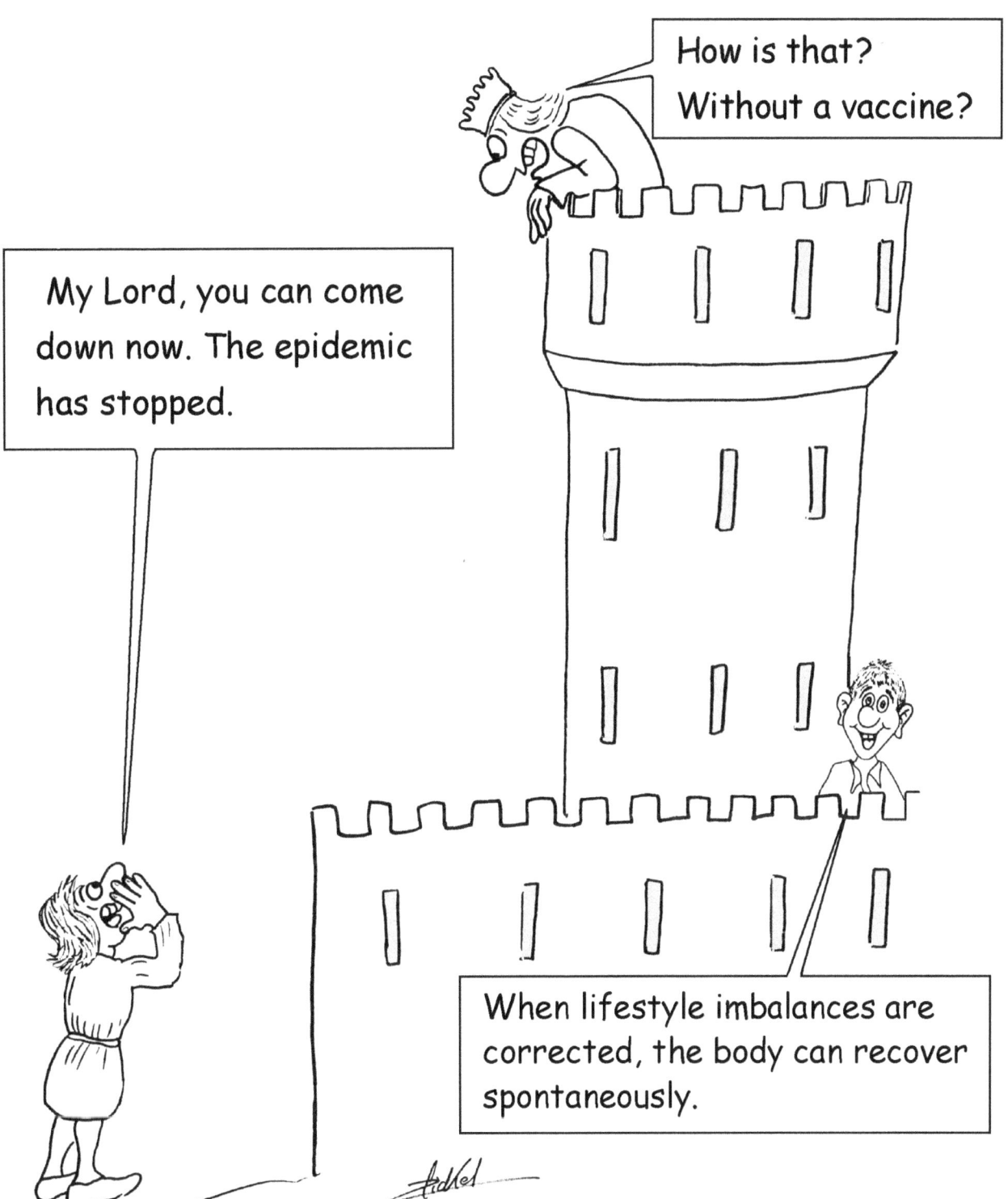

The scientists and the doctors take credit for the glory of an evolution which is due in fact to the plumbers and to the farmers! It is thanks to them that a better hygiene has developed and that we could get a better food. (...)
With good nutrition, you can ensure a good immune system and you are no longer vulnerable to diseases.

Peter Duesberg
Professor of cellular and molecular biology at the University of Berkeley

Vaccination Theory

Vaccinations consist of stimulating the immune system by introducing a microbial aggressor—either attenuated, killed or manufactured by genetic engineering—into the body.

Vaccinating against an infectious agent supposedly causes the immune system to keep a memory of that agent for a certain —rather an uncertain— period of time.

However, that theory is undermined by the discovery and observation of modern immunology.

Watch out! We're keeping our eyes on you.

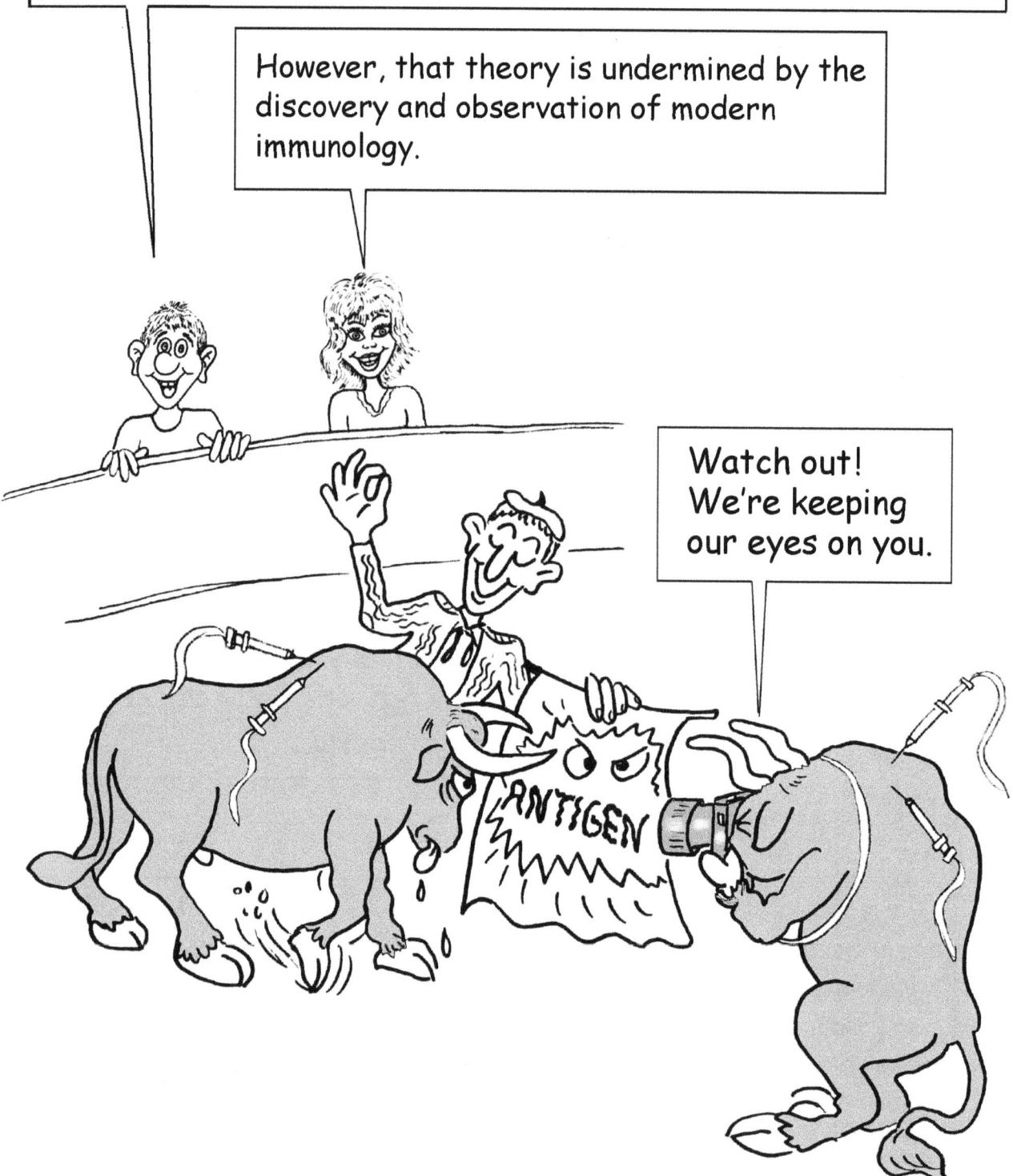

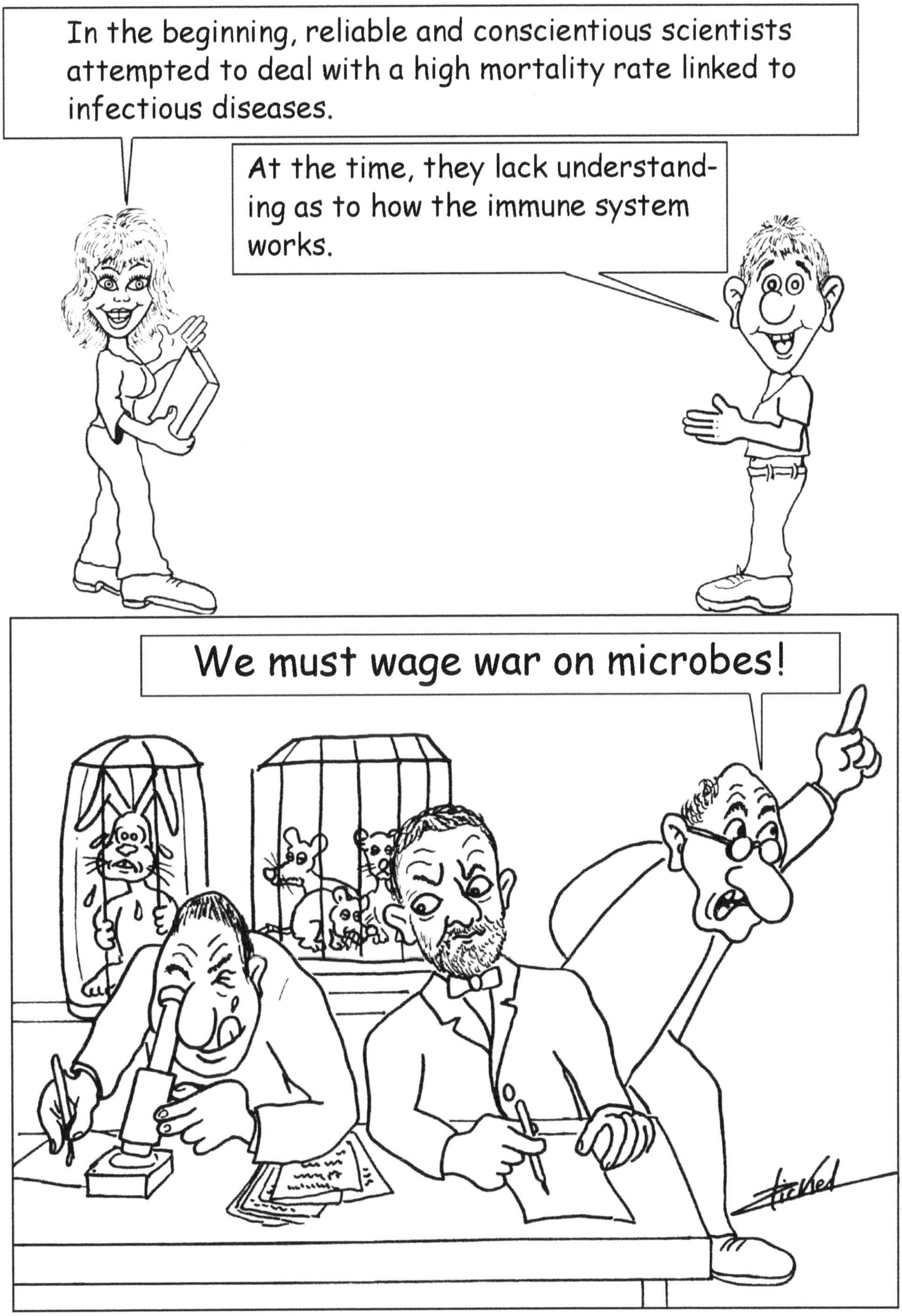

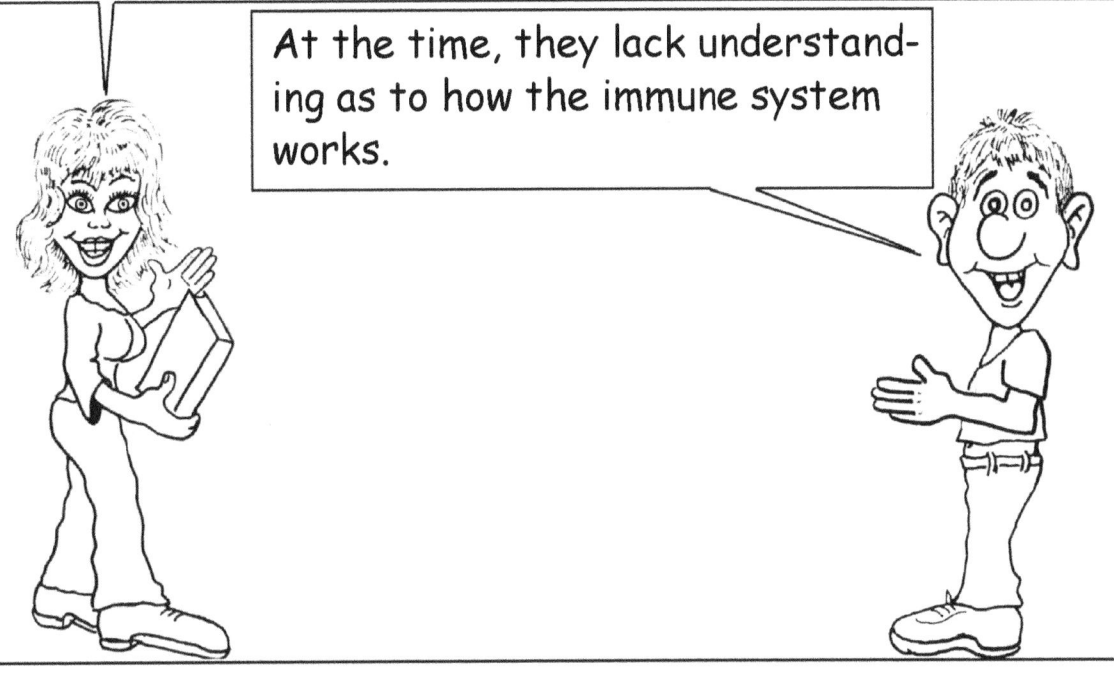

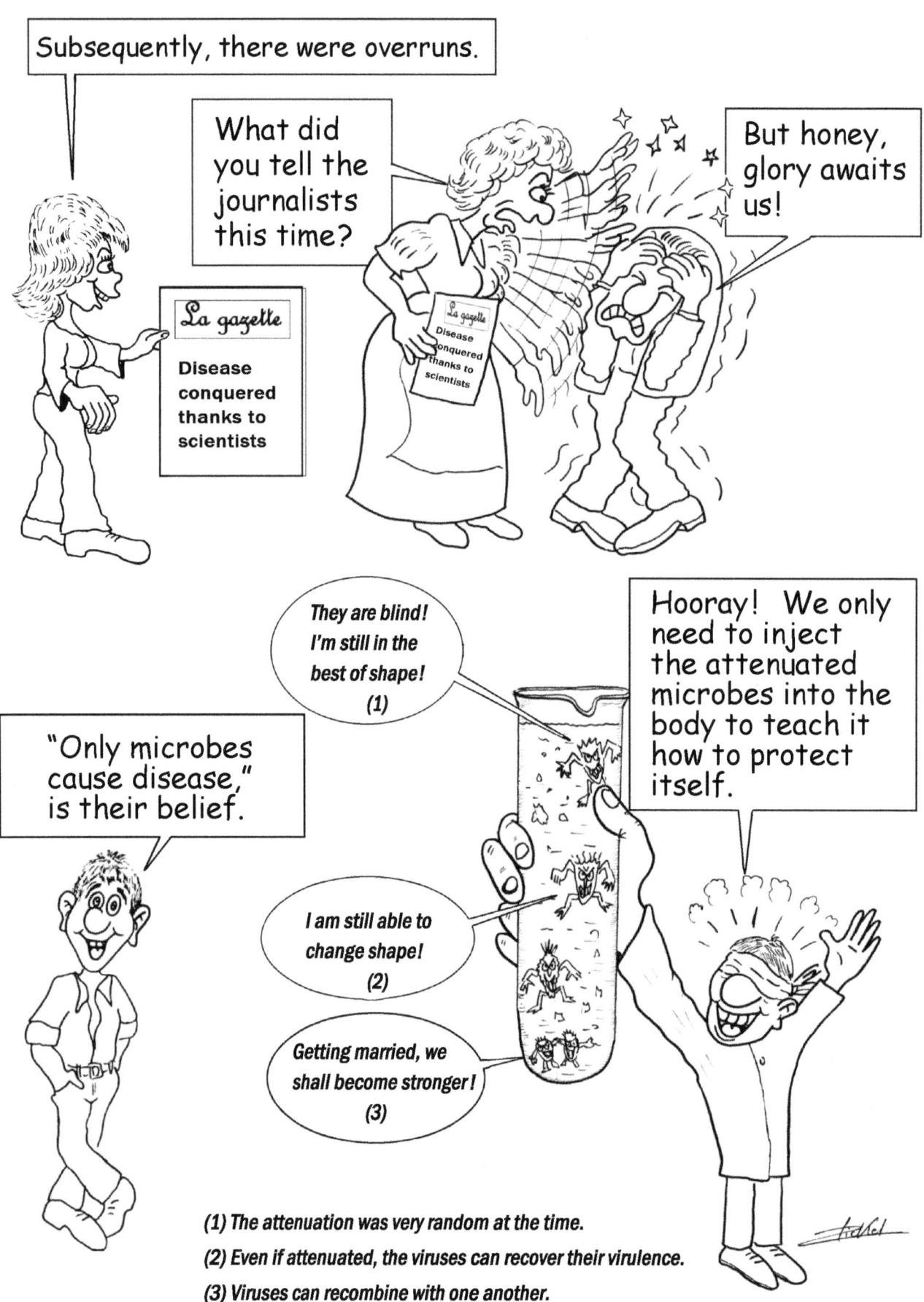

COWination

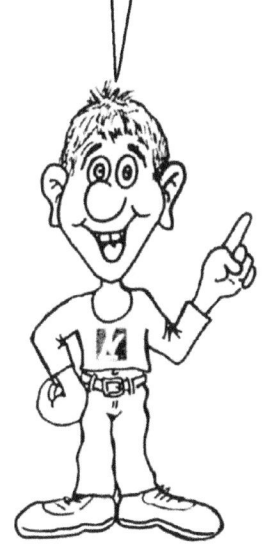

Vaccination comes from an old and unproven technique consisting of injecting pus from patients infected by a mild form of smallpox. That technique was aborted because it reactivated and amplified epidemics.

Jenner, an English pseudo doctor of the 18th century, applied a new method, using pus from sick cows.

I always thought vaccination was a COWardice act.

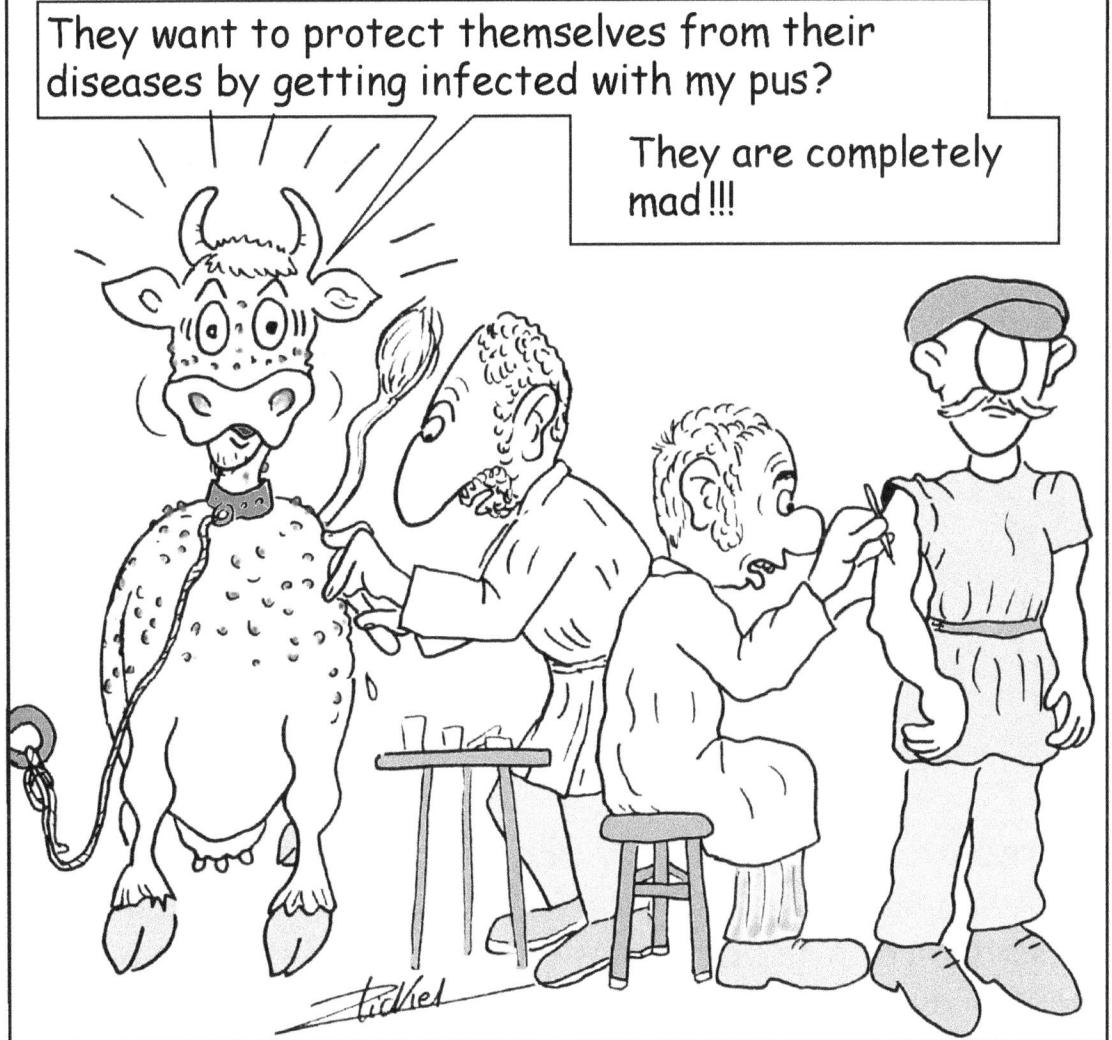

They want to protect themselves from their diseases by getting infected with my pus?

They are completely mad!!!

In the 1880s, a chemist, Louis Pasteur, became famous plagiarizing the works of his contemporary, Prof. BÉCHAMP. [1] BÉCHAMP's work is considerable but remains ignored because it does not fit in with the pharmaceutical industry's theory for making money and profiting from disease.

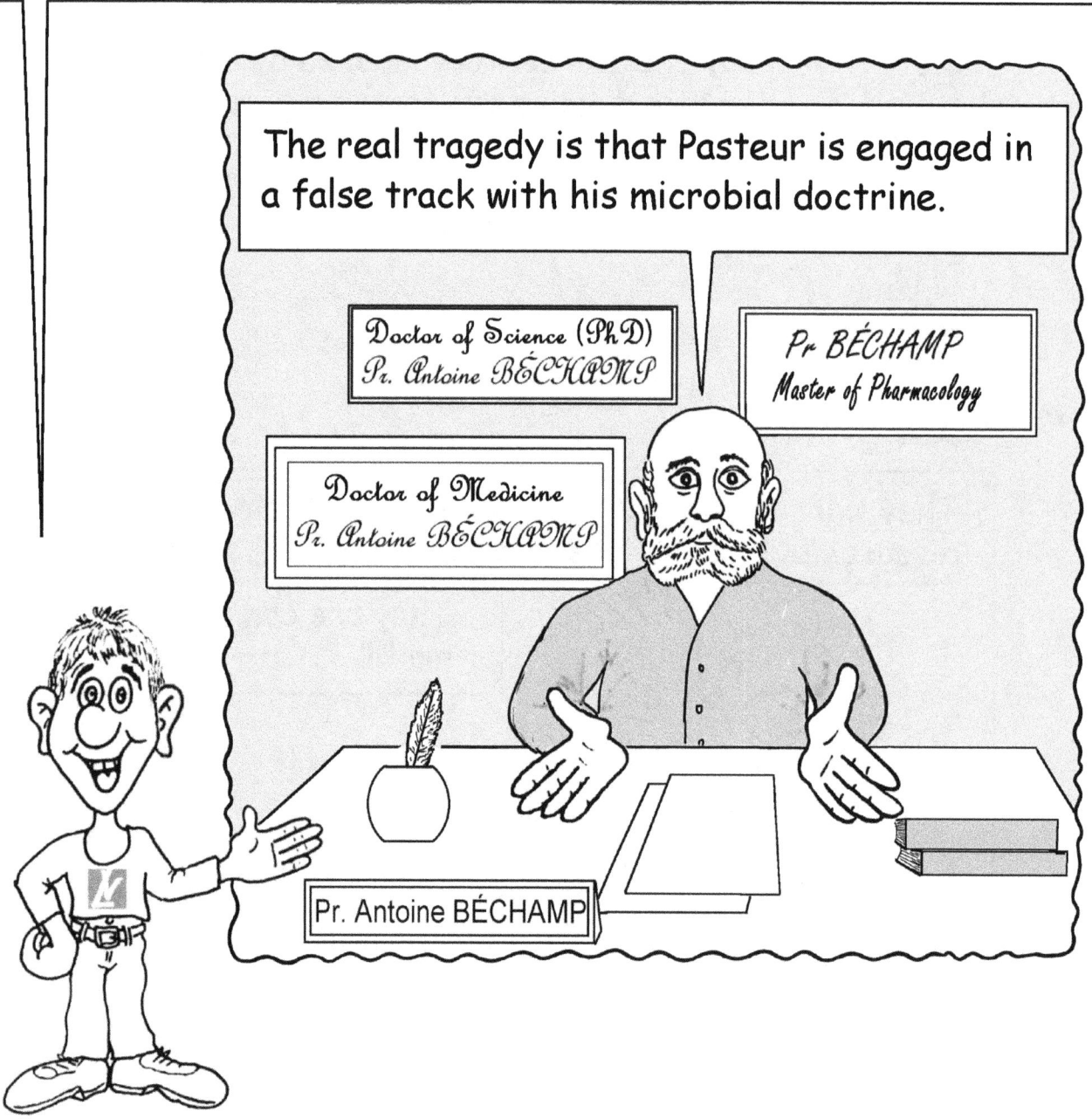

The real tragedy is that Pasteur is engaged in a false track with his microbial doctrine.

Doctor of Science (PhD)
Pr. Antoine BÉCHAMP

Pr BÉCHAMP
Master of Pharmacology

Doctor of Medicine
Pr. Antoine BÉCHAMP

Pr. Antoine BÉCHAMP

(1) Professor at the School of Pharmacy in Strasbourg.
Professor at the Faculty of Medicine in Montpellier.
First dean of the Faculty of Medicine and Pharmacy in Lille.
Master of Conference at the Academy of Medicine in Paris.

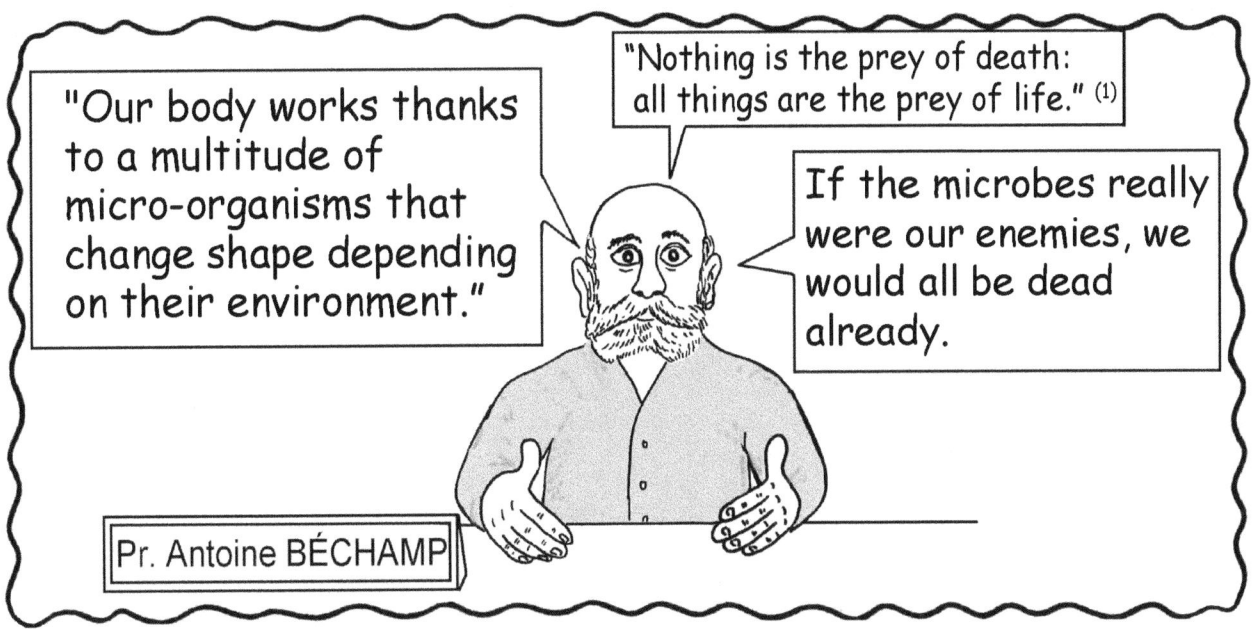

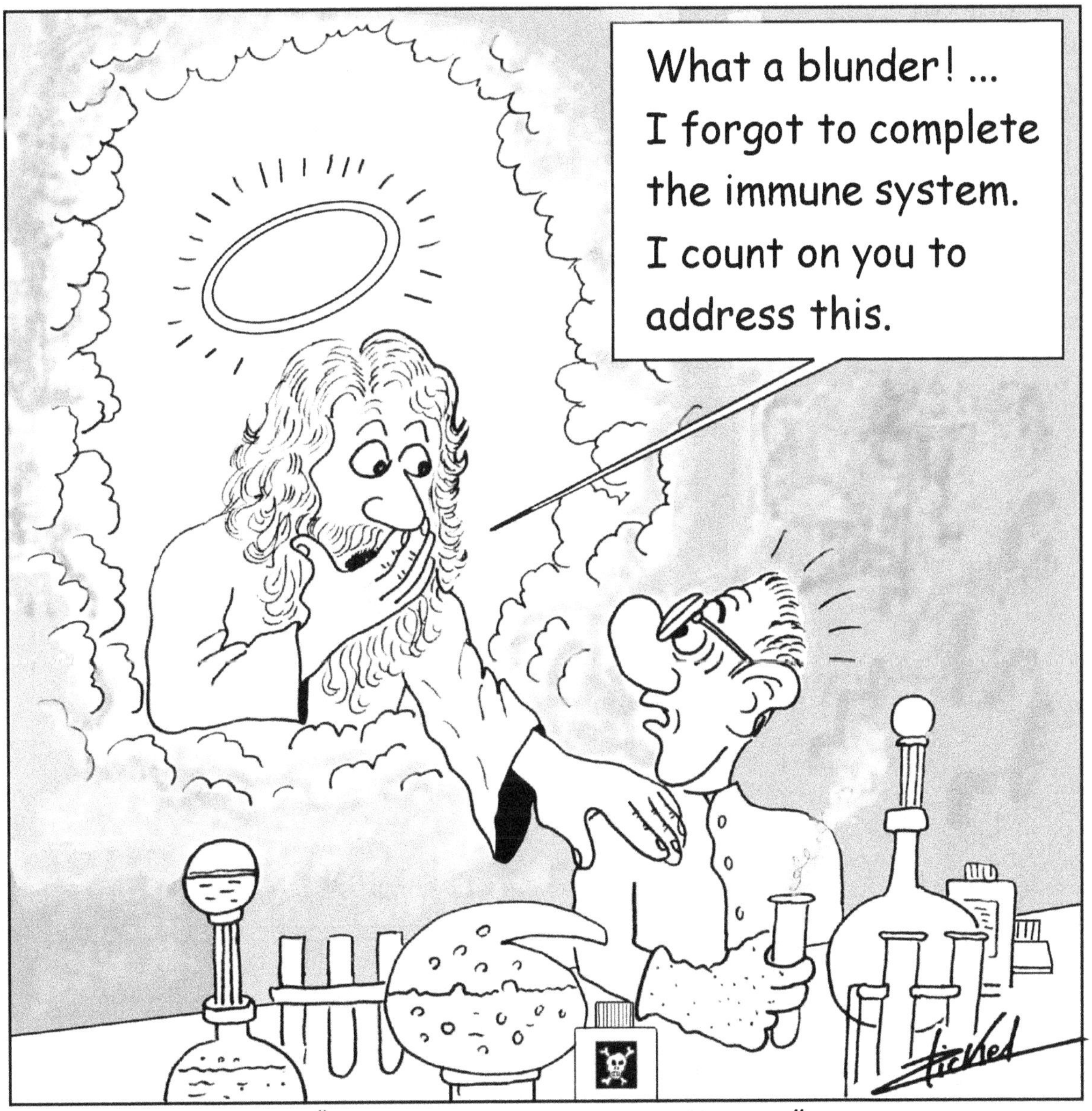

(1) Béchamp, Antoine, "The Blood and its Third Element" [1912]

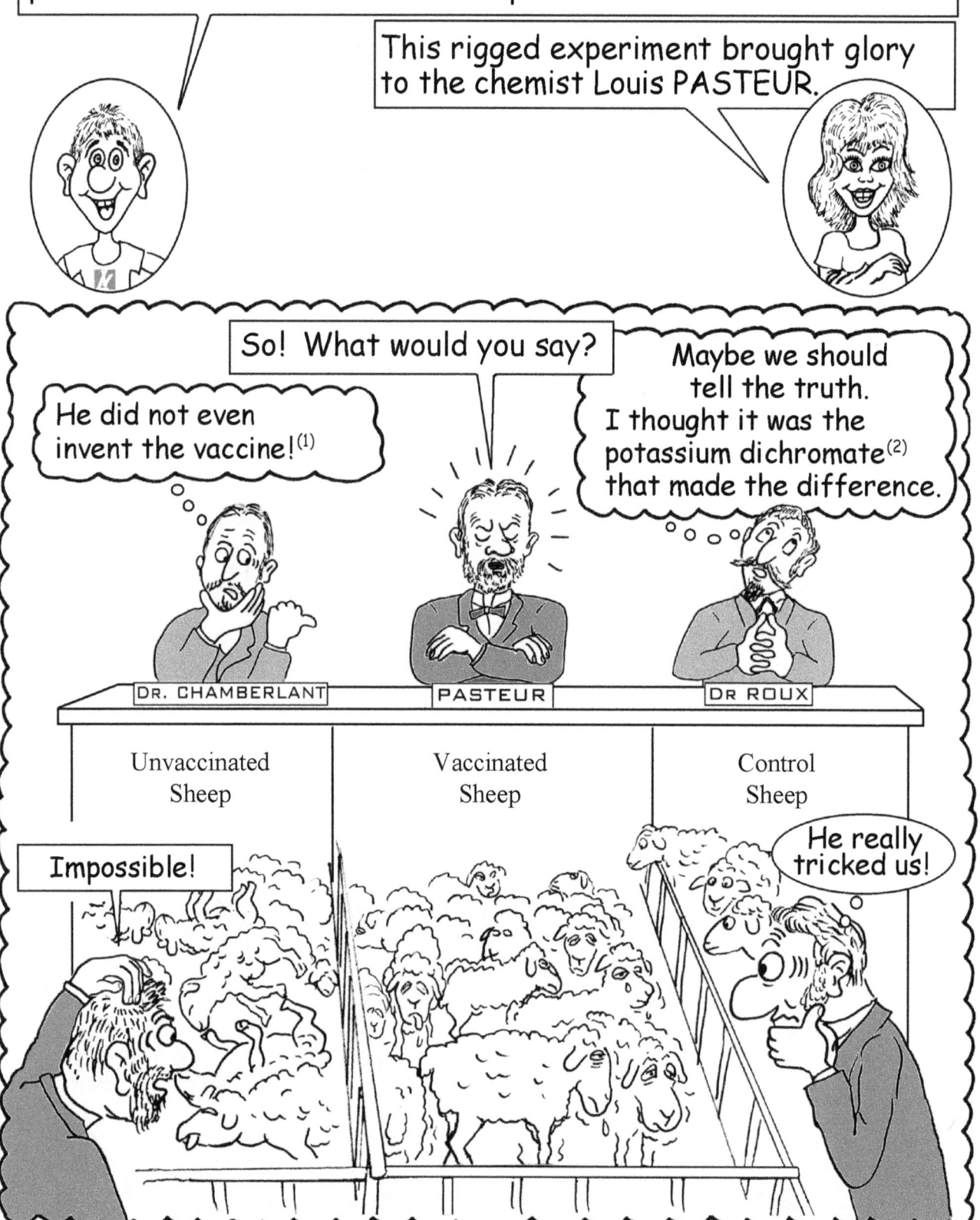

(1) Dr. TOUSSAINT of Toulouse was the inventor.
(2) Very toxic product altering the internal environment and finally leading to degeneration (Professor Louis Claude VINCENT)

After the experiment at Pouilly Le Fort, other countries embarked on creating an anthrax vaccine. That was a total failure. Approximately 200,000 sheep perished as a result of the vaccine prepared according to Pasteur's formula.[1] But it was not attenuated like the vaccine used at Pouilly Le Fort.

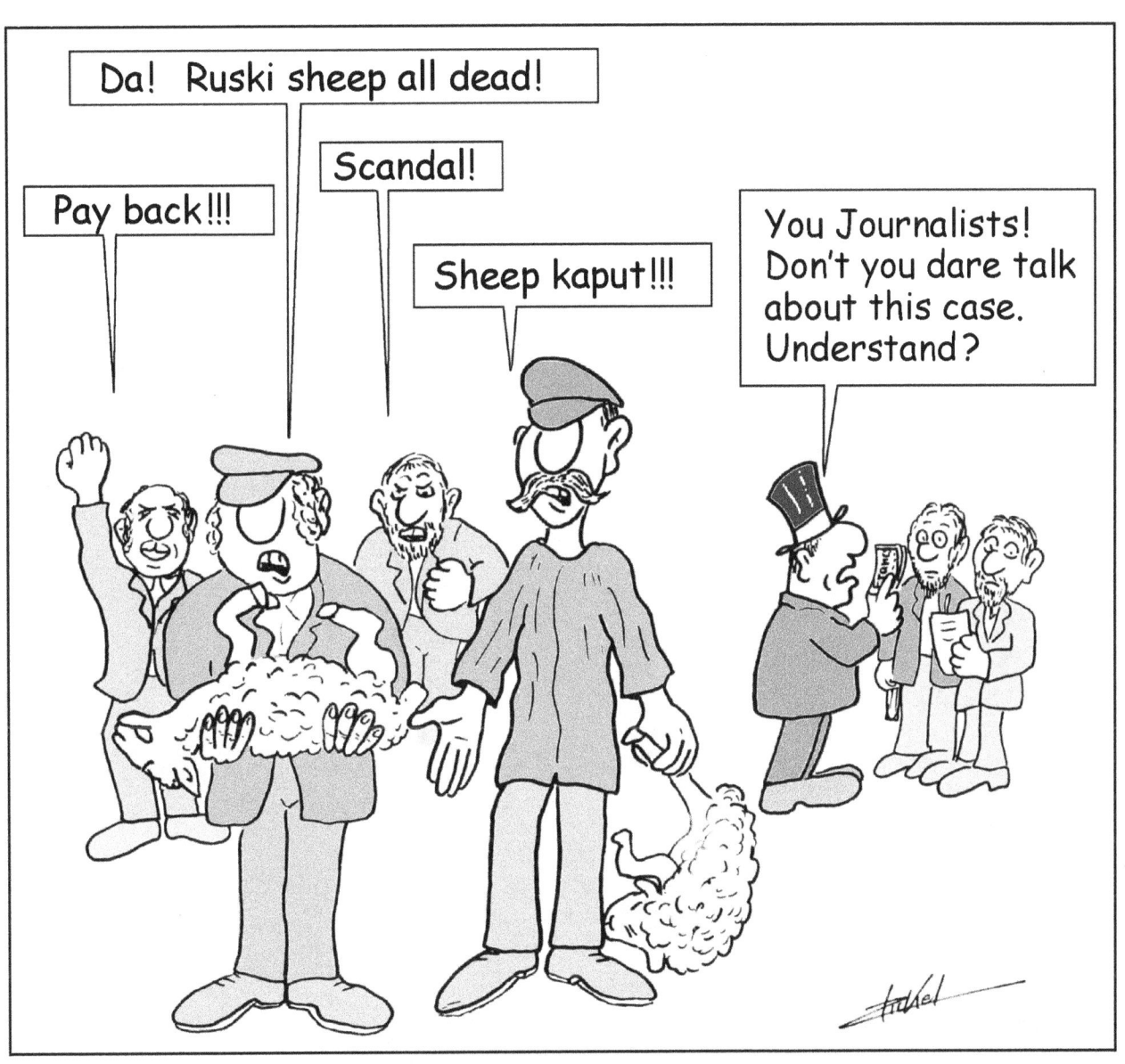

(1) *Pasteur Exposed,* by Ethel Douglas Hume [1923]

Lucky Guinea Pigs

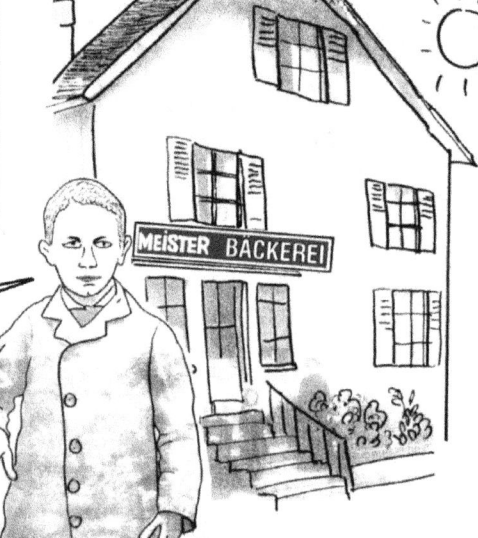

On the evening of July 6, 1885, Pasteur experimented with a rabies vaccine by using the Dr. Galtier (of Lyon, France) process. Pasteur vaccinated a nine-year-old boy, Joseph Meister, from Alsace, France.

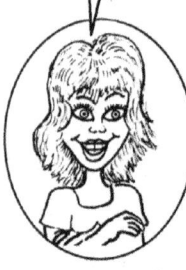

I am Joseph Meister. On the morning of July 4th while out looking for yeast for my father, who is a baker in Steige, I was bitten by a dog.

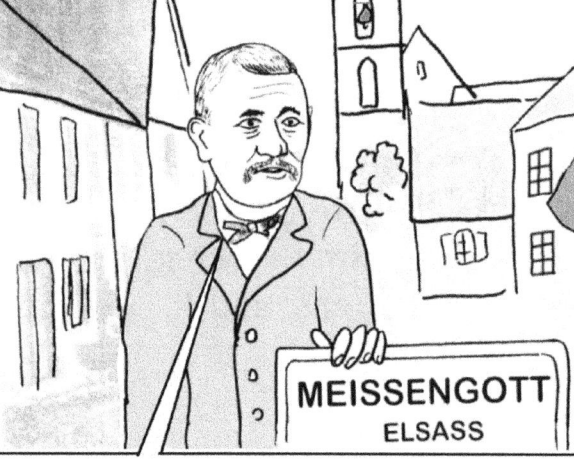

Nobody knows if the dog really was rabid.

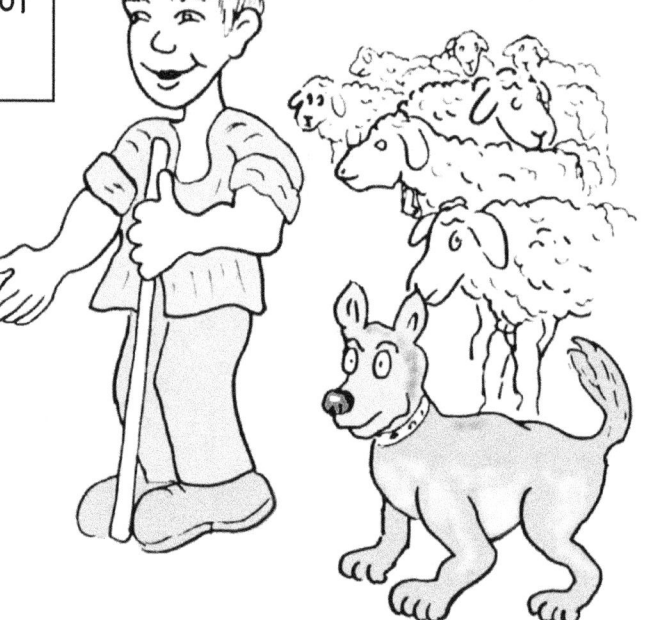

I am Jean Baptiste Jupille who, according to official records, was saved from rabies by the vaccine. However, the dog that bit me was not rabid.

I am Theodore Voné, and my dog bit Joseph Meister. My dog has bitten two other boys, including me. None of us have received any treatment.

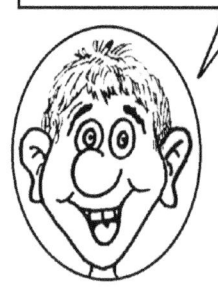

After these two cases, Pasteur rushed to present "his" vaccine procedure to the Academy of Sciences.

Vaccines: The Great Illusion

False Testimony

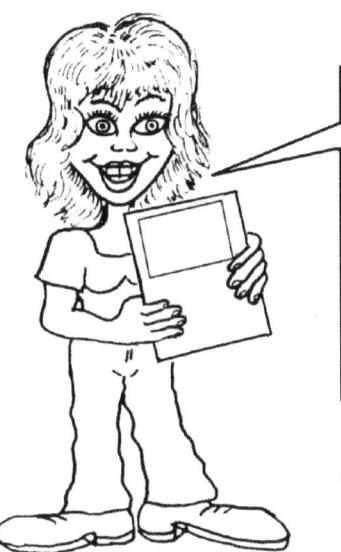

While the news of the "apparent victory over rabies" began to spread over the world, Pasteur treats a third child bitten by an unidentified dog. The child died of rabies symptoms, which was termed "laboratory rabies."
The dead child's parents filed a complaint.

Dr. Adrien LOIR (nephew and close associate of Pasteur):
"A l'ombre de Pasteur : Souvenirs personnels" (1938)

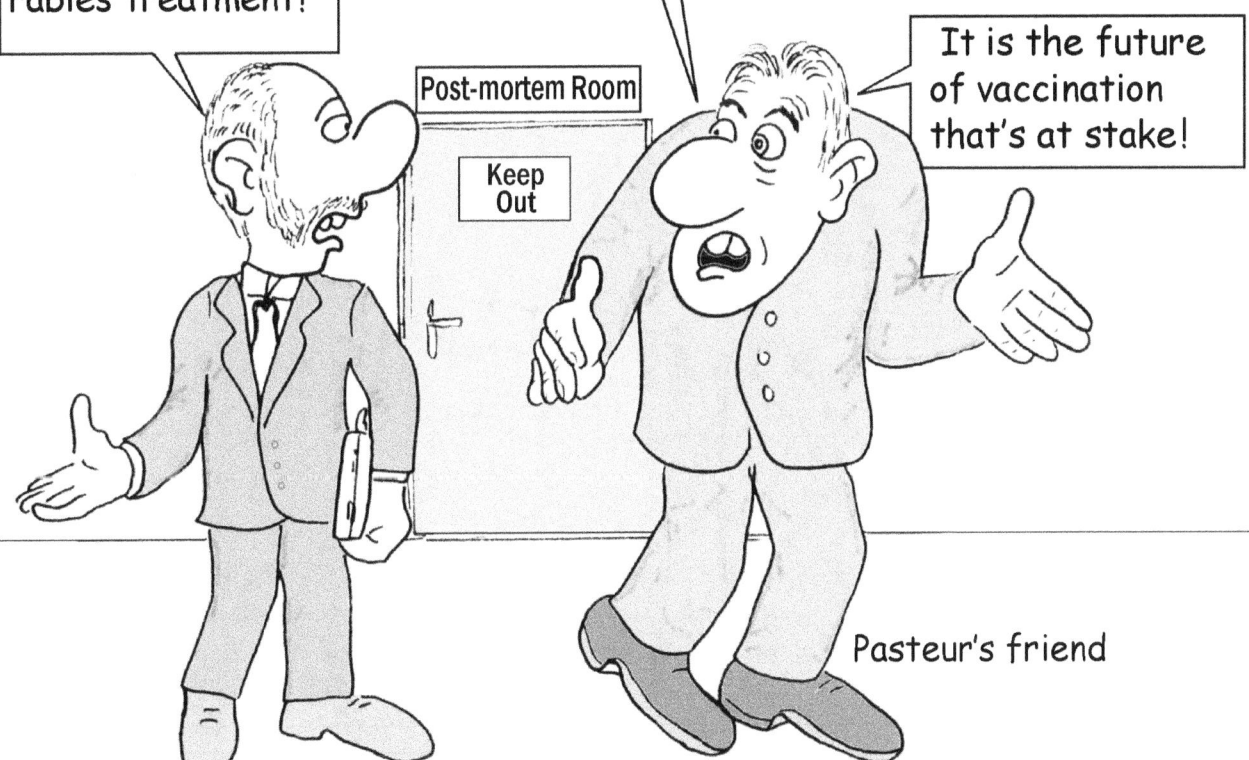

Professor Brouardel, the young Jules Rouyer then did die from the rabies treatment!

Ah yes! ... But in the autopsy report, I noted "Death following a uremia crisis."
Otherwise, it would mean a fall back of 50 years in the evolution of science. We must avoid that.

It is the future of vaccination that's at stake!

Pasteur's friend

Mr. PASTEUR does not cure rabies : he gives it.
  Dr. LUTAUD (Study on rabies and the Pasteur Method)

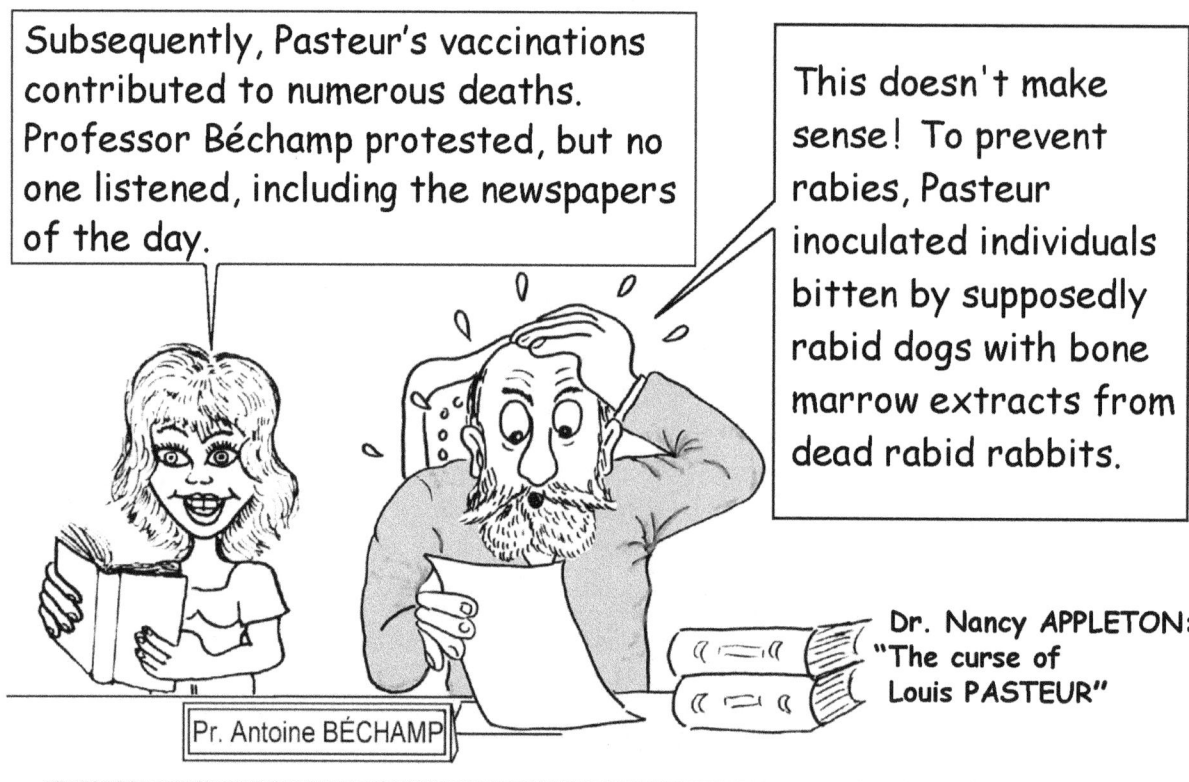

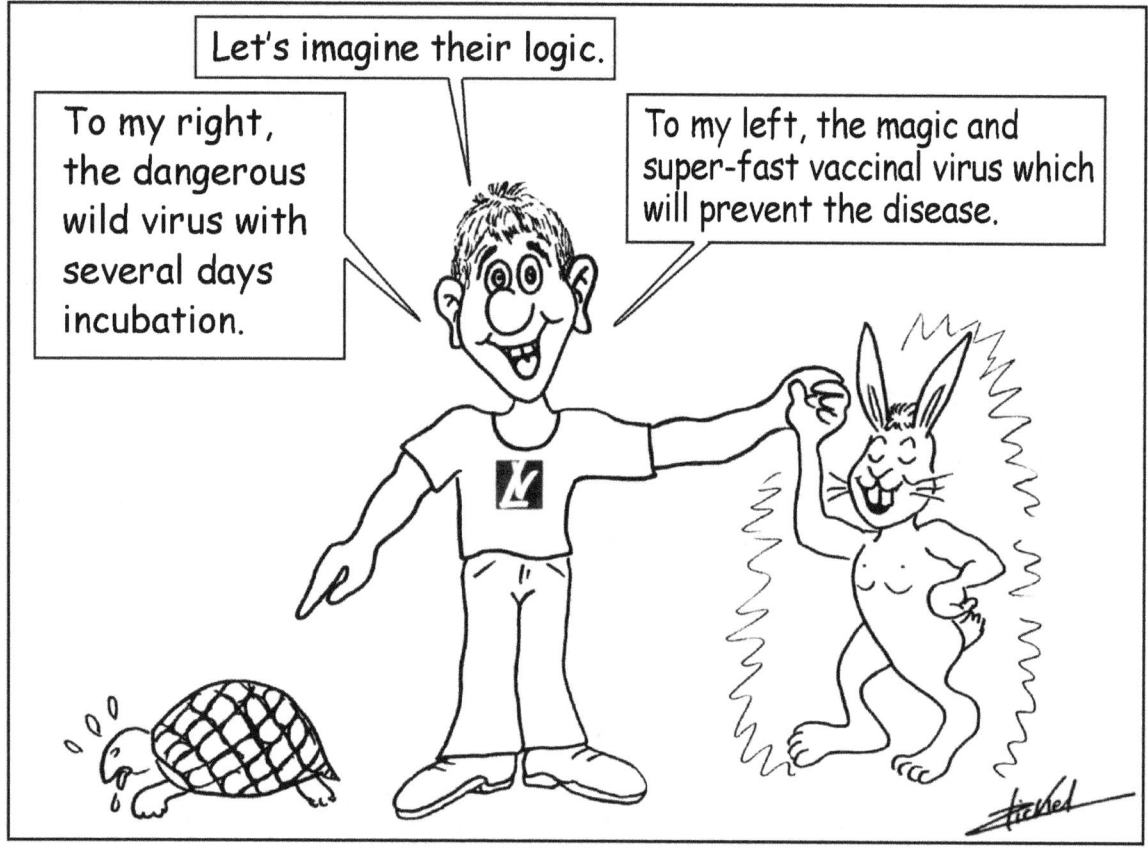

> *The pasteurian ideas, spread and taught as a catechism for altar boys, are pushing back the intelligence and accordingly the civilization.*
>
> **Dr. René DUFILHO**

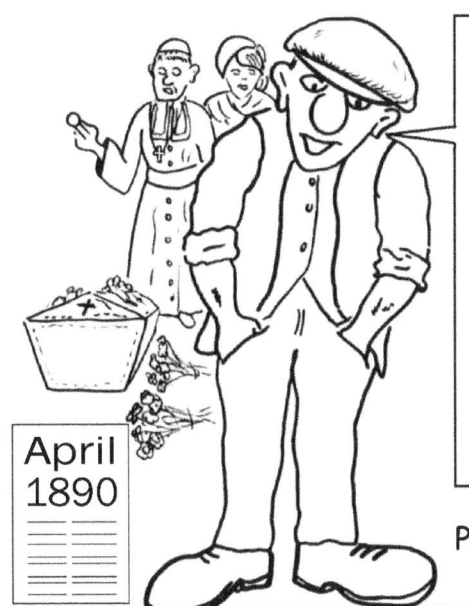

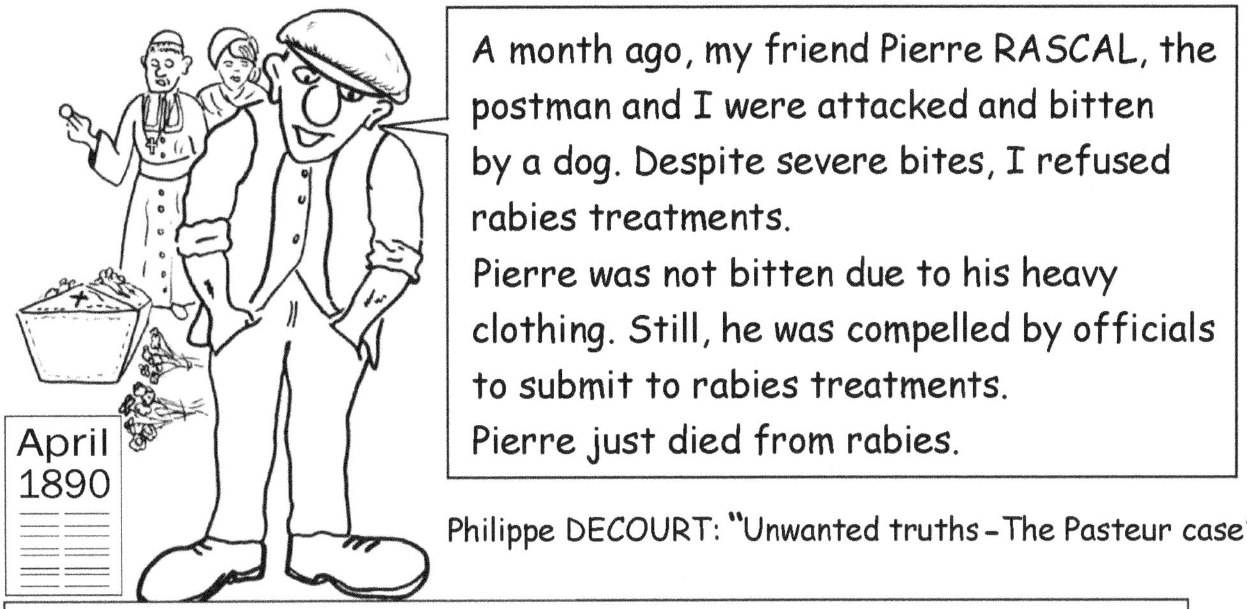

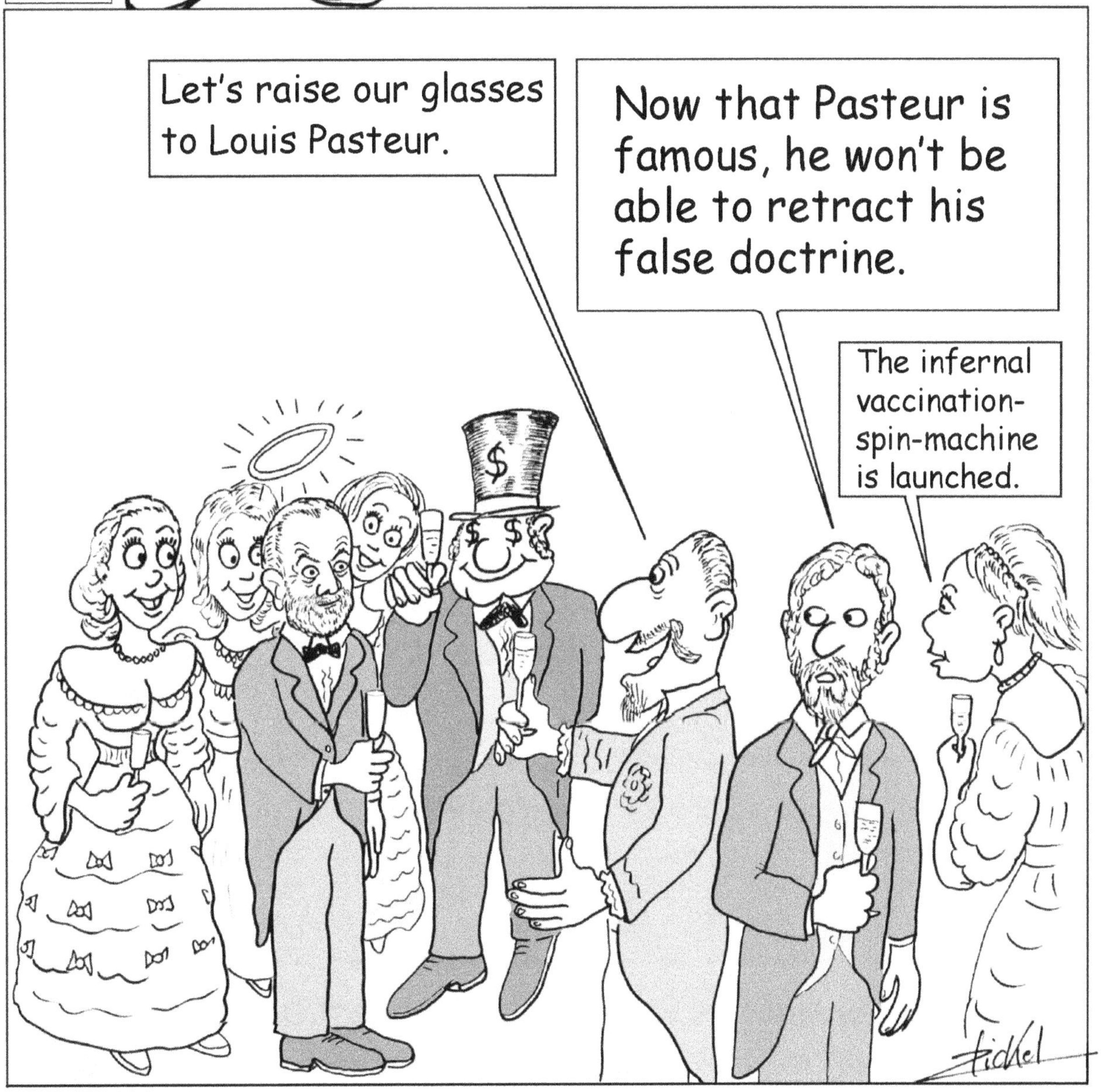

> *Any vaccination is a scandal when considered on a scientific level.*
> **Dr. Jacques KALMAR**

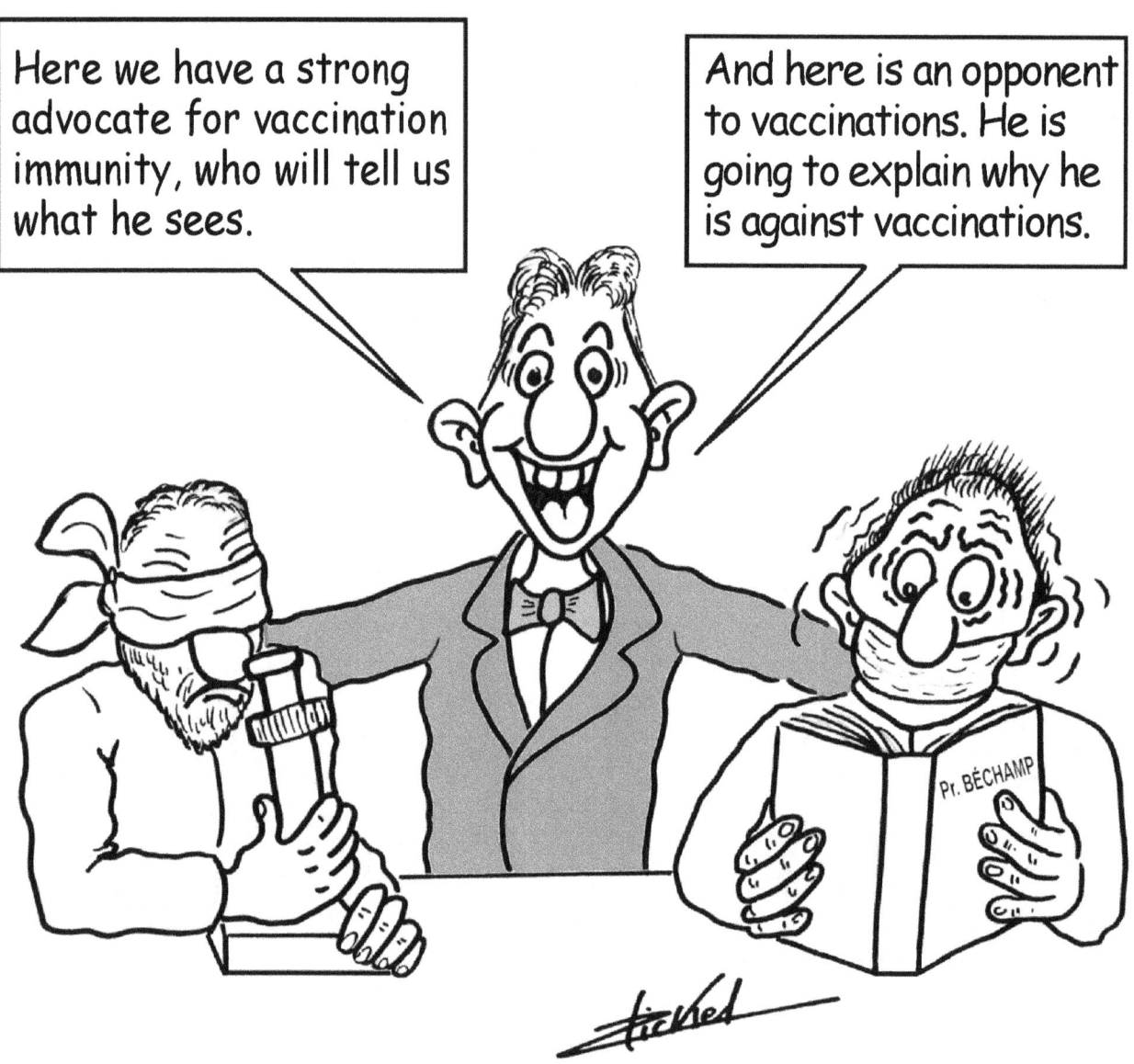

> *Monstrosities such as vaccinations are not based on science but on money.*
> **Professor Jules TISSOT**

Vaccines: The Great Illusion

> **The Immunizations are nothing but abominable hygienic mystifications which have brought the science and practice of the art of healing into disrepute, while decimating humankind to enrich the vaccinators.** — Dr. Hubert BOENS

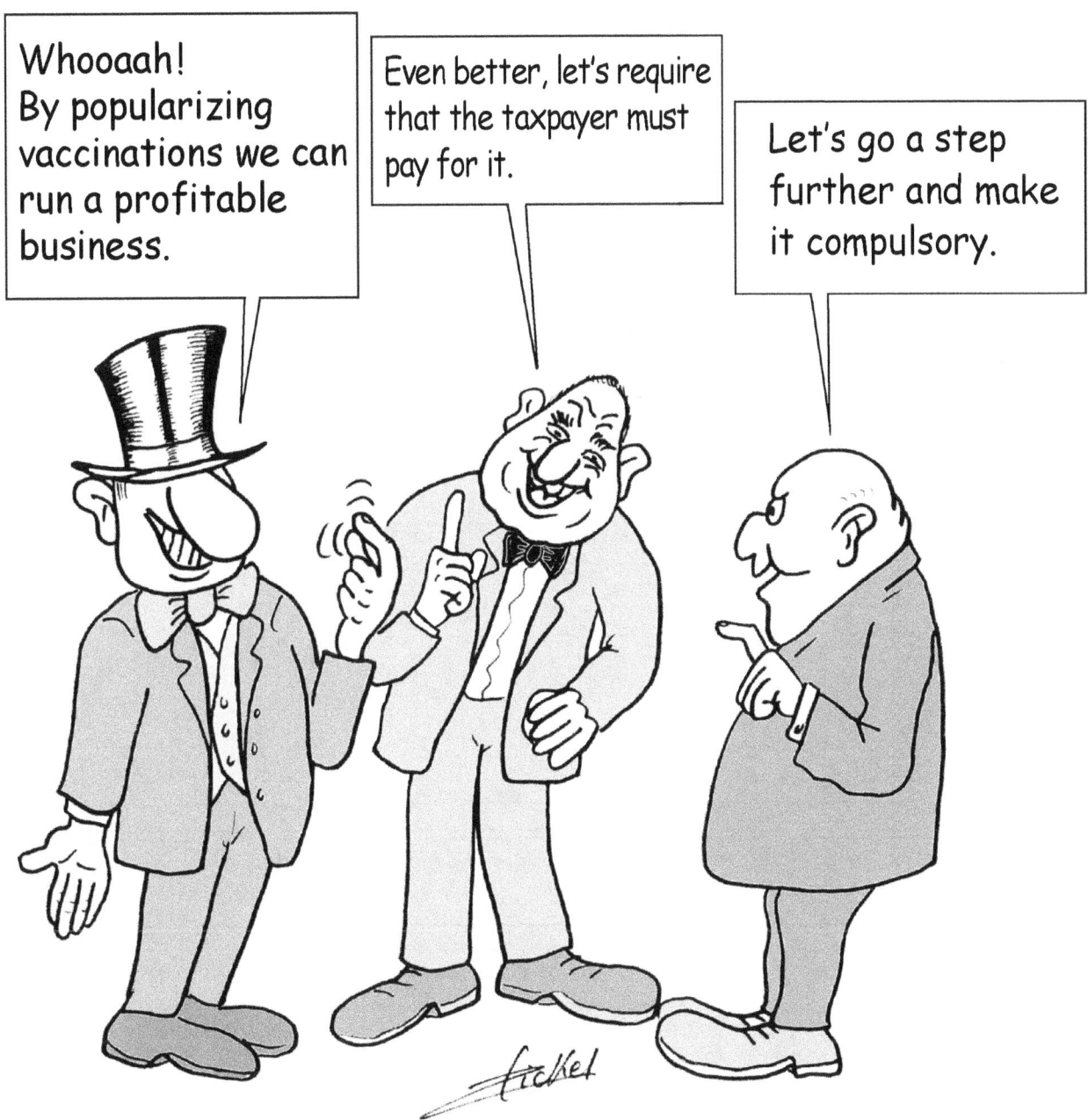

> *We are invited to consume, ignoring the manipulation of scientific facts to justify.* — Dr. Didier TARTE

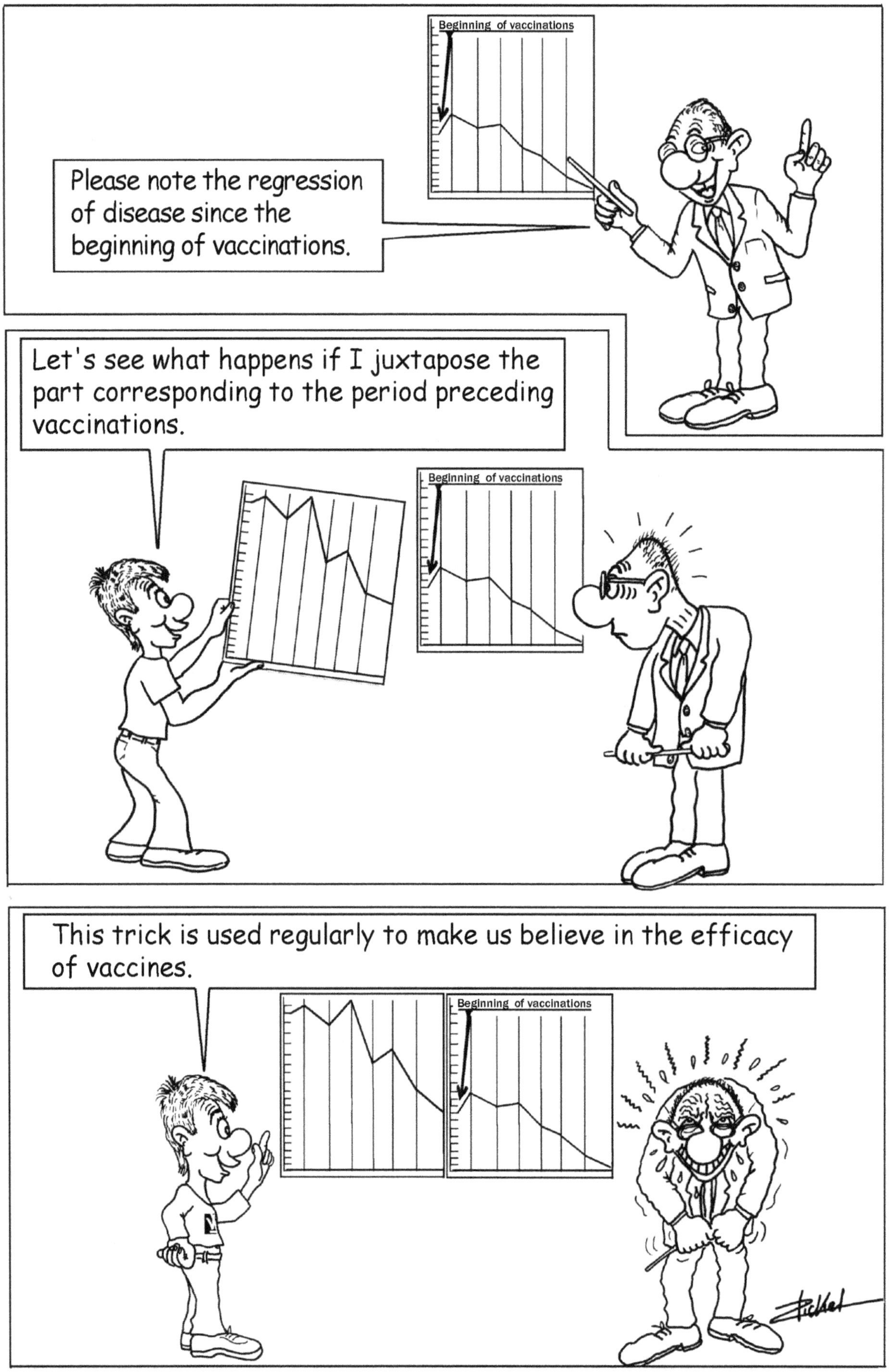

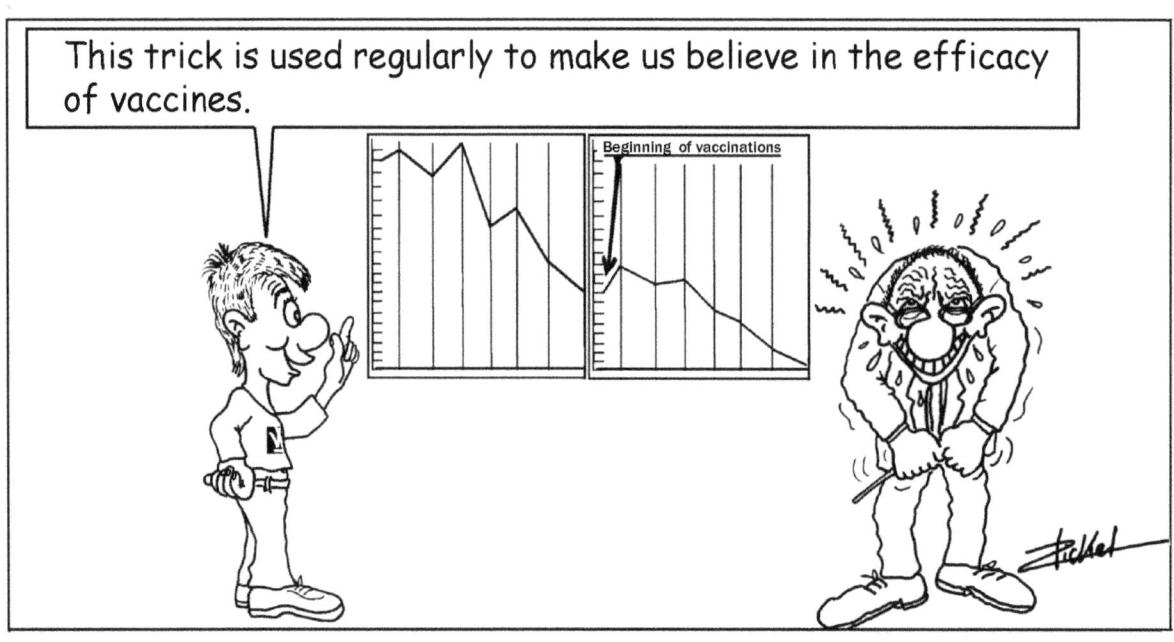

Vaccines: The Great Illusion

The Magic of Statistics

"Vaccine laboratories, with the help of public health officials, are skillful magicians who are adept at demonstrating vaccine efficacy."

"Vaccines were introduced at a time when mortality rates for various diseases were plummeting and for which vaccines took the credit."

Progression of Tuberculosis Mortality Rates in France.
Figures from INSERM (Med. Lab. Research)

Rabies, a Scourge?

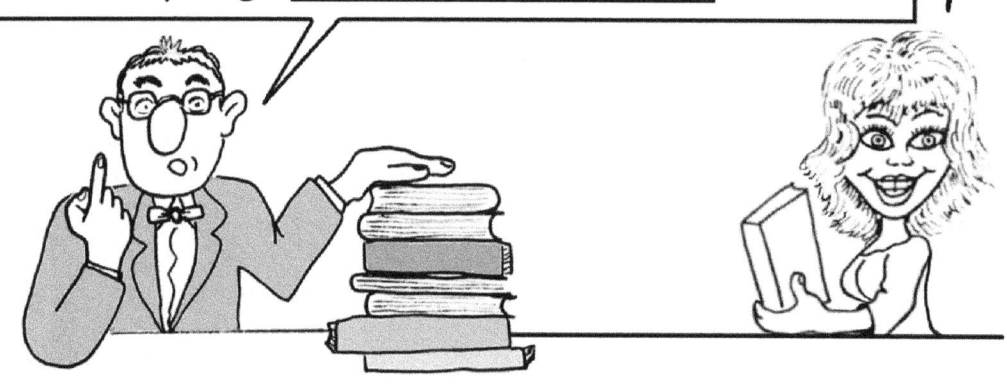

Compared with other diseases that raged at the time, rabies was a marginal phenomenon. The introduction of the Pasteur vaccine resulted in an increase in deaths due to a form of rabies called "laboratory rabies."[1]

When we cross-check scientific studies, we find only 5 to 16 percent of individuals bitten by a rabid animal actually contract rabies.
However, Pasteur "cured" (or killed) individuals bitten by dogs **assumed to have been** rabid.

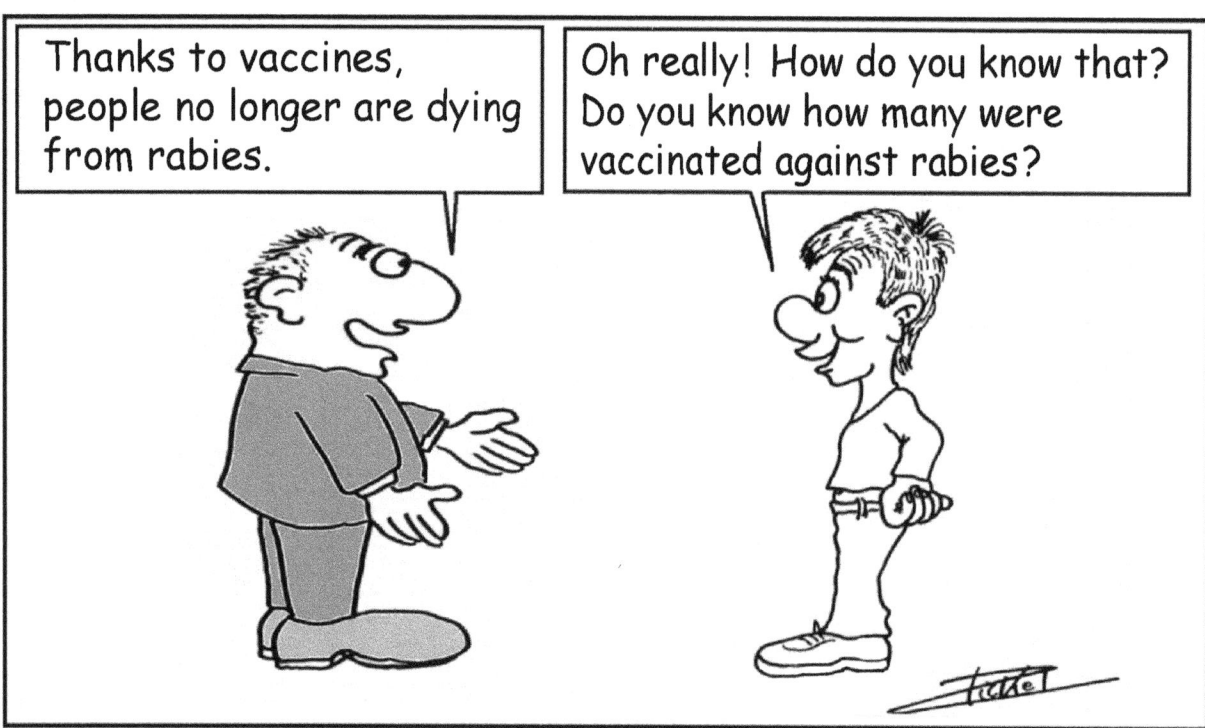

Thanks to vaccines, people no longer are dying from rabies.

Oh really! How do you know that? Do you know how many were vaccinated against rabies?

(1) Ethel Douglas HUME : "Béchamp or Pasteur?" [1923]
Dr. Eric ANCELET : "Pour en finir avec Pasteur"

DIPHTHERIA: Yet another deceiving vaccine

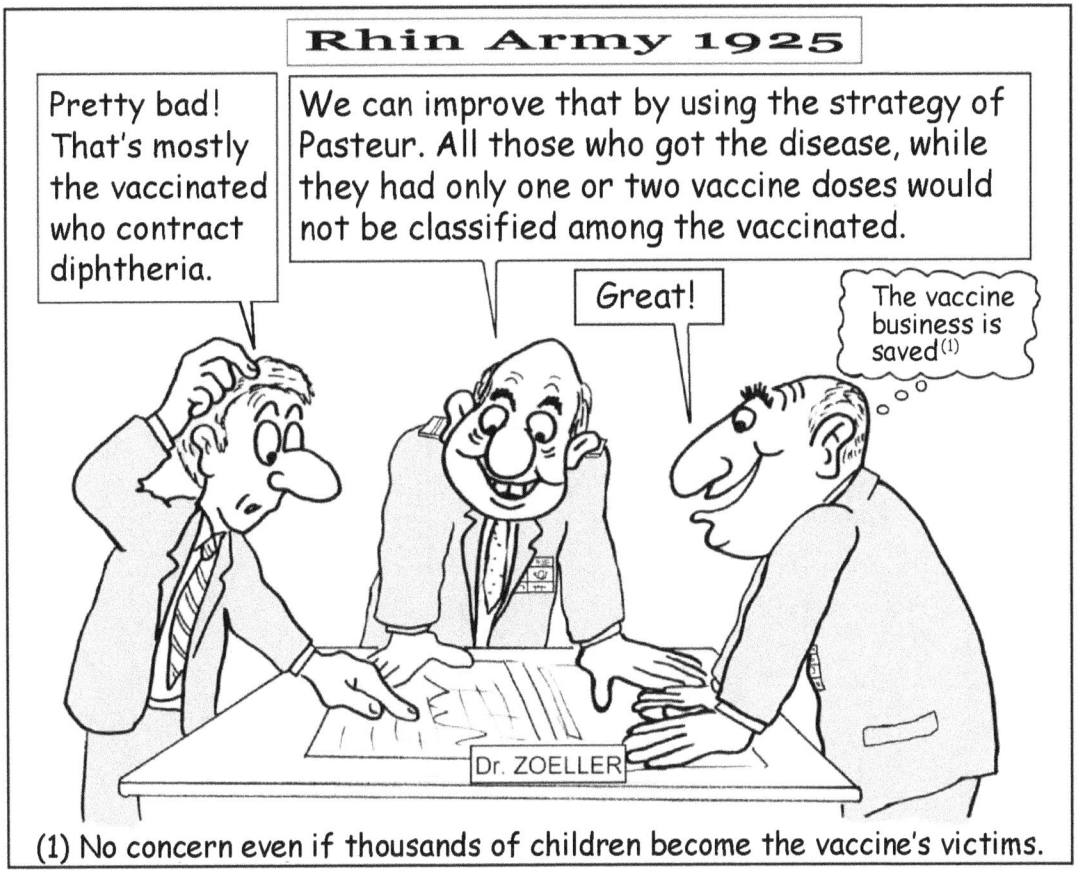

(1) No concern even if thousands of children become the vaccine's victims.

In 1941 children in France were vaccinated against diphtheria, which did not prevent diphtheria cases from tripling in 1943.

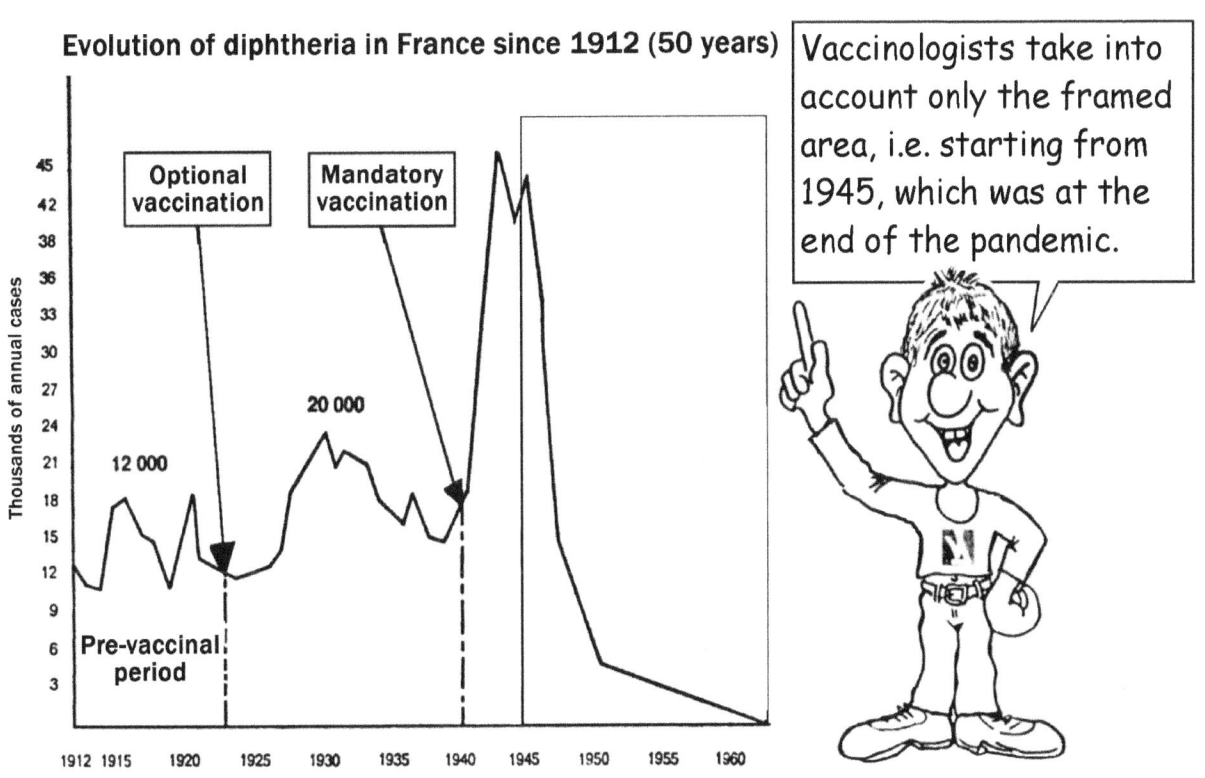

Diphtheria Statistics in Berlin, 1938 to 1950

Connection with vaccinations. Mortality Rates per 100,000 inhabitants. Logarithmic scale.

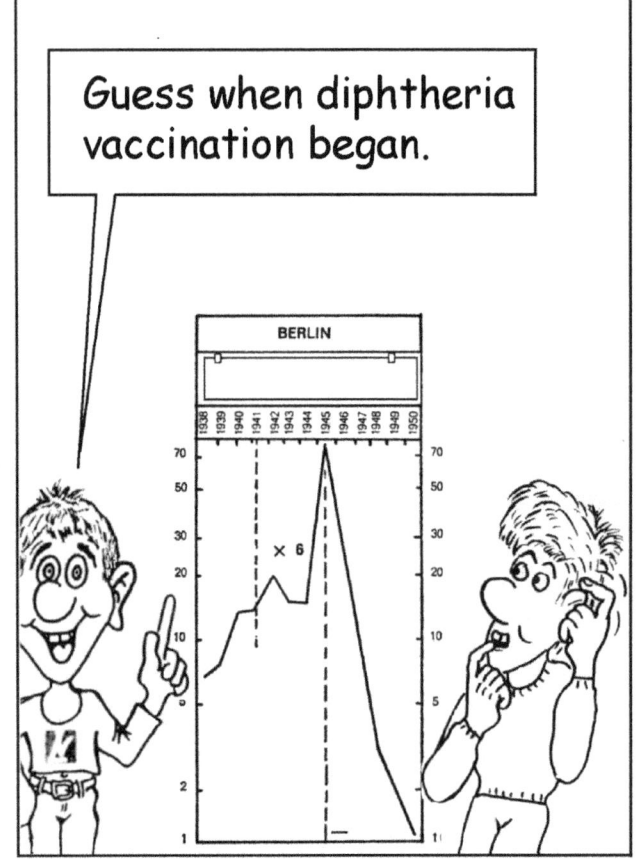

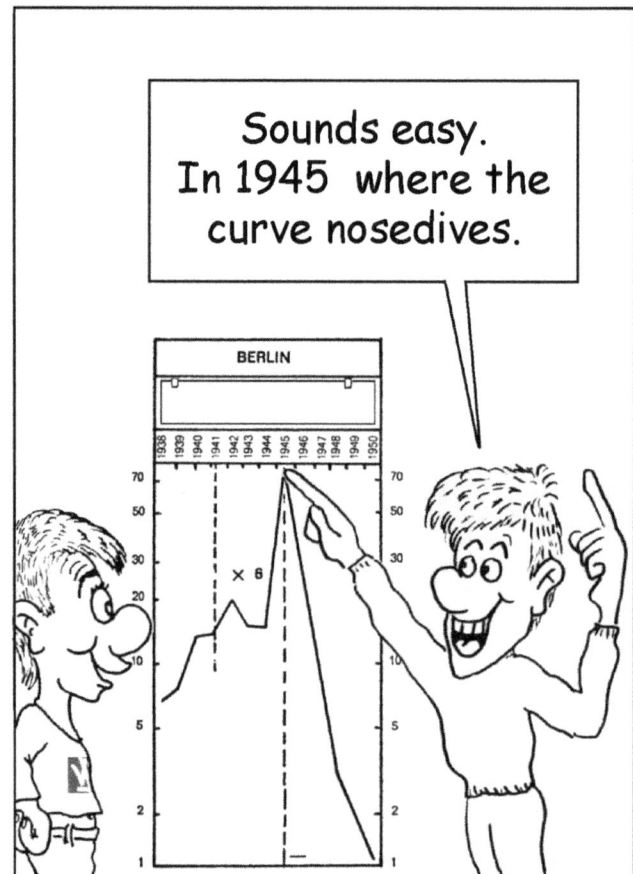

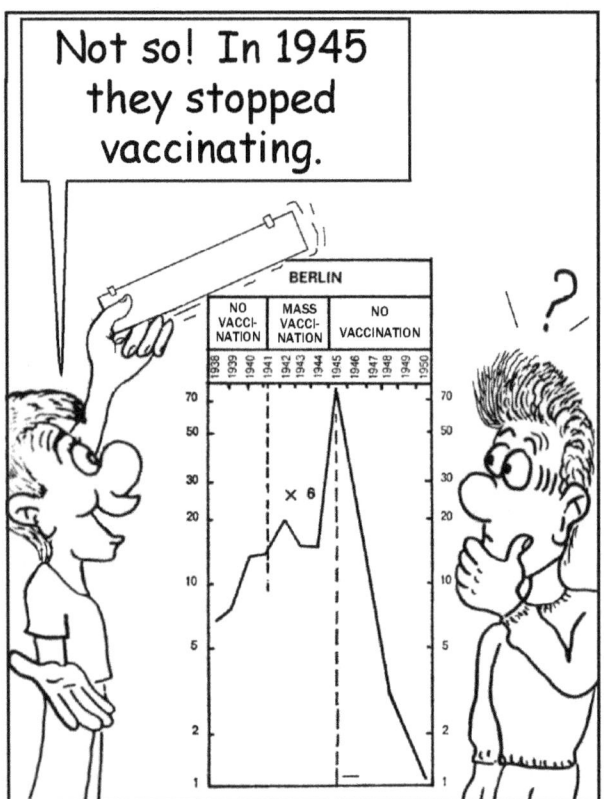

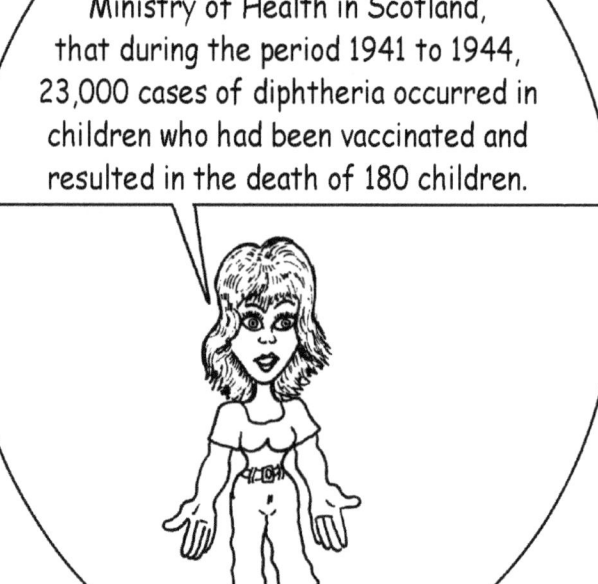

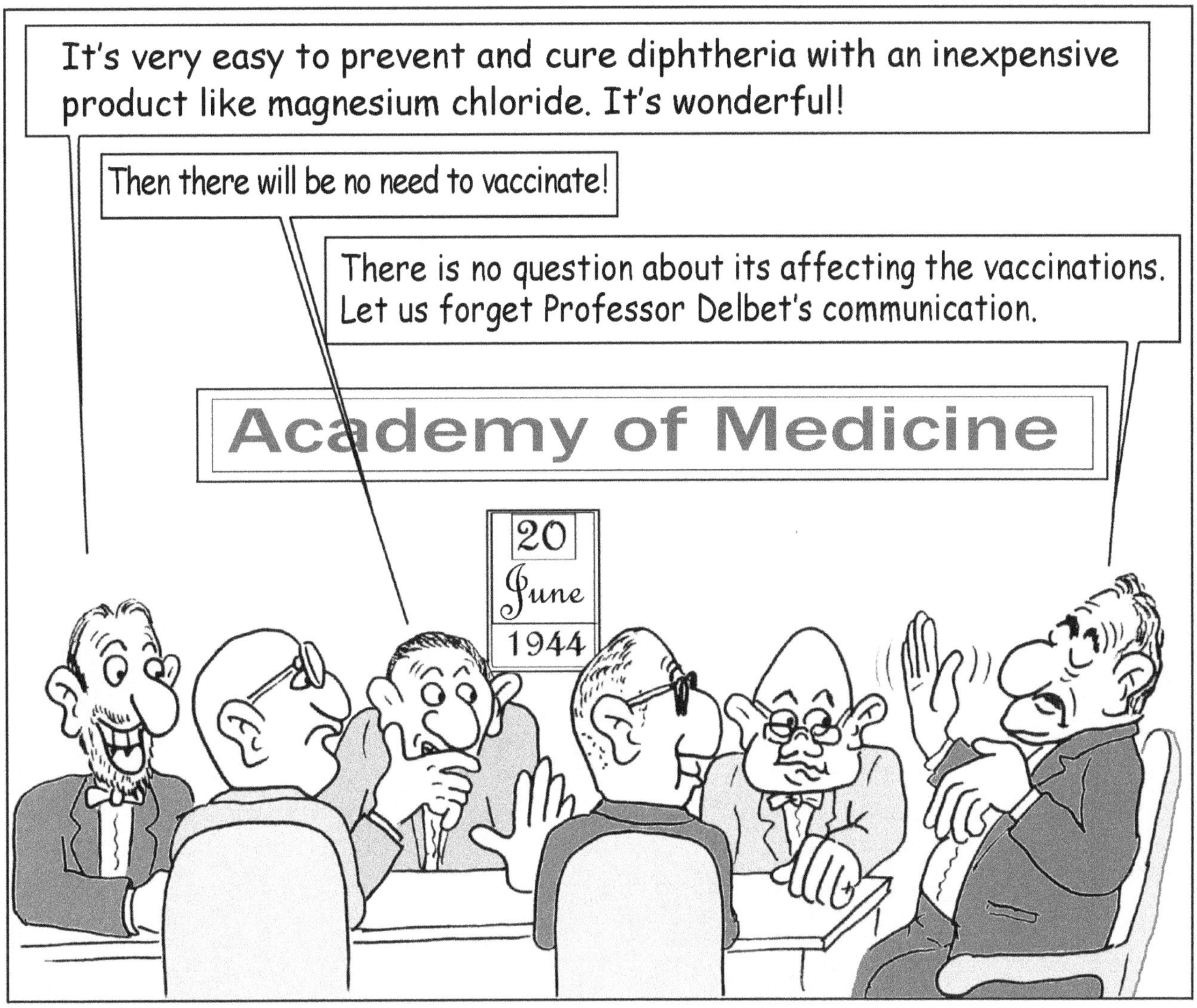

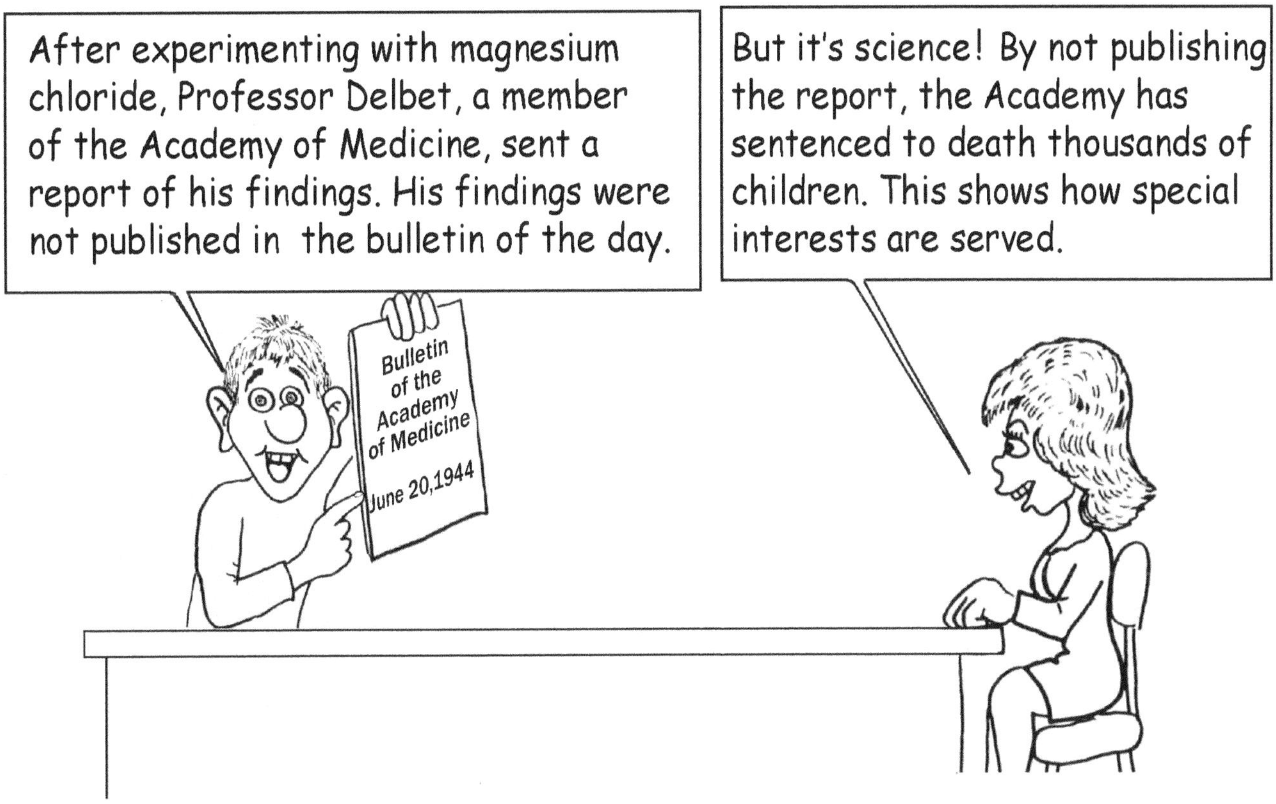

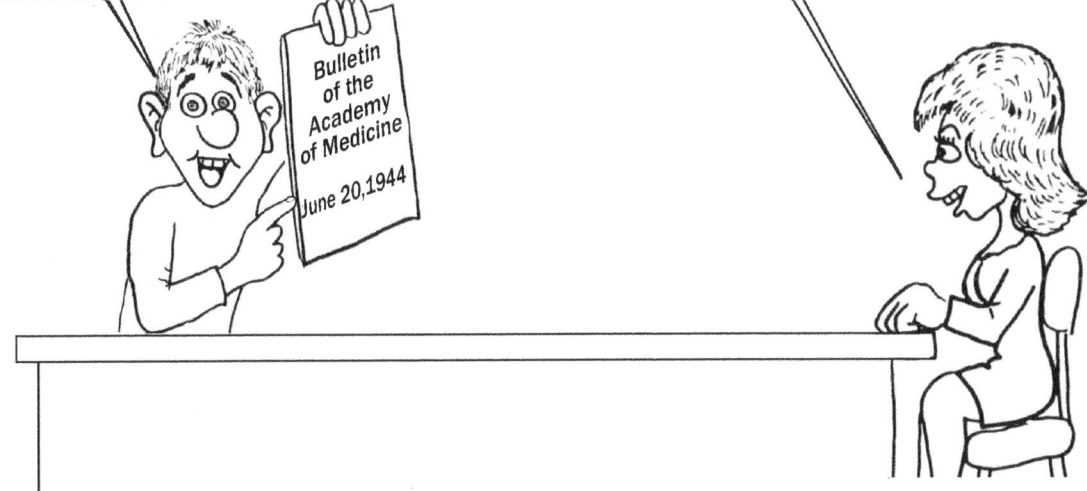

Vaccines: The Great Illusion

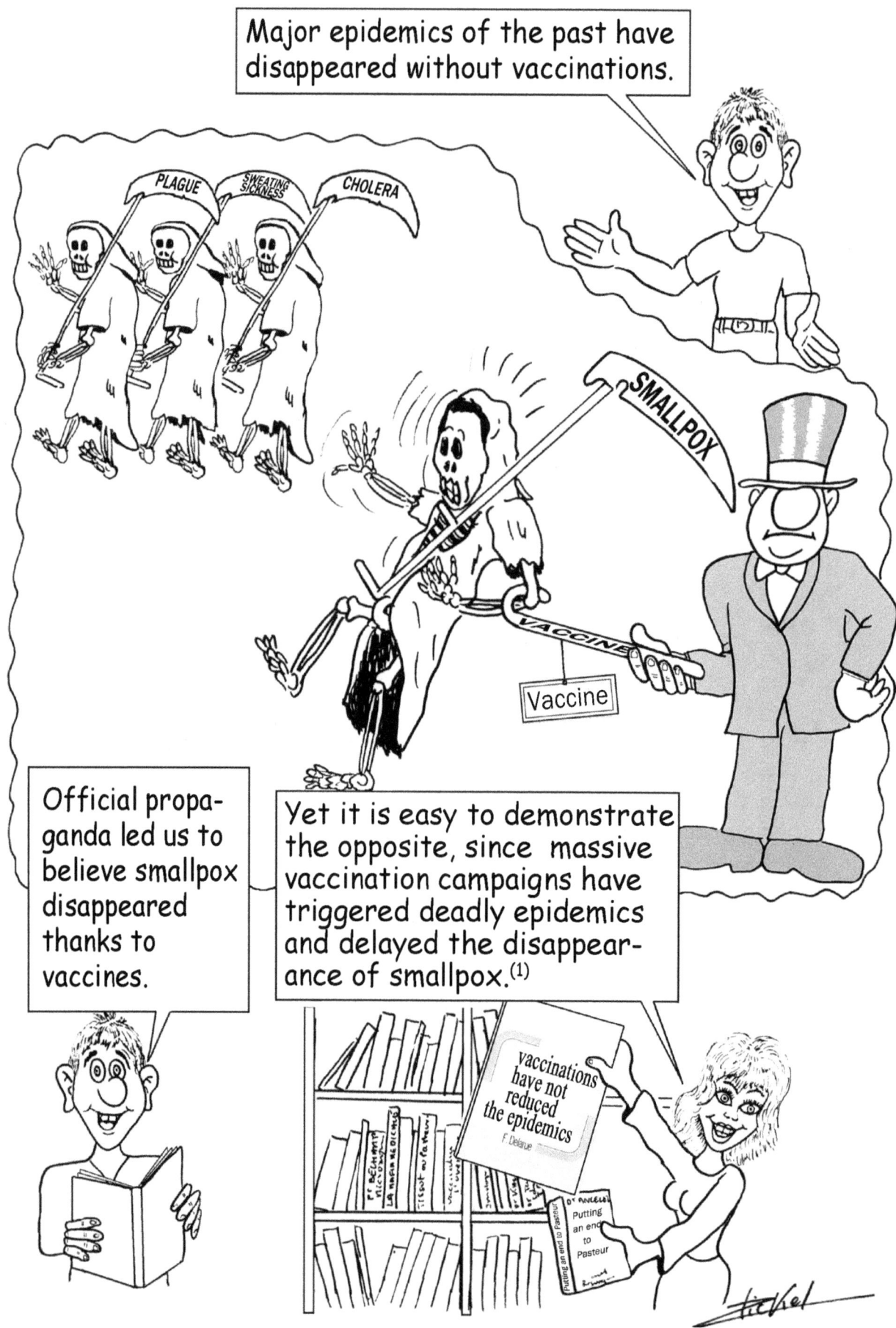

(1) DELARUE, Fernand : "Vaccinations have not reduced the epidemics."

Vaccines: The Great Illusion

Smallpox: Some facts among many

In May 1871 English medical authorities claimed that 87.5 percent of the population were vaccinated. Yet the following year, England experienced the worst epidemic in history, which ended with 44,840 deaths.

In Scotland, the most vaccinated country in the world at that time, more than 9,000 vaccinated children died from smallpox between 1855 and 1875.

Smallpox killed 120,000 people in Germany between 1870 and 1871. 96 percent of them were vaccinated!

These examples document that vaccination increased the number of smallpox cases.[1]

Nearly a century later, the WHO was forced to admit that mass vaccination was unable to eradicate smallpox, and without isolation of patients and monitoring of contacts, epidemics persisted.

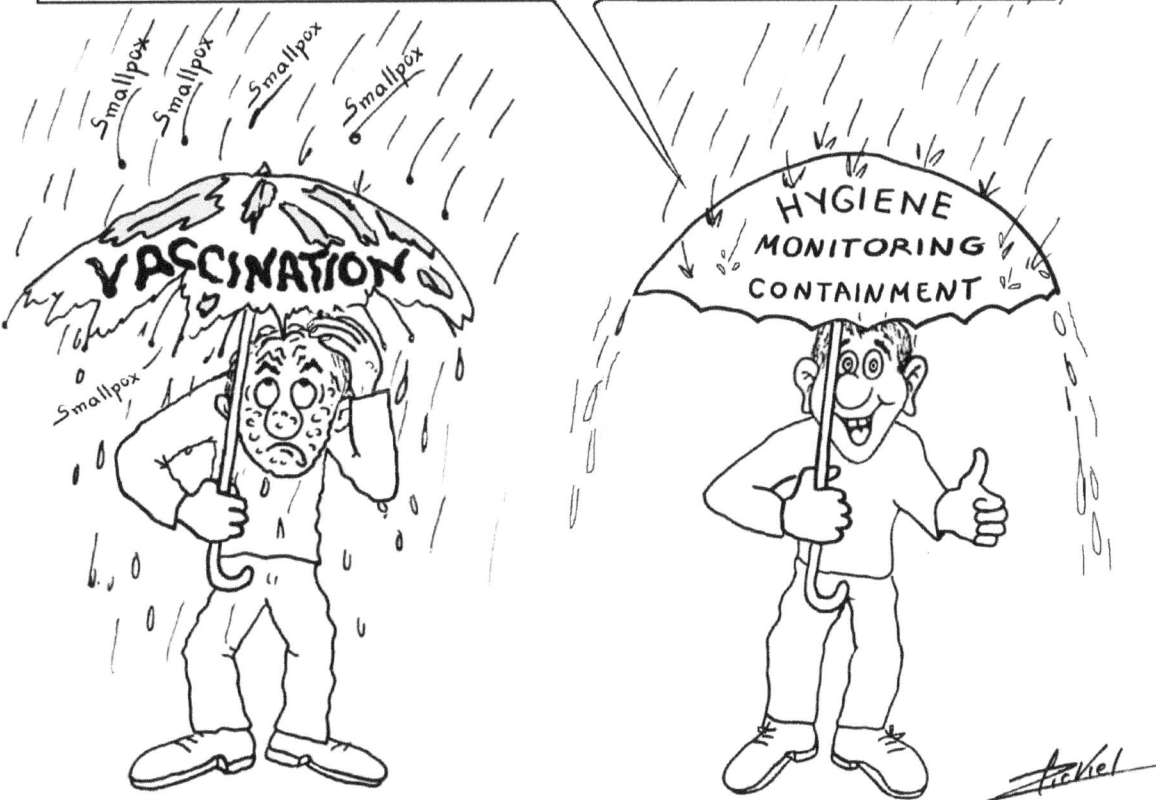

(1) DELARUE, Fernand: "Vaccinations have not reduced the epidemics."

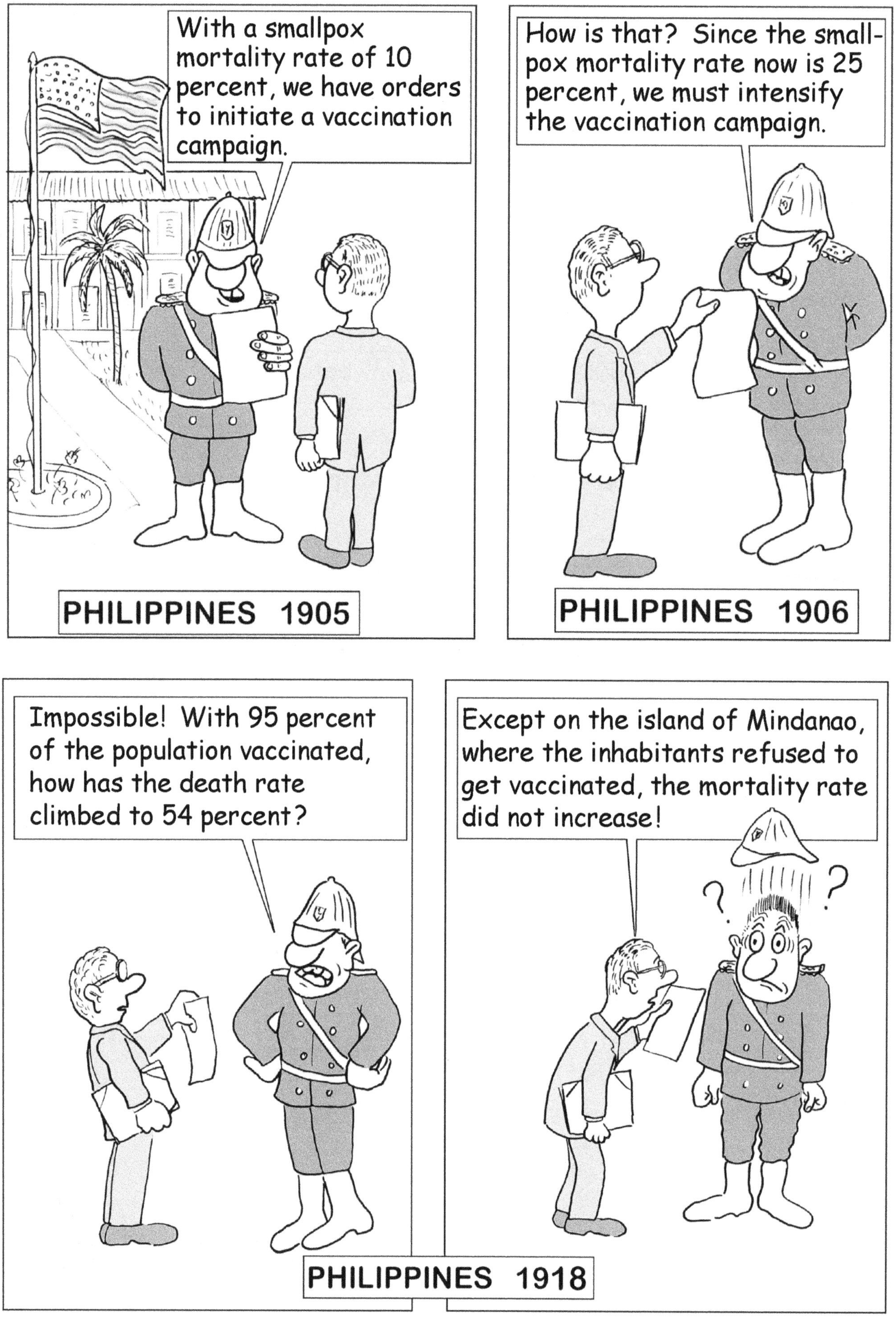

Vaccines: The Great Illusion

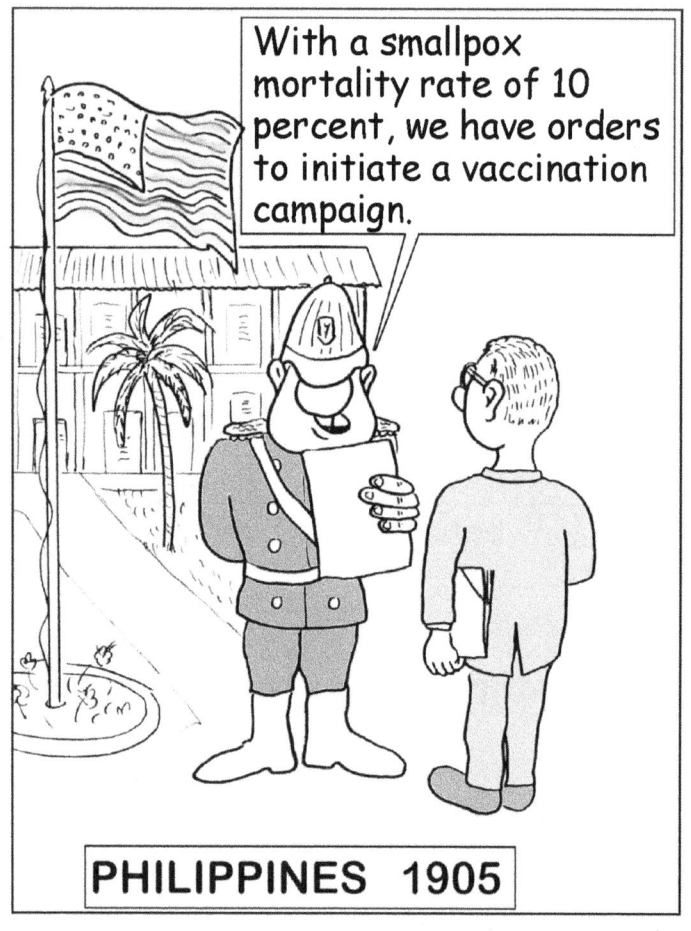
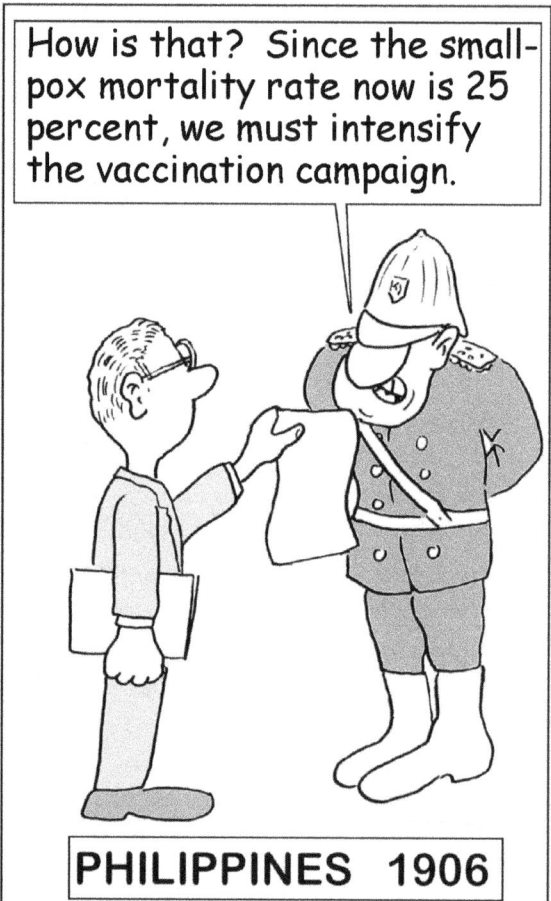

Vaccines: The Great Illusion

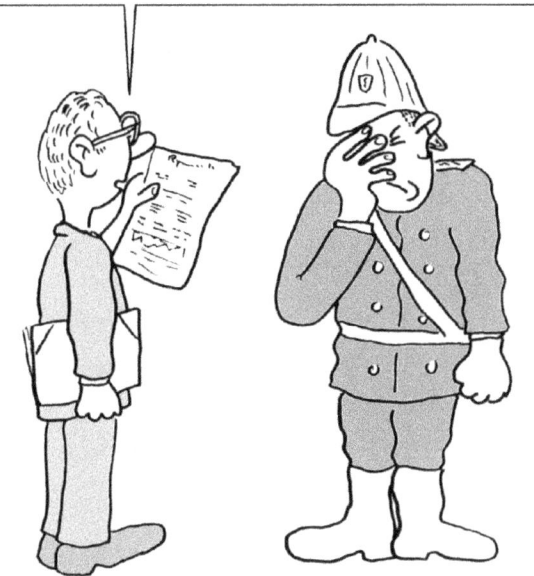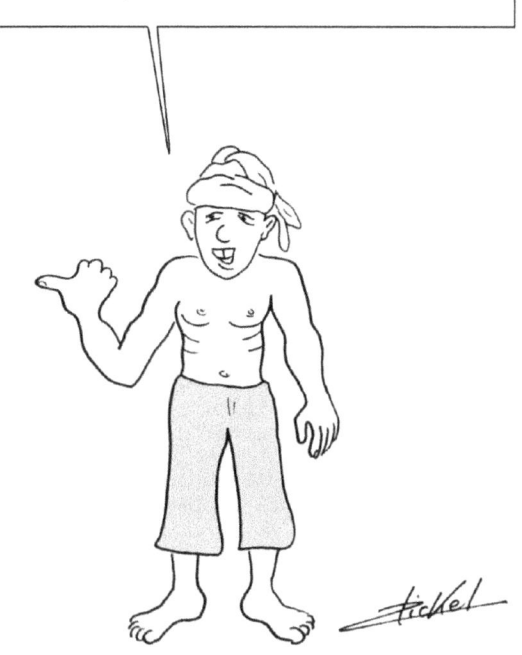

According to the Official Report of the Mission of Inquiry in the Philippines, headed by Inspector General Leonard WOOD of the USA.

I am firmly convinced that vaccination cannot be shown as having any logical relationship with a decrease in the number of cases of smallpox. Most of the people died of smallpox they contracted after being vaccinated.

Dr. J. W. HODGE (*The Vaccination Superstition*)

The studies that are quoted endlessly by these elite members of academia and government agencies and used to close the door on the vaccine connection to neurodevelopmental problems are purposefully designed so as to suggest no link between vaccines and any complication. This falsified research is protected by academia, the media, and government agencies.

Dr. Russell BLAYLOCK

Tuberculosis and the BCG Vaccine

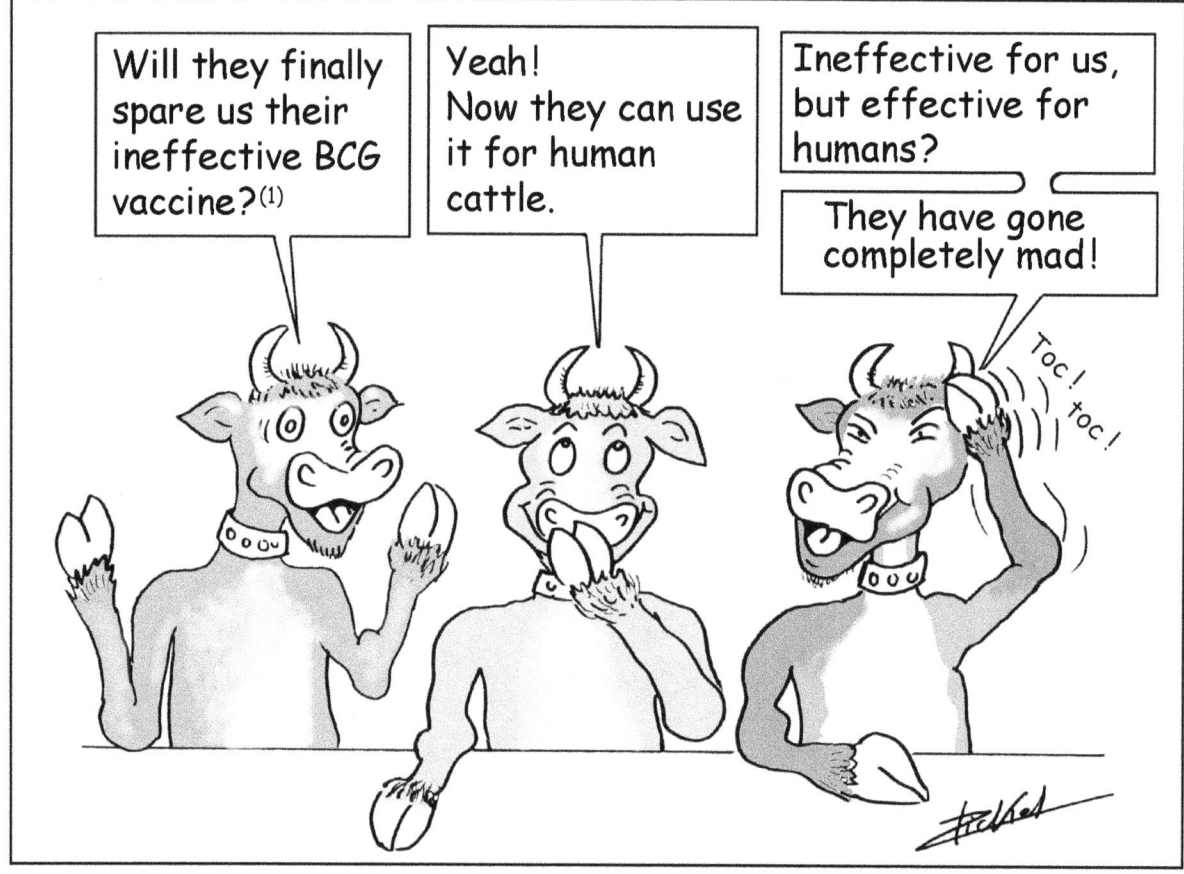

(1) The BCG vaccination of cattle was prohibited in 1955 due to tuberculine contamination making the meat unfit for consumption.

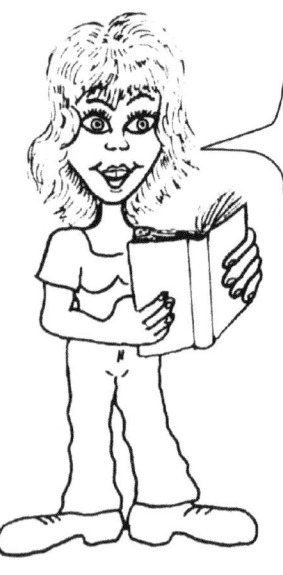

The French will have to become cannibalistic before prohibiting the BCG vaccine.

In a major trial, carried out in India with 260,000 people, more cases of tuberculosis occurred among the vaccinated than in the placebo control group.

I was amazed that the legend of security of the BCG vaccination has been established so easily.
Dr. JAMES

The BCG Mafia

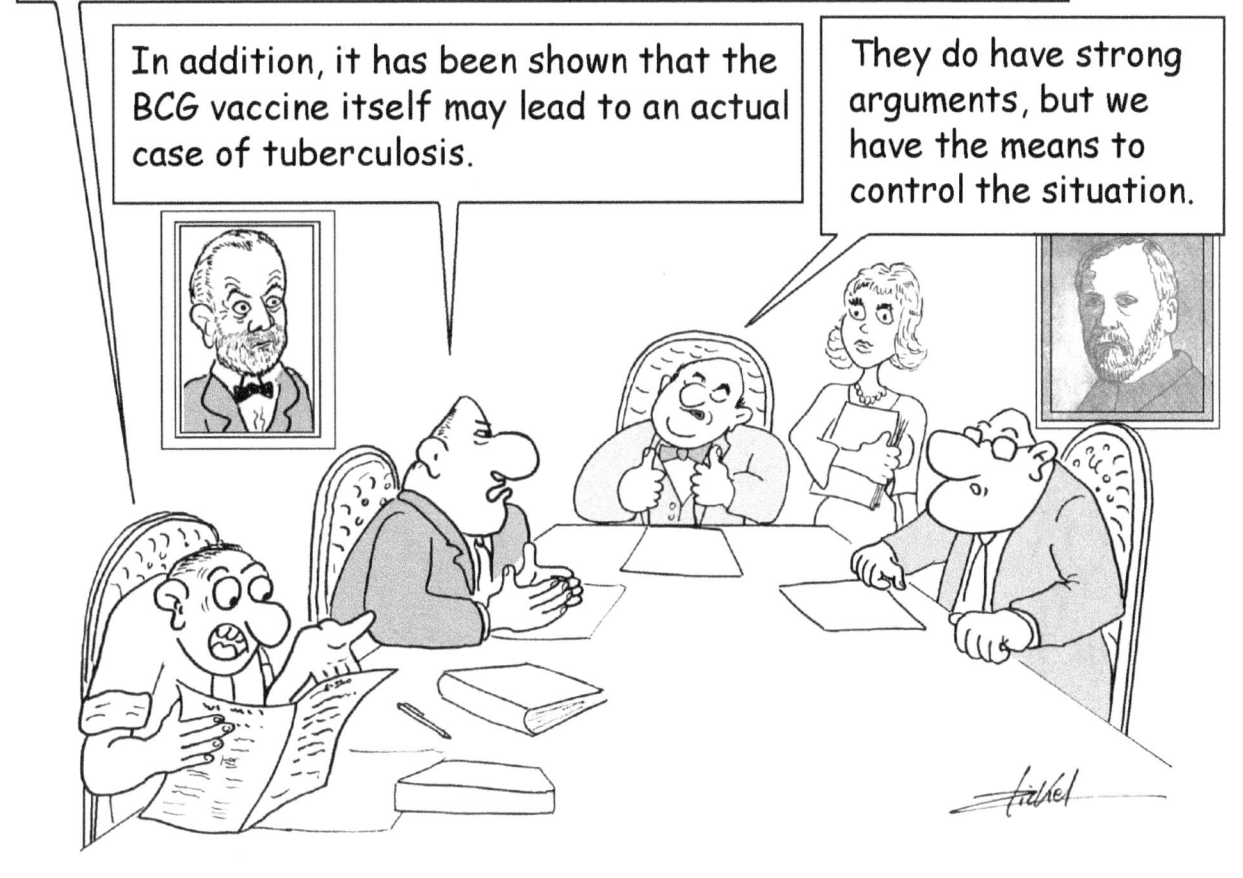

... When a bus drops down a ravine, loaded with 40 pupils, the tragedy makes the headlines in the newspapers all around the world.
The hundreds of children killed each year by the BCG vaccine remain anonymous ... The goose that lays the golden egg at the Pasteur Institute would end up in a sauce pan ! The medical profession should in no case be informed ...

... Learn here a terrible truth: each time you hear about the terrible death of a child, felled in the first few weeks of his life, by a "viral meningitis", you have the right to suspect the BCG vaccine, even if the autopsy confirmed the classical diagnosis of "viral encephalitis" blistering ...

... If the doctor responsible for such a horror is aware of the cause-effect relationship, then he is a brilliant murderer, or a coward for keeping it secret. If he does not understand this relationship, then he is a dangerous fool, ready to do it again...

Dr. Jean ELMIGER "La Médecine retrouvée"

The WHO does not recommend the BCG vaccine. It was not recommended in Germany since 1973. However, French authorities continued mandating it until July 2007.

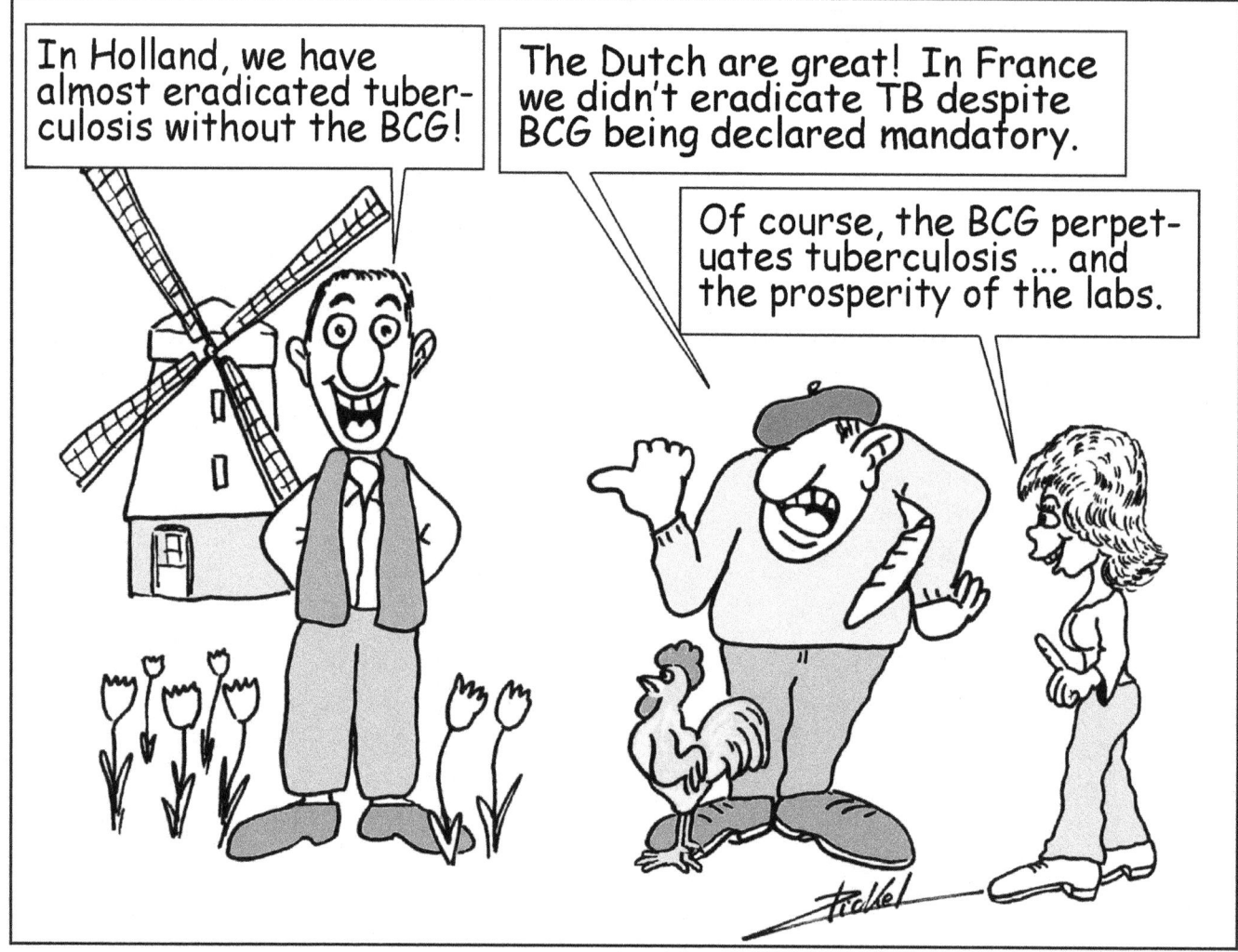

In 1945, Holland was the country of Europe the most affected by the scourge of tuberculosis. In 1974, without ever having made use of the BCG vaccine, the disease was virtually eradicated. In contrast, the scourge of tuberculosis regained strength wherever the BCG was still practiced.

Statistical Bulletin of the Department of Public Health and Social Security (# 1 - 1974)

The BCG hampers the fight against tuberculosis

Professor Michel REY

> The vaccination with BCG without particular indication has only drawbacks and involves dangers. (...) This vaccination must therefore be crossed off our catalog of tuberculosis control measures, without replacement. According to us, the vaccination with BCG is no longer scientifically based, and medically, it is no longer relevant.
>
> **Professor FREERKSEN**
> Cited in the "Concours Médical" by
> Dr. GOUDREAU, Director of the National Committee Against Tuberculosis,
> Professor PARIENTE, Pulmonologist

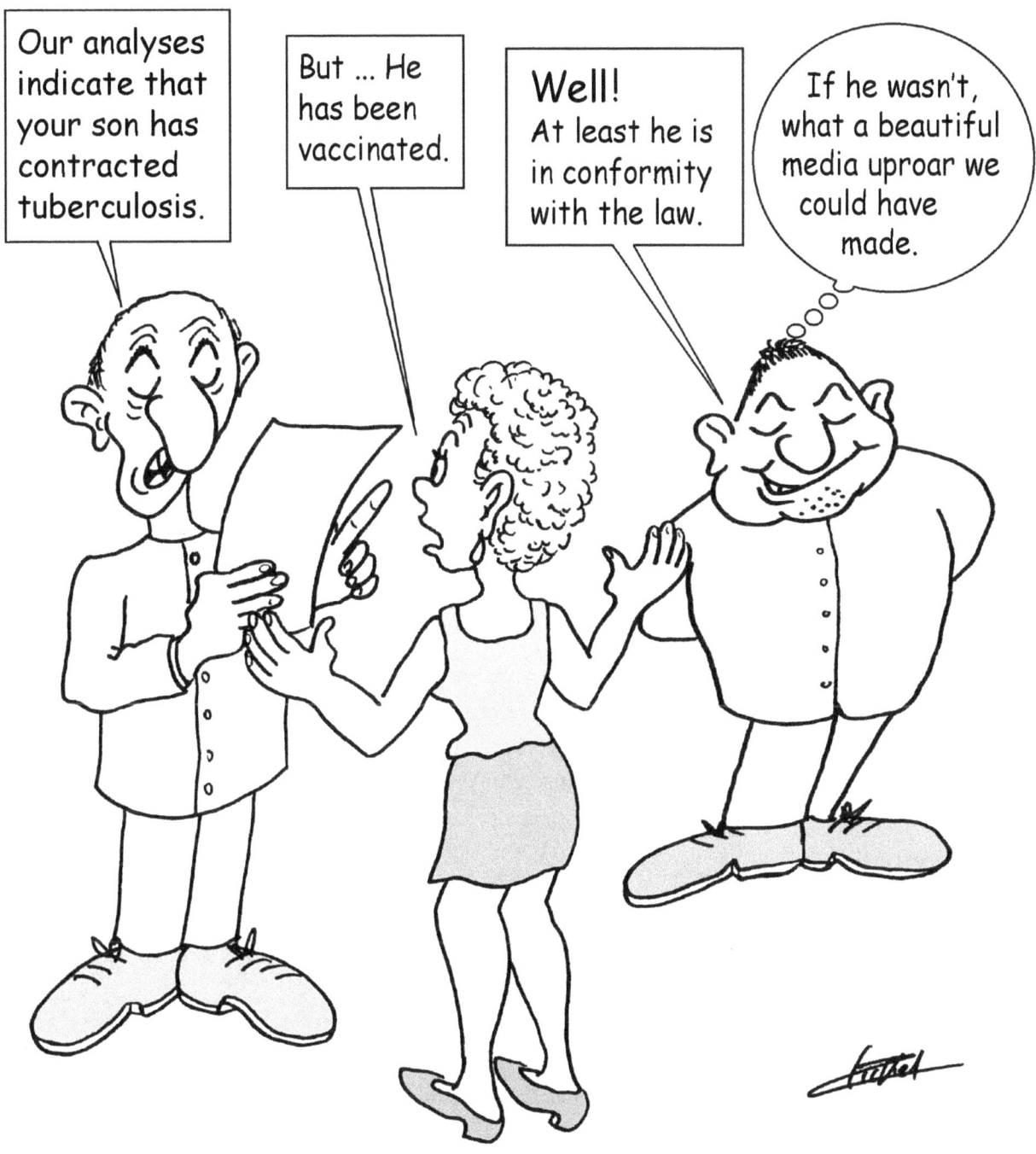

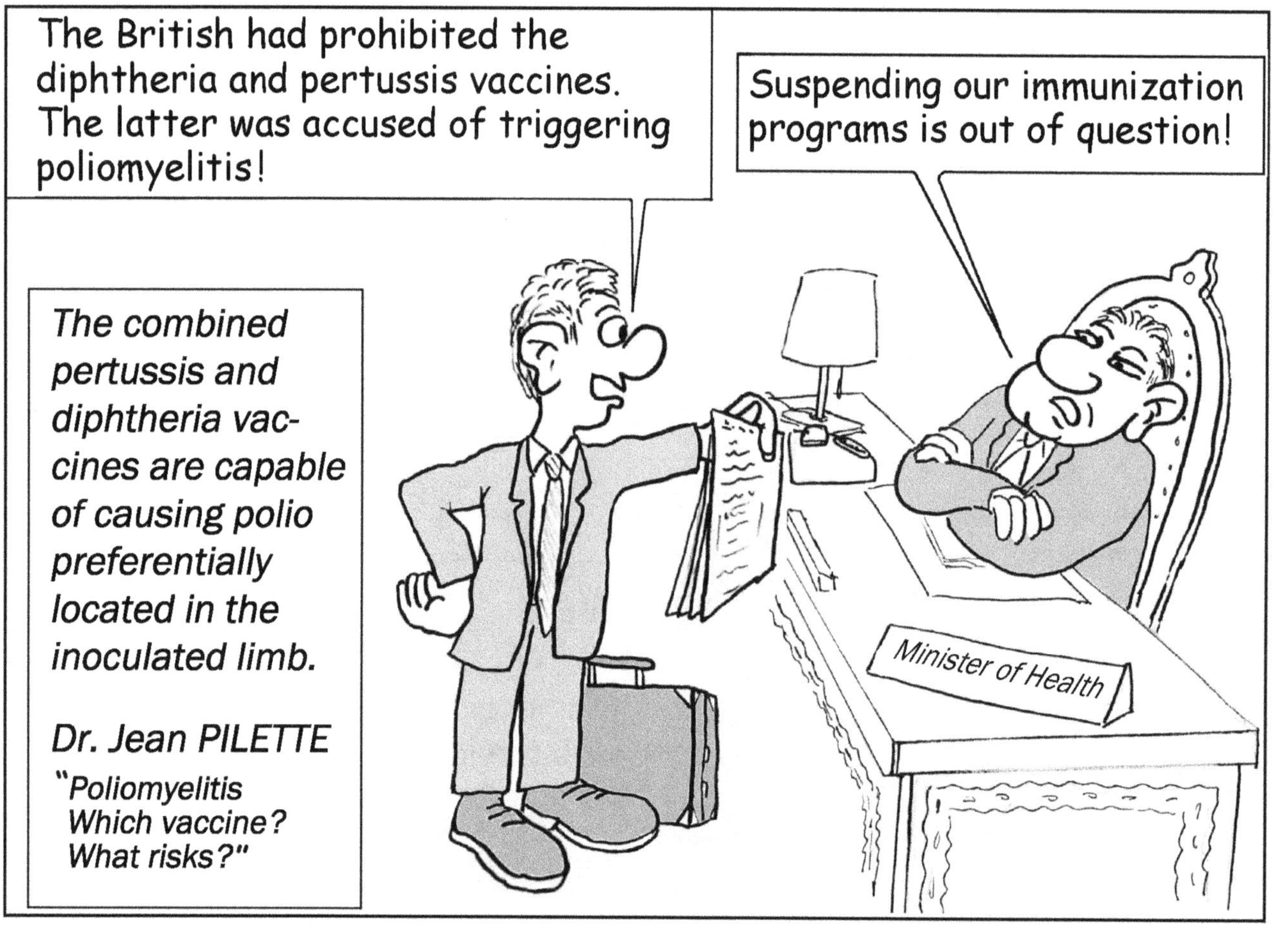

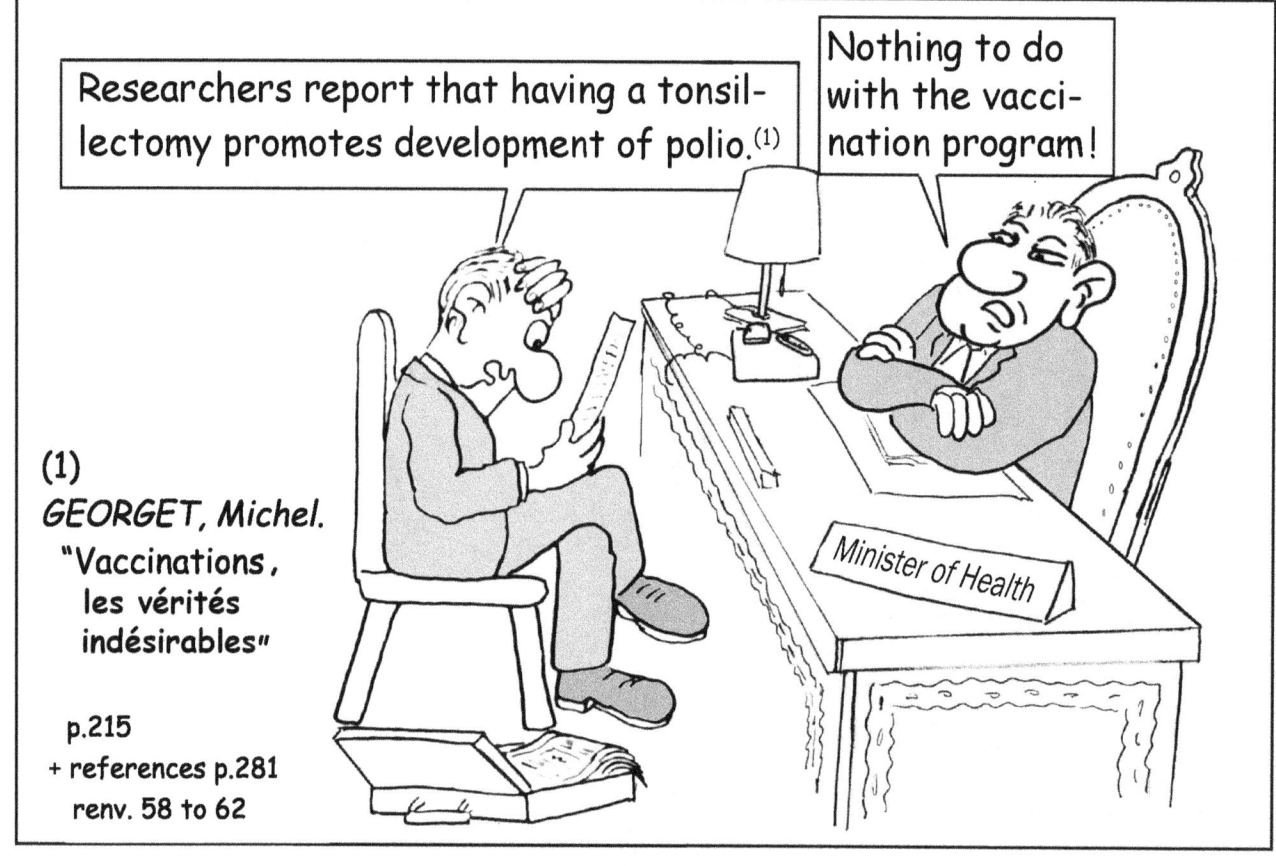

Poliomyelitis: the vaccine at any cost (cont'd)

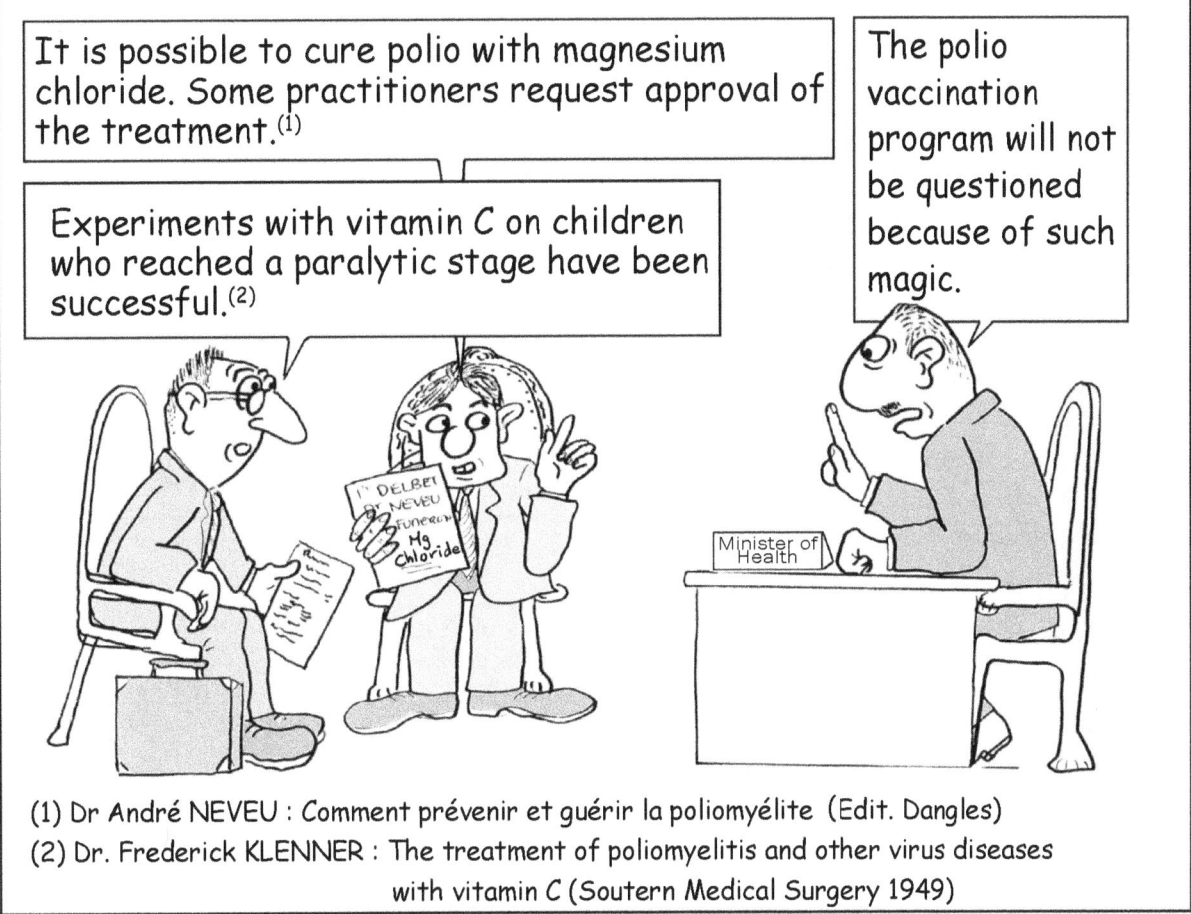

(1) Dr André NEVEU : Comment prévenir et guérir la poliomyélite (Edit. Dangles)
(2) Dr. Frederick KLENNER : The treatment of poliomyelitis and other virus diseases with vitamin C (Soutern Medical Surgery 1949)

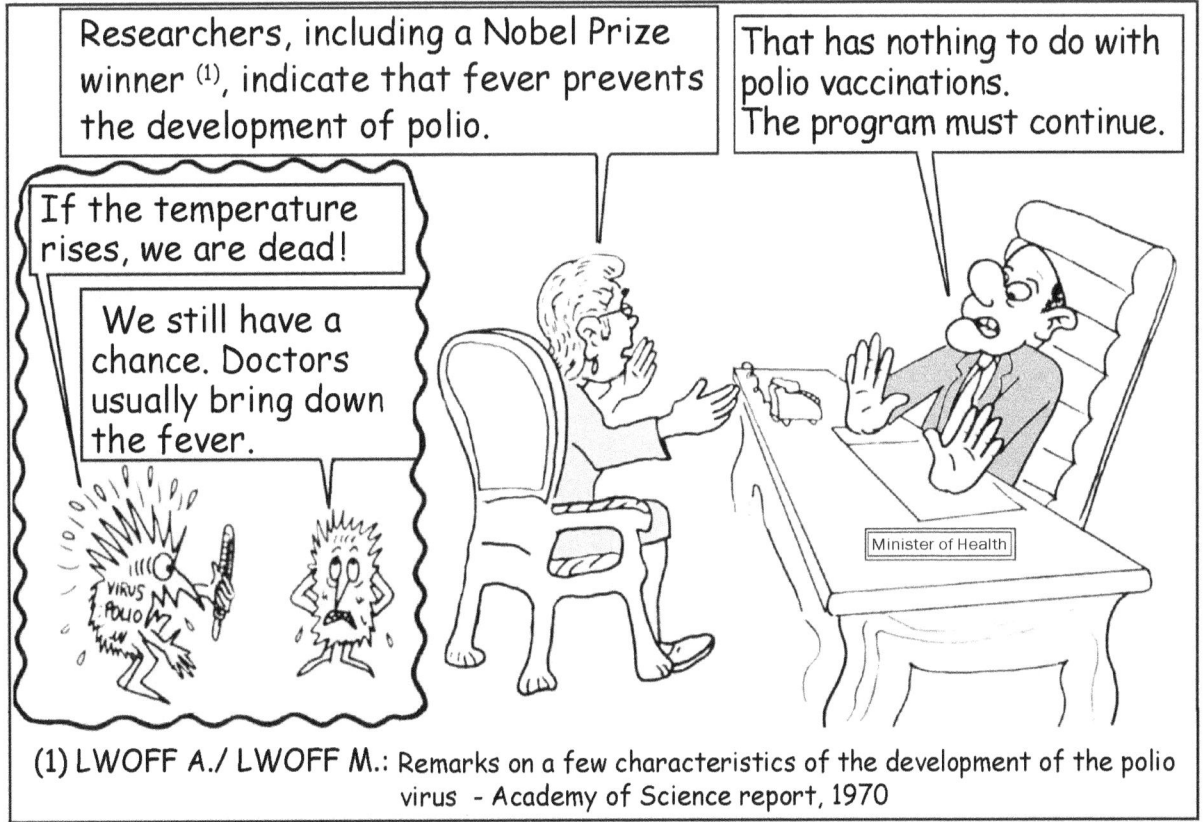

(1) LWOFF A./ LWOFF M.: Remarks on a few characteristics of the development of the polio virus - Academy of Science report, 1970

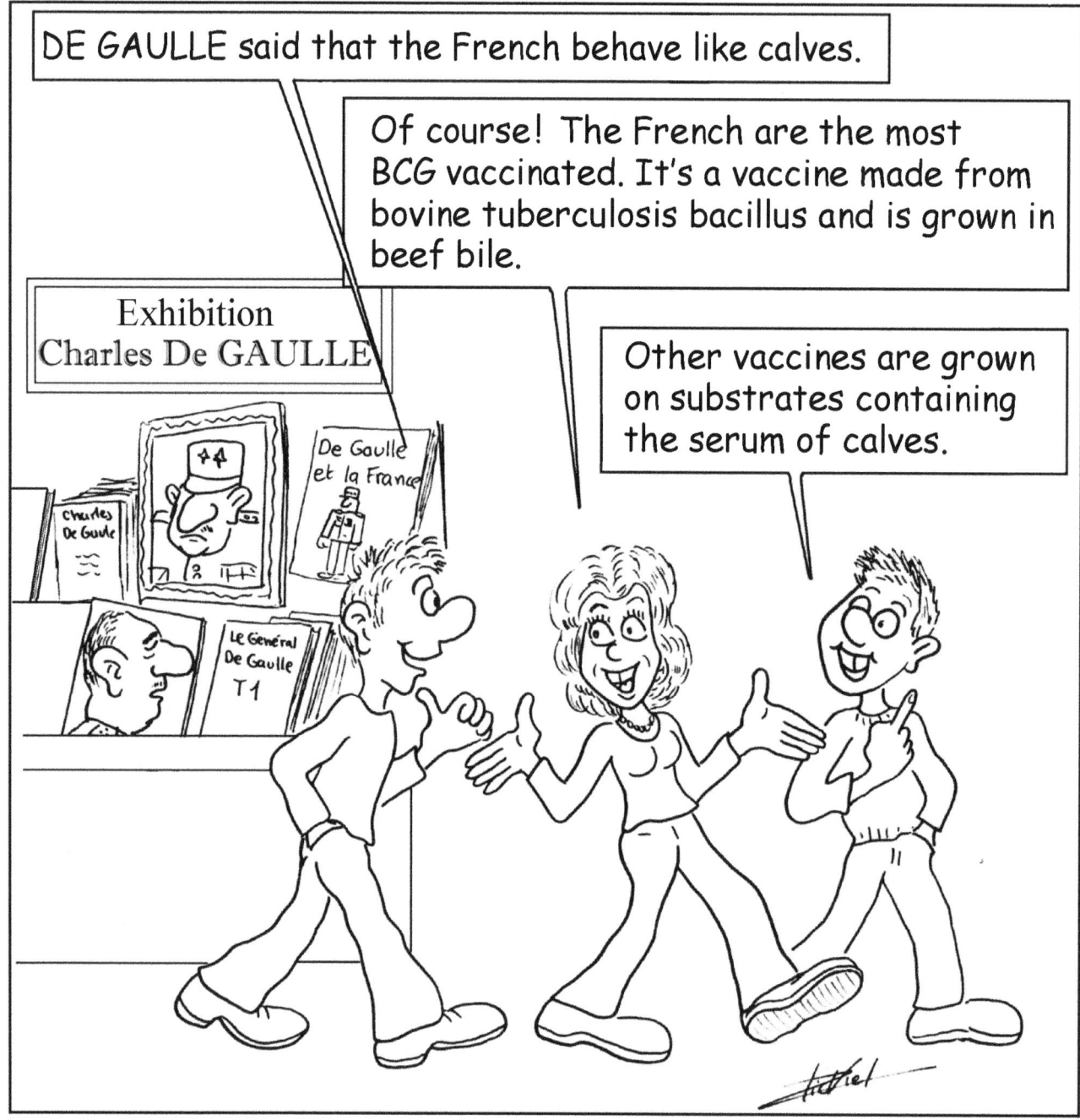

... The Vegetarians have always claimed that ingesting the flesh of animals gradually introduces in humans the bestiality of the slaughtered animal ... Who is talking here of ingestion? ... It is injected through the skin, beyond one's control ... The C. & G. (Calmette and Guérin) partners did not choose the animal at random. They chose the cow. This peaceful bovine is slowly but surely becoming the analog and quasi-parental link between the large family of the French ...

Dr. Jean ELMIGER "La Médecine retrouvée"

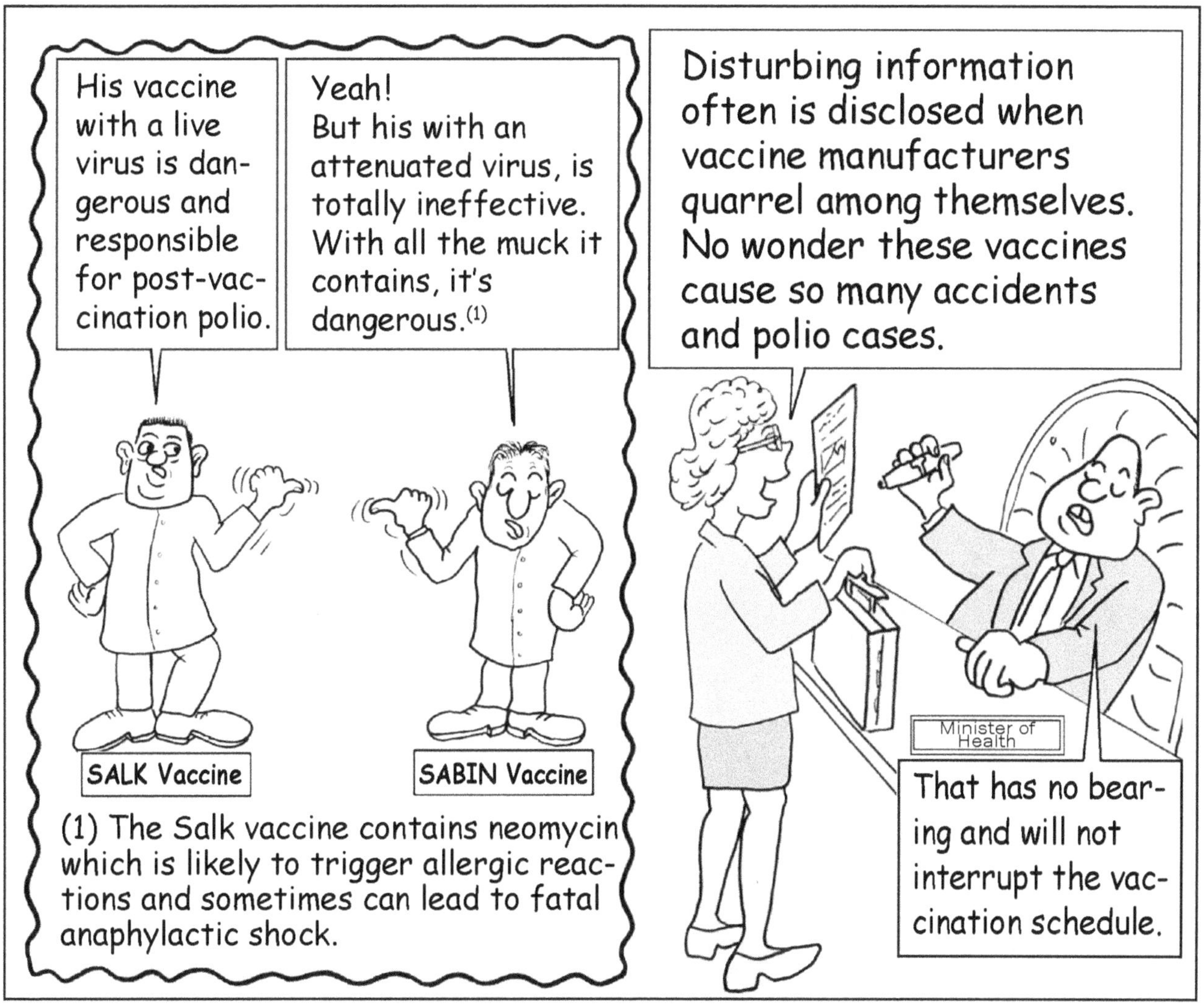

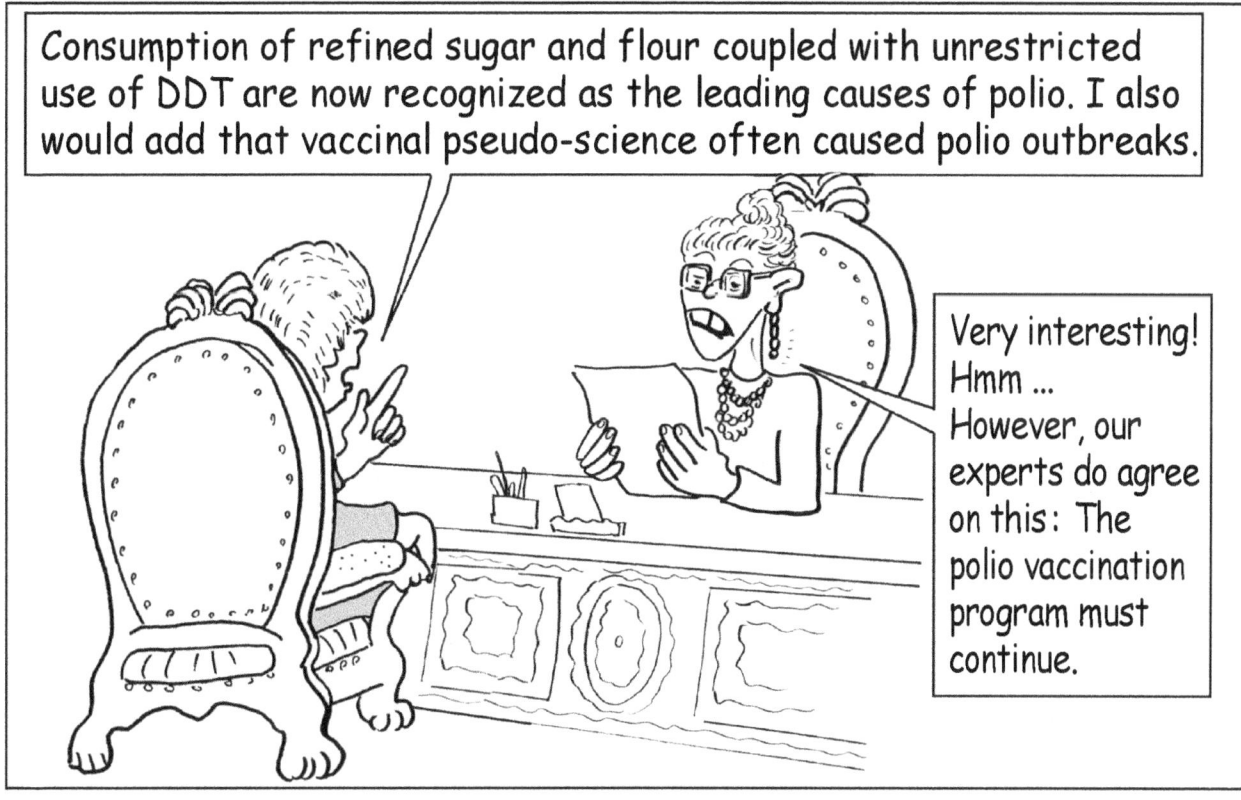

Vaccines: The Great Illusion

> *Almost all the polio cases registered in the U.S.A., between 1980 and 1994, were caused by the administration of the attenuated oral vaccine.*
> AFP dispatch, February 1, 1997

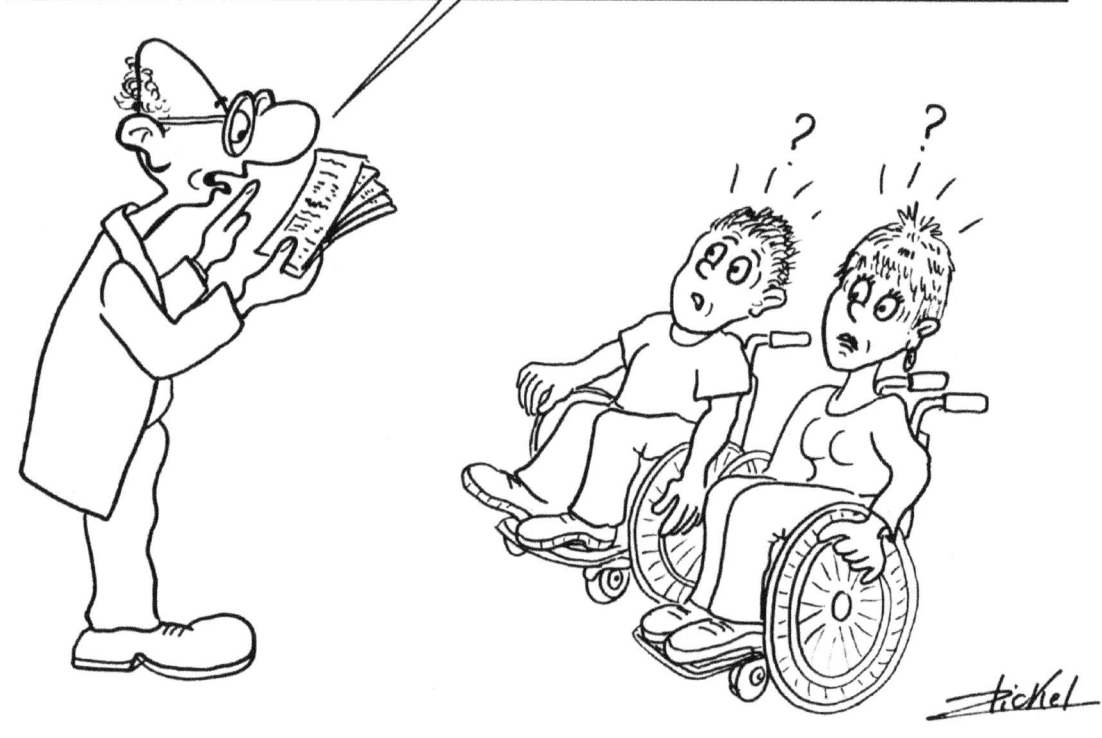

> *Since 1957, the WHO registers in the statistics only the paralytic forms of poliomyelitis, whereas before the vaccination, all forms of polio were included, which seems to show a regression of the cases, which is far from being the truth.*
> Viera SCHEIBNER, PhD (Australian expert)

> *Unlike previously established beliefs about polio virus vaccines, evidence now exists that the live vaccine cannot be administered without risk of producing paralysis. The live viral polio vaccine carries the risk of producing paralytic polio in vaccinated individuals and in their contacts.*
>
> Dr. Jonas SALK
> (SALK produced the original polio vaccine in the 1950s.)

Whooping Cough

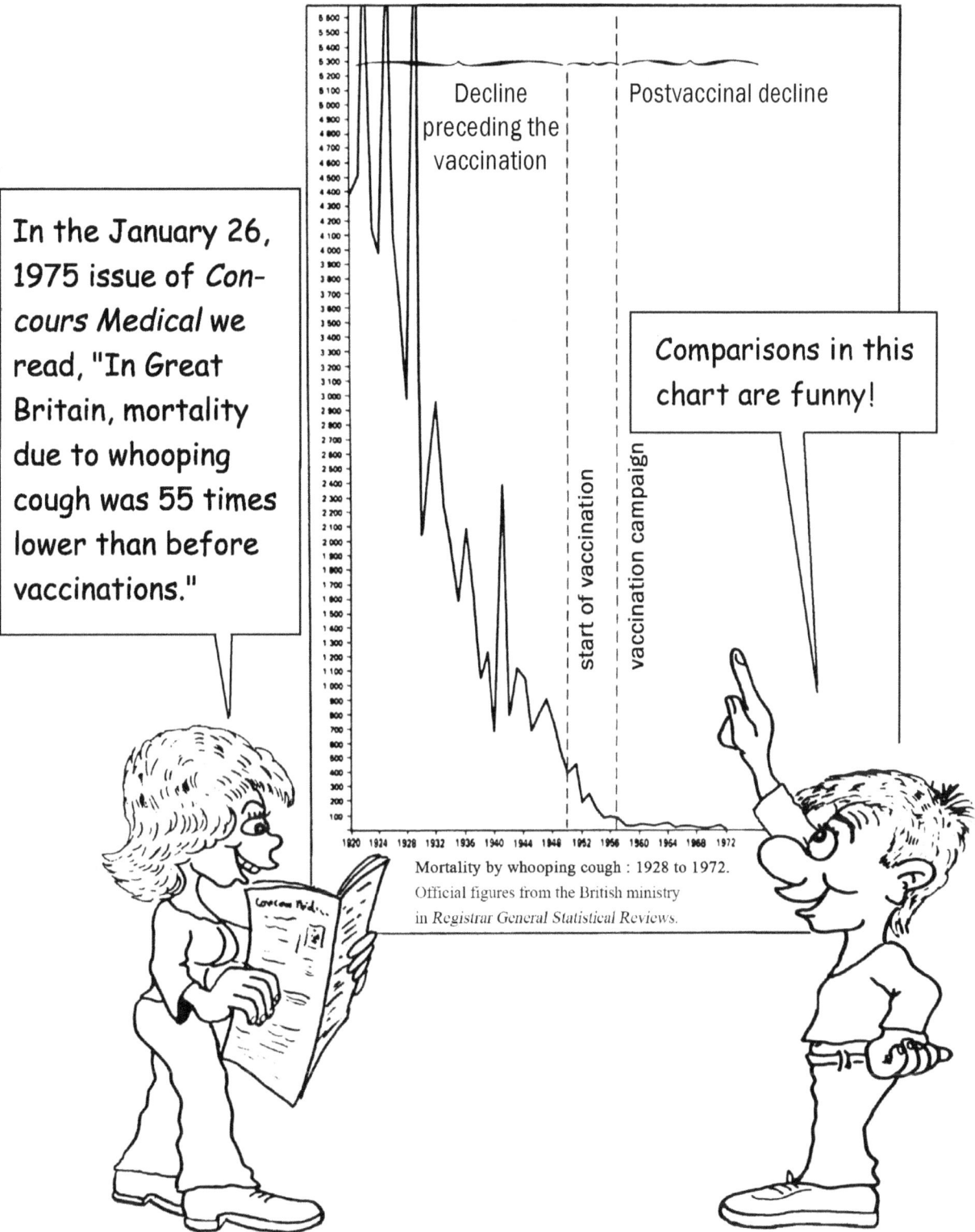

Mortality by whooping cough: 1928 to 1972.
Official figures from the British ministry in *Registrar General Statistical Reviews*.

In the January 26, 1975 issue of *Concours Medical* we read, "In Great Britain, mortality due to whooping cough was 55 times lower than before vaccinations."

Comparisons in this chart are funny!

> The worst of all vaccines is that one against whooping cough. (...)
> It is responsible for a large number of deaths and a large number of irreversible brain damage in newborns.
> Dr. KALOKERINOS *(May 24, 1987 Sunwell Tops)*

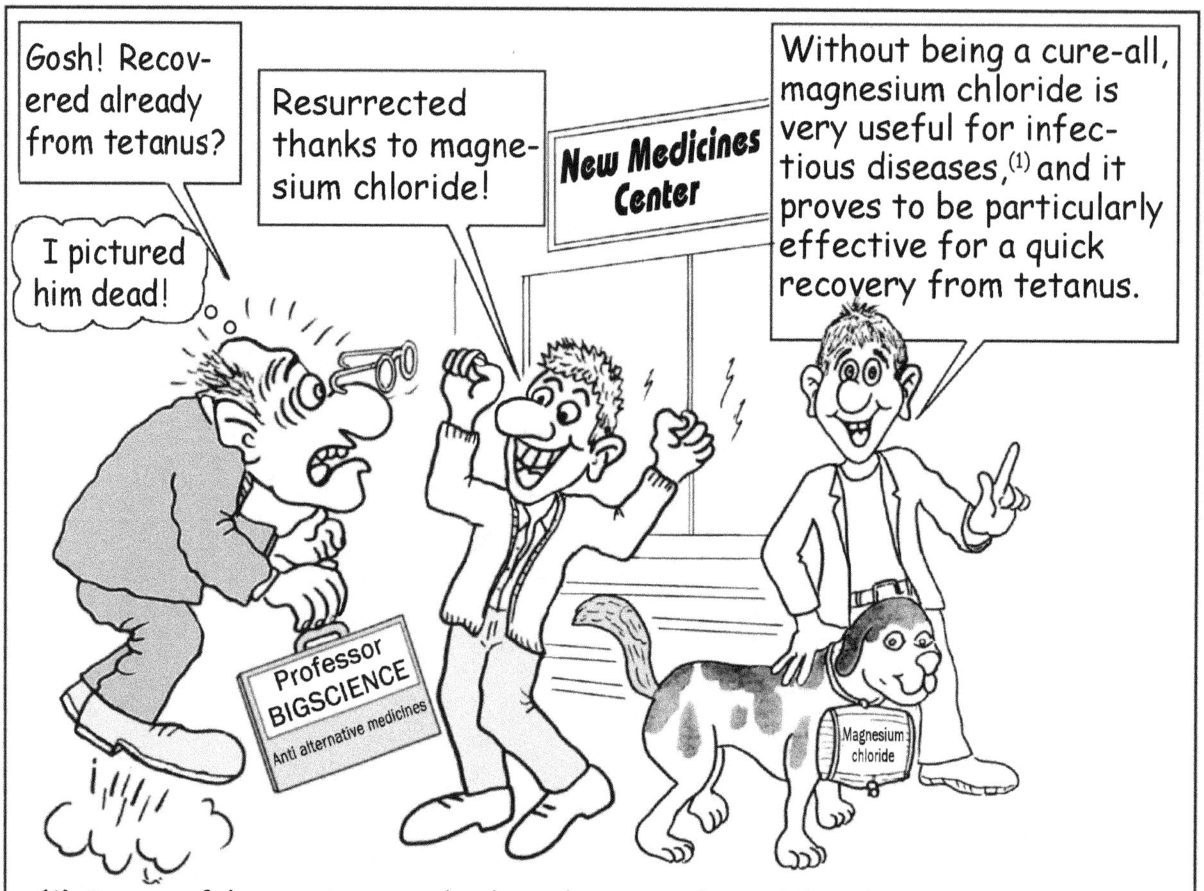

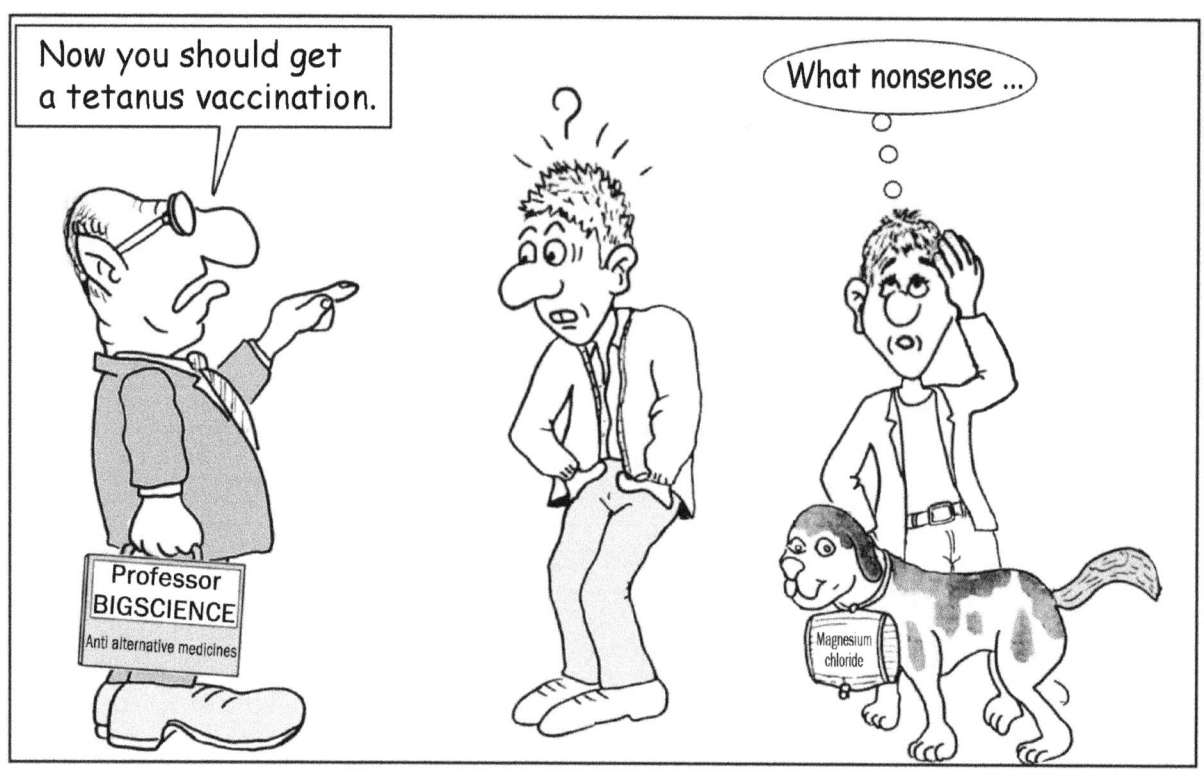

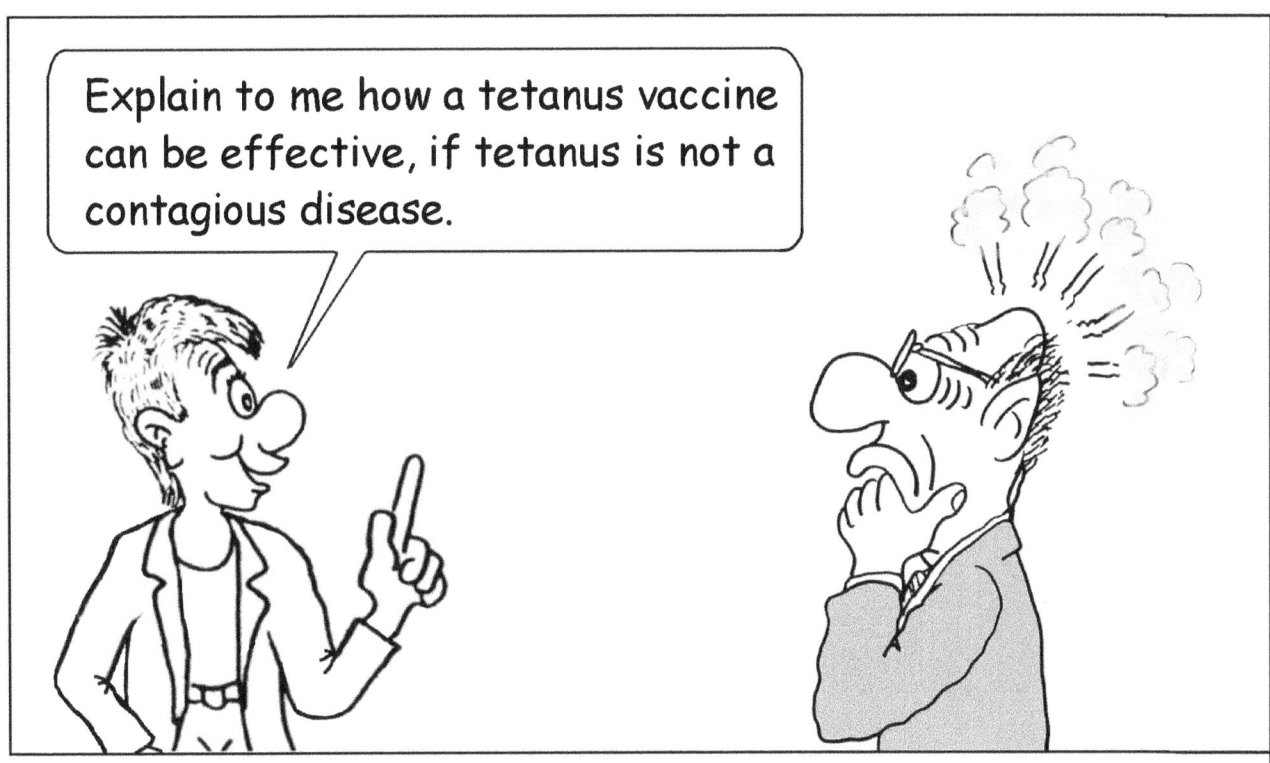
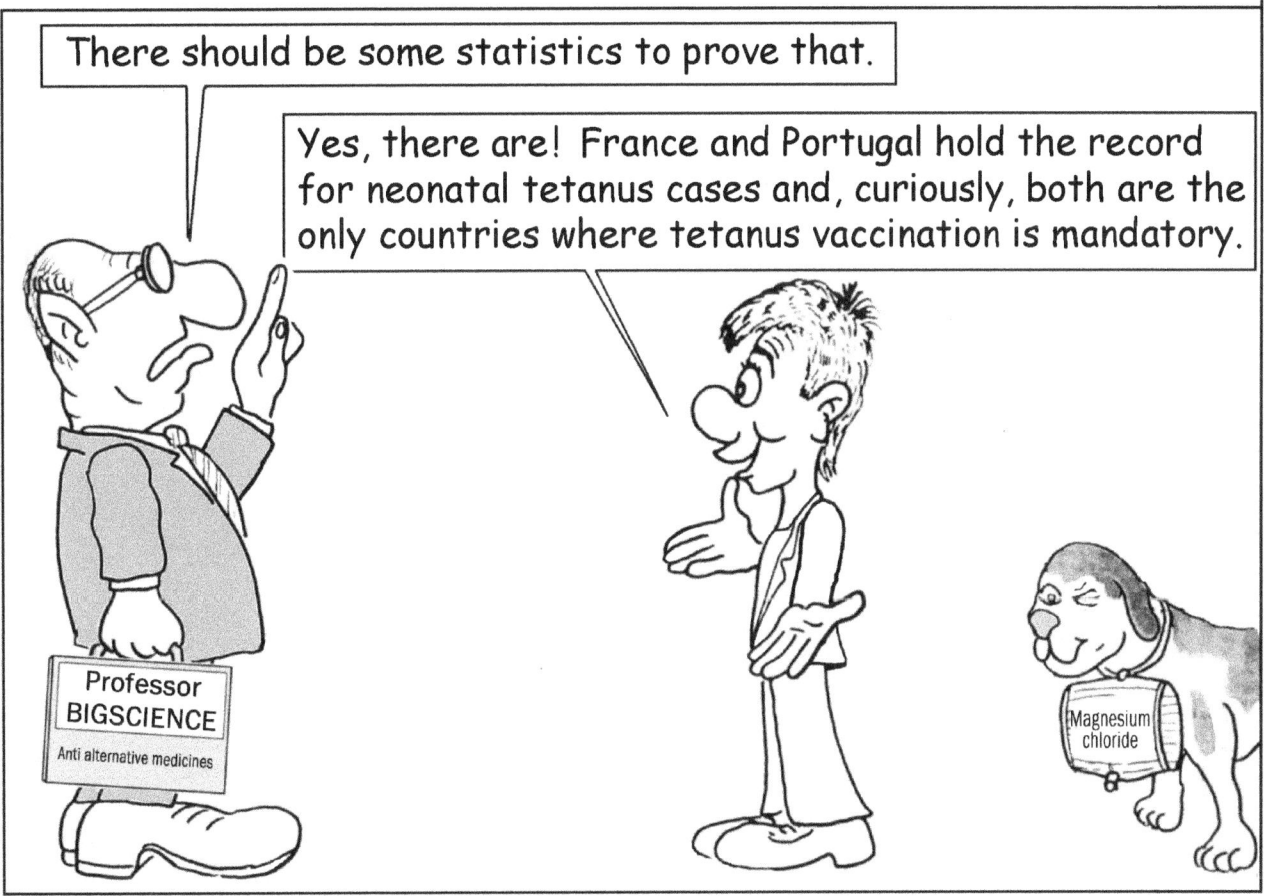

The decline of tetanus as a disease began before the introduction of the tetanus toxoid in the population.
                               Medical Journal of Australia 1978

Hepatitis B: a ghost epidemic

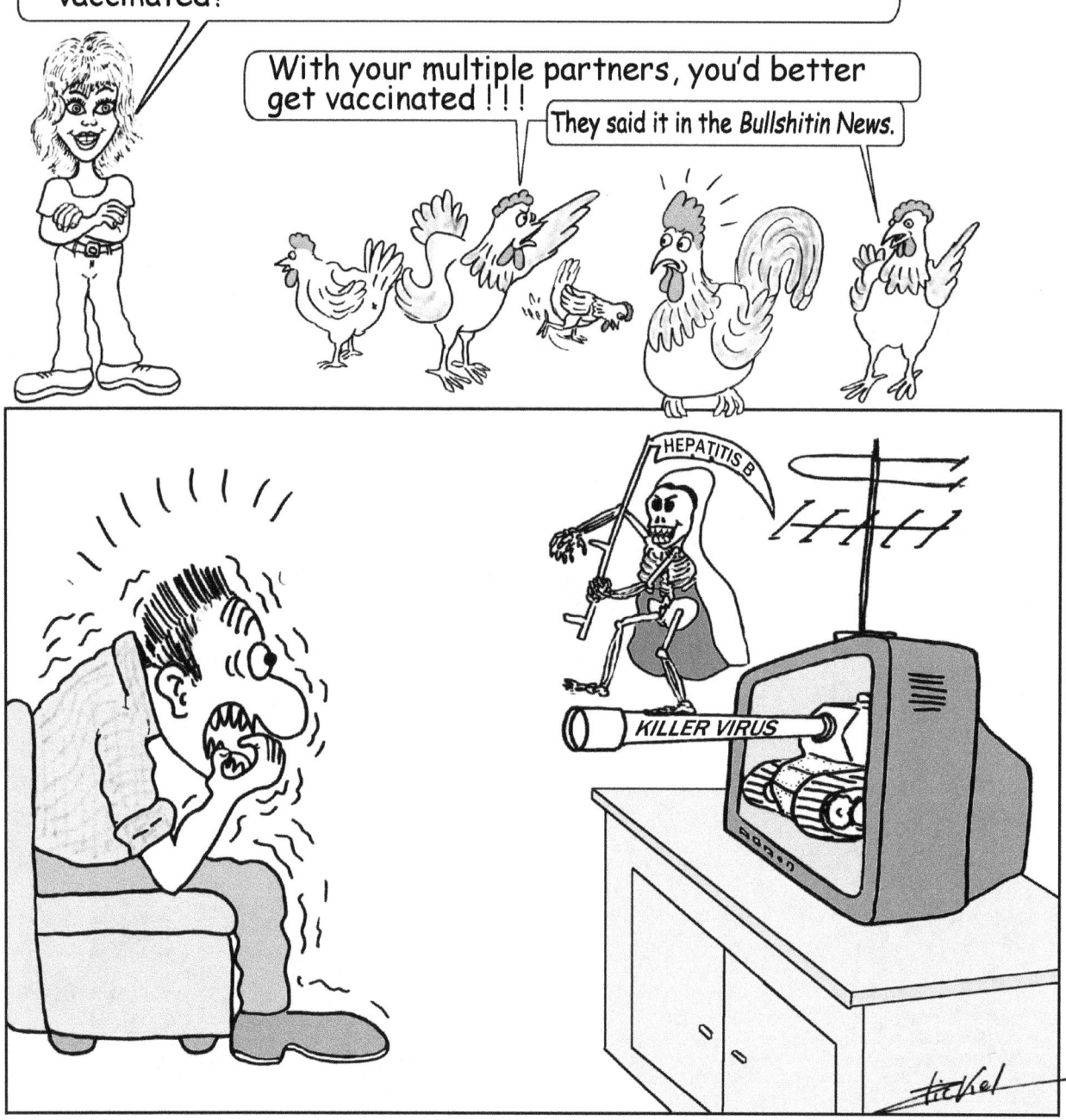

Inventing an epidemic by emphasizing the potential gravity of a disease while exaggerating its transmission capabilities, is now a classic scare tactic to get everyone vaccinated!

With your multiple partners, you'd better get vaccinated!!!

They said it in the *Bullshitin News*.

We led a rough campaign. We violated the conscience of people. Even 80-year-old grandmothers came to claim their vaccine!

Professor Alain FISCH

Hepatitis B: the Massacre

> This vaccine seriously damaged the health of some of those who were inoculated.
> Studies report severe autoimmune and neurological complications.

> Twenty years old and already in a wheelchair!
> Thank you Big Pharma, for protecting me from hepatitis B.

> Don't mention it.

The presence of cerebral edema in very young children who die soon after vaccination against hepatitis B is disturbing ...
Children under age 14 have a greater chance of dying or suffering from the hepatitis B vaccine than contracting the disease itself.

Jane ORIENT, MD,
Director of the Association of American Physicians and Surgeons

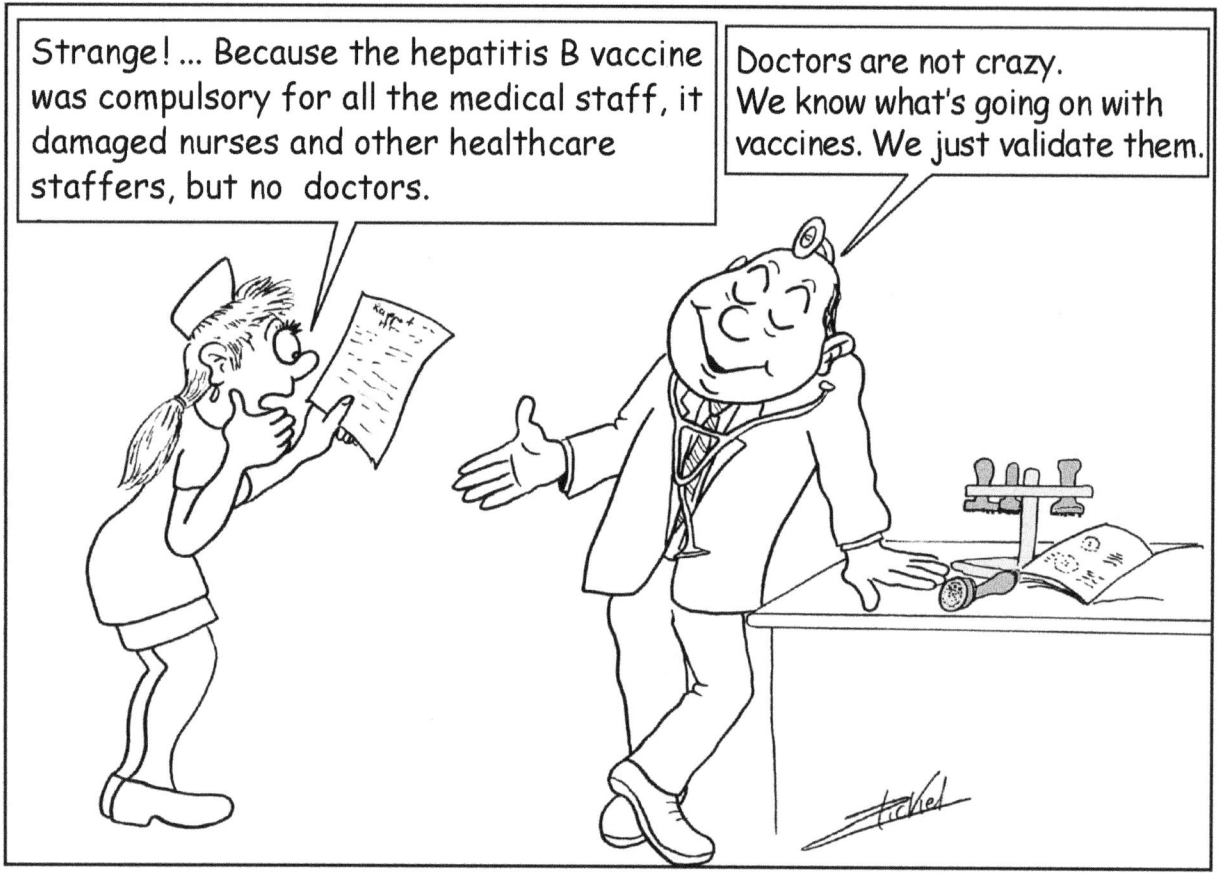
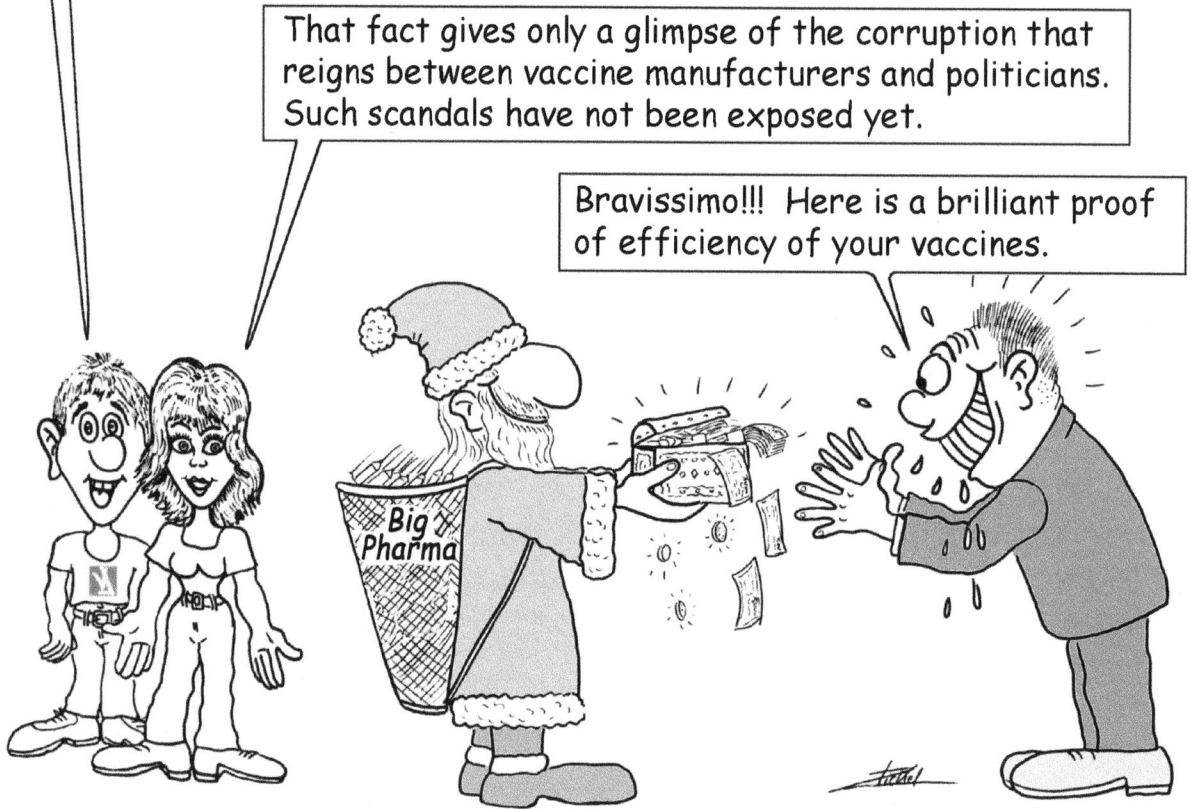

Vaccines: The Great Illusion

Hepatitis B incidence fell dramatically before introduction of the vaccine. The good news is that hepatitis B, as with other liver diseases, can be cured with simple lifestyle changes.

You'd better not say that. If people aren't afraid of getting hepatitis B, that will be bad for business.

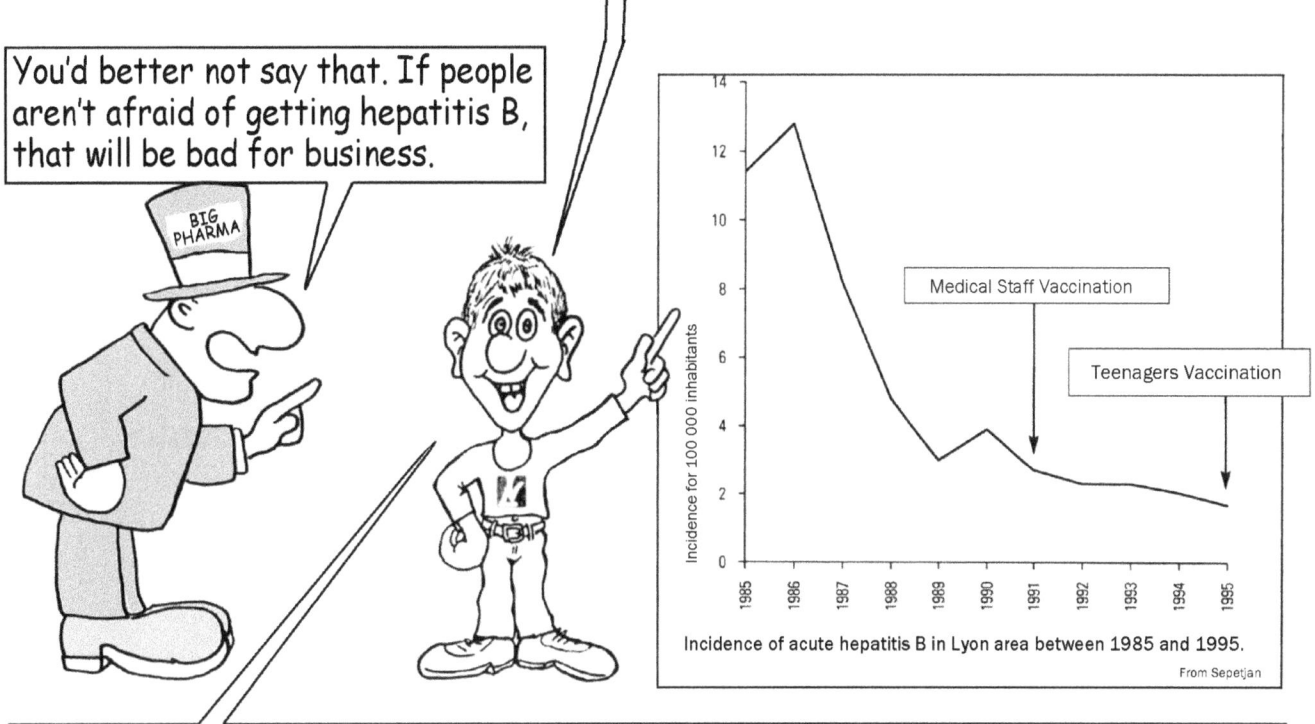

Incidence of acute hepatitis B in Lyon area between 1985 and 1995.
From Sepetjan

Reduce or eliminate fatty foods such as meats, and dairy products while also decreasing sugars and starchy foods. Eat plenty of raw fresh fruits and vegetables, take vitamin C, and try fasting for a little while.

Most liver diseases are alcohol or drug-related.

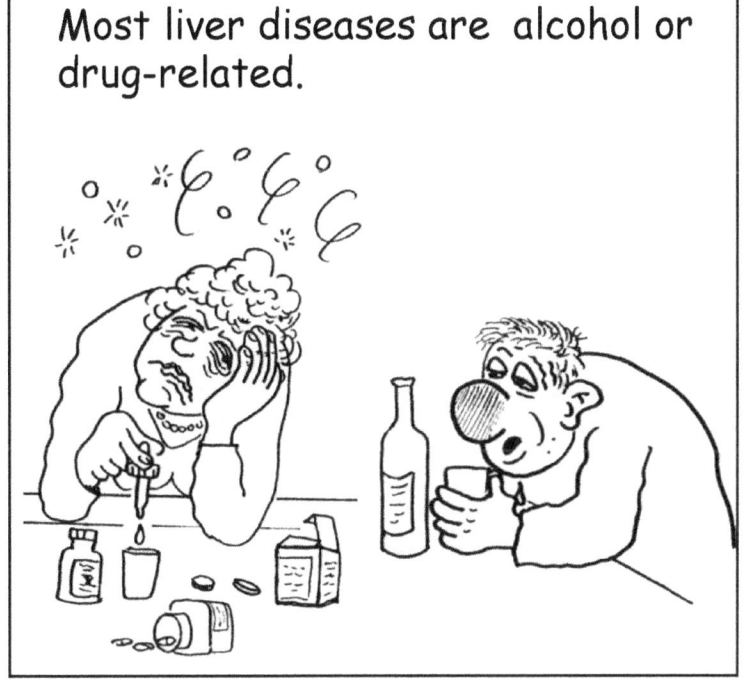

Anger is the liver's enemy!

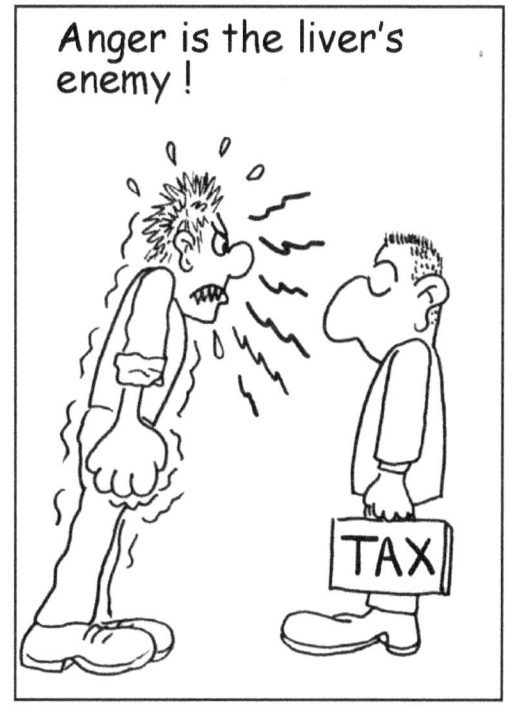

Measles

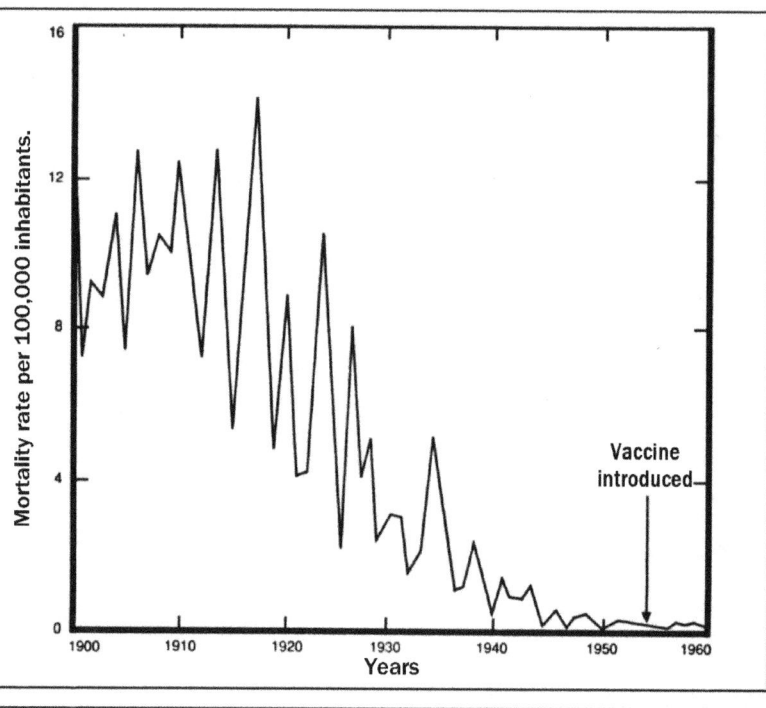

**United States
Measles Mortality Rate:
state death rates
1900-1932 and 1933-1960**

Rate for 1,000,000 inhabitants.

(Cf. IAS Newsletter, vol 10, # 1 and 2).

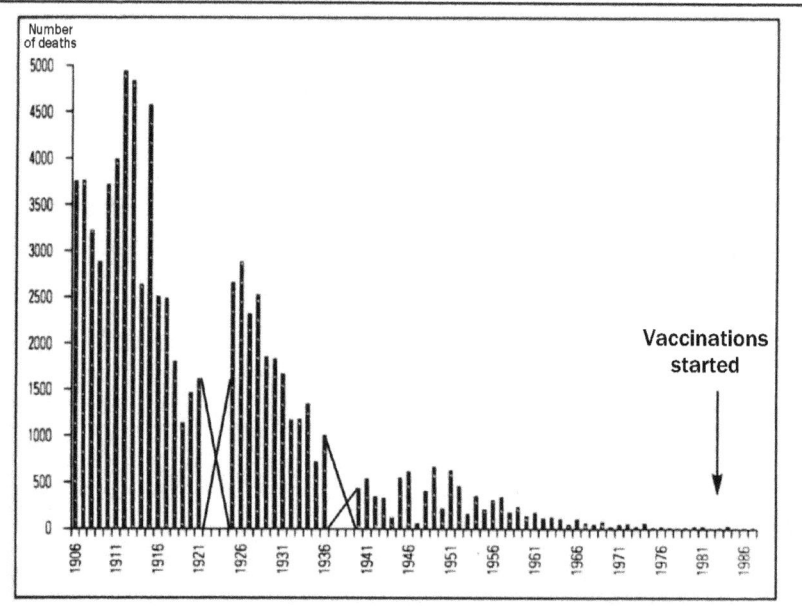

**Measles Death Rate
in France**

(Absence of data for years
1922-1924 and 1937-1939.)

(Statistical directory of France)

Studying these charts, no one can say there are fewer measles deaths thanks to vaccinations.

It is important to know that measles, as well as other infectious infant diseases, strengthen and improve children's immune systems with natural, life-long immunity.

Any measles deaths can be attributed only to compromised immune systems and inadequate treatments.

Influenza: a flawed vaccine

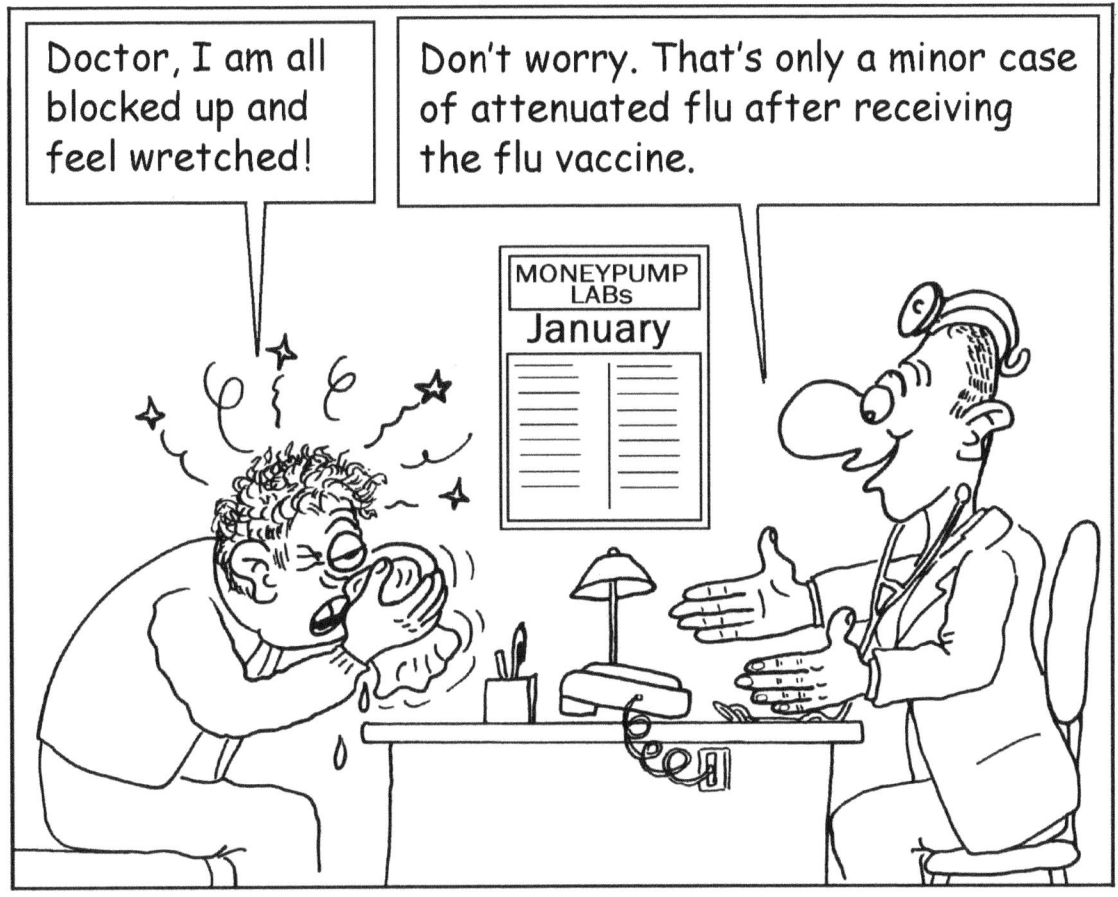
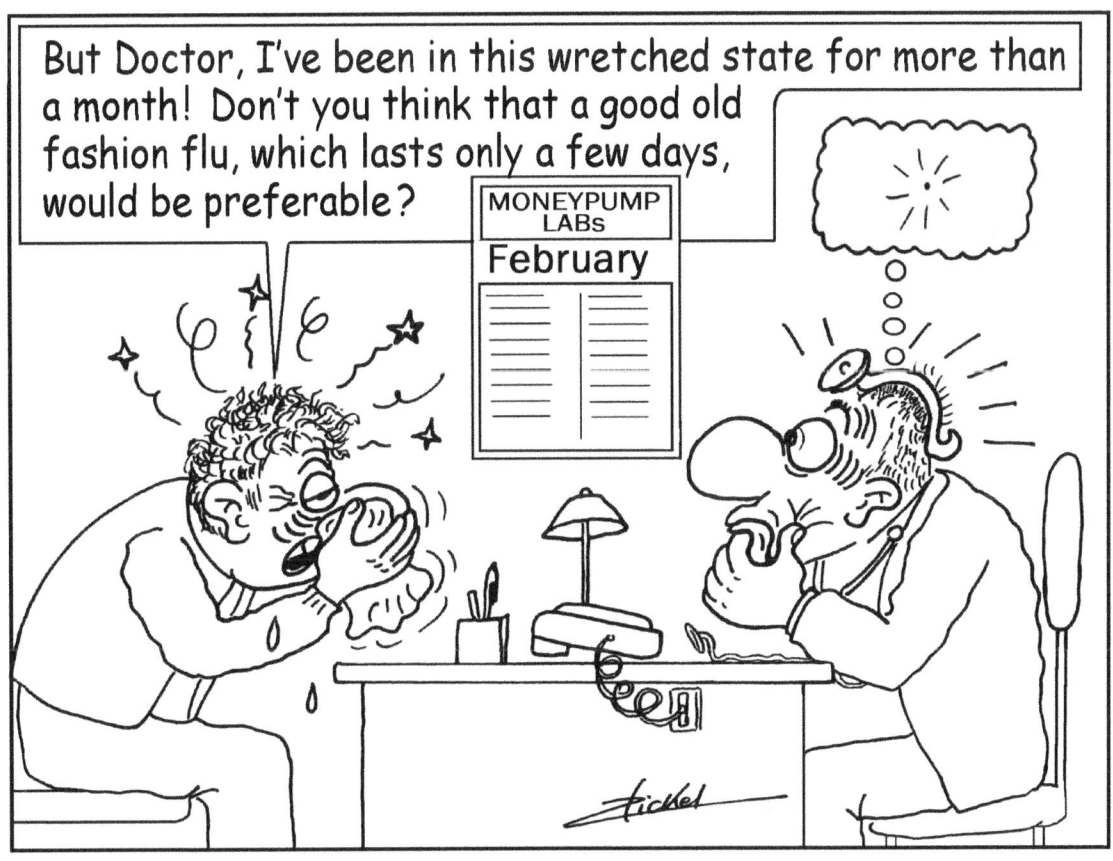

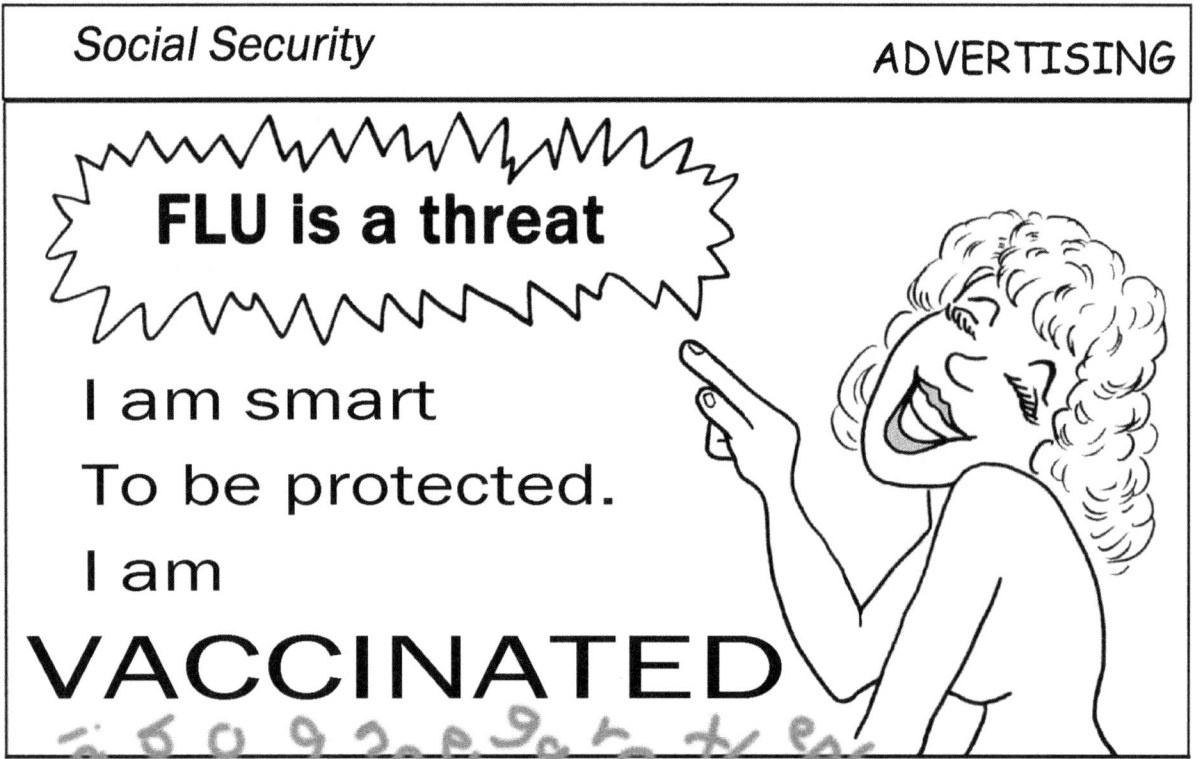
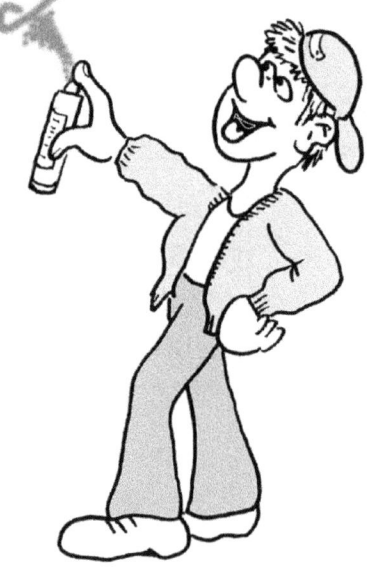

> There is no evidence that any influenza vaccine thus far developed is effective in preventing or mitigating any attack of influenza.
> The producers of these vaccines know they are worthless, but they go on selling them anyway.
>
> *Dr. J. Anthony MORRIS*
> *Chief Vaccine Control Officer, U.S. FDA, until 1976*

Vaccines: The Great Illusion

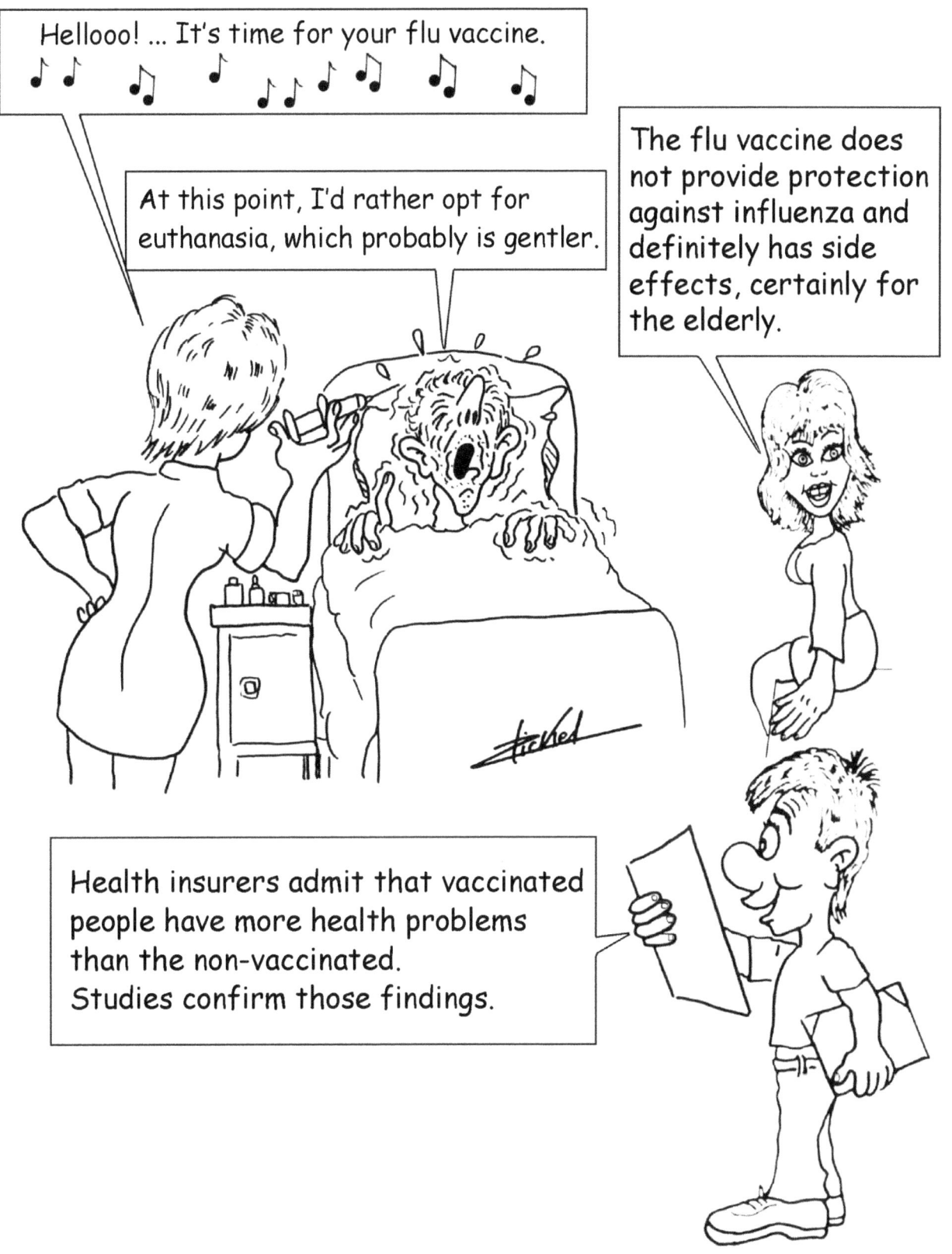

Vaccines: The Great Illusion

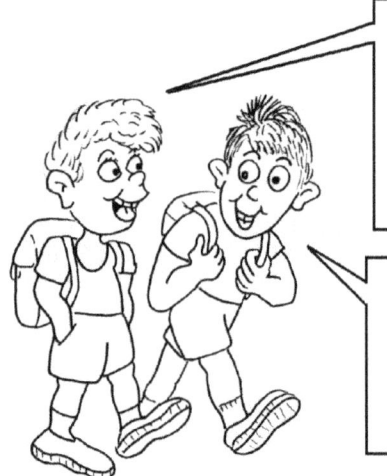

I'm lucky! My parents practice natural health and healing methods.
They taught me that viruses are not necessarily the cause of the flu.

And I learned that even if viruses were involved, the vaccine still would not work.

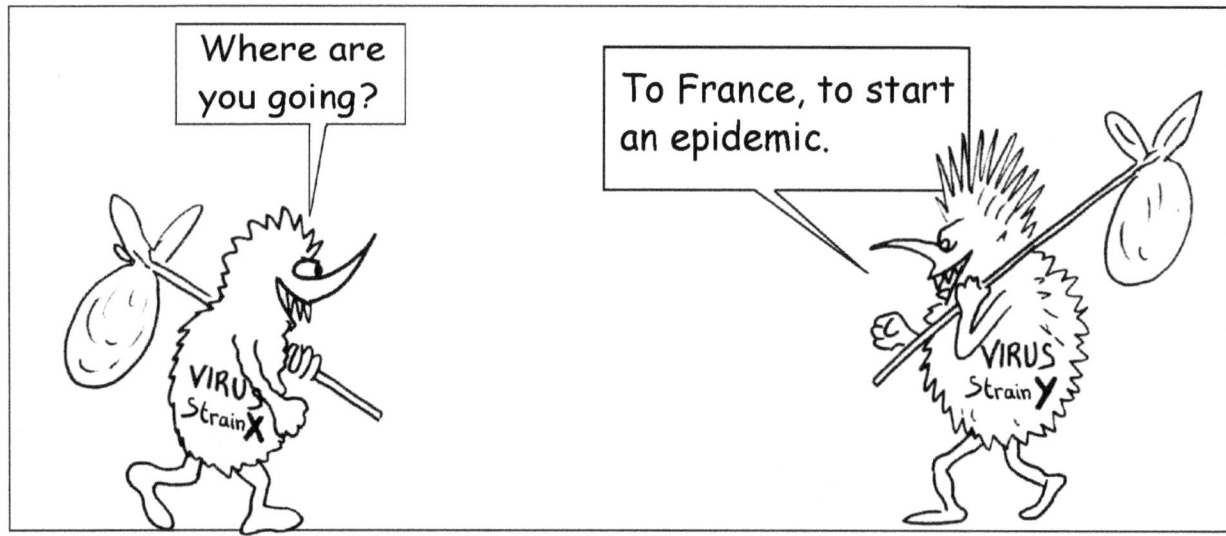

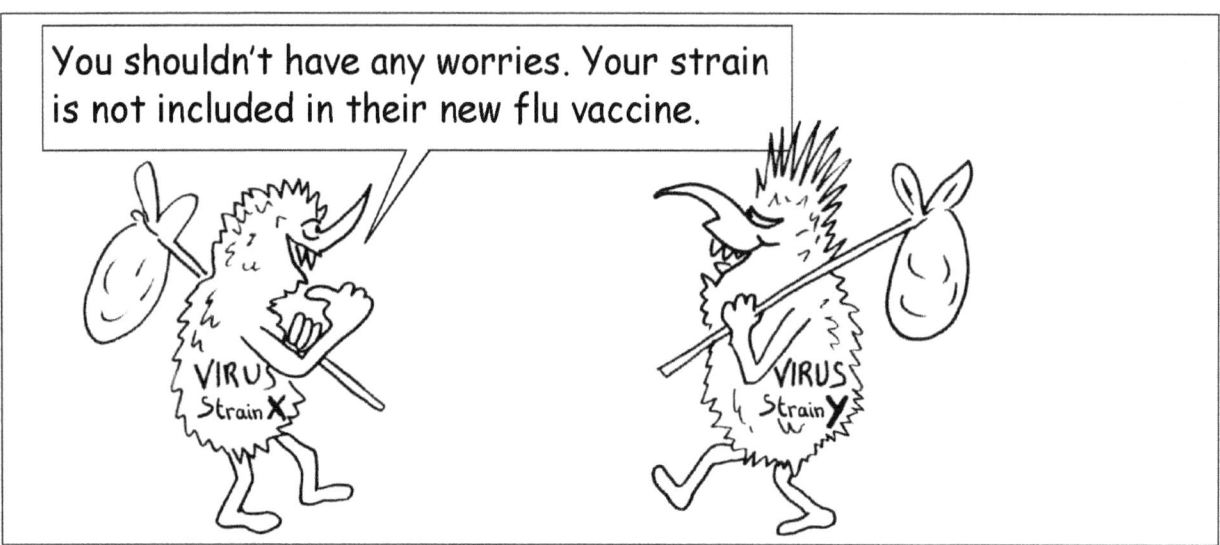

The flu virus is as shifting as a chameleon.

Professor John OXFORD
(Courrier International, February, 1998)

Influenza: aggression or liberation?

An acute disease is nothing more that an effort of nature which tries hard with all its power to restore the health of the patient, by eliminating the pathogenic element.

Thomas SYDENHAM, 1692.
Physician, the father of English medicine, called the English Hippocrates

The flu is a vital process, a wholesome cleansing crisis, that you should not hinder.

Most of the medicines and other inadequate treatments result in all those dreaded complications.

No antibiotics, they are useless. They do not touch viruses. I prescribe rest, fresh air, sunlight, a glass of water and thoughts about wellness and joy.

Dr. COMMONSENSE

Natural forces within us are the true healers of disease.

HIPPOCRATES

HPV vaccine: just another vaccine with sad effects

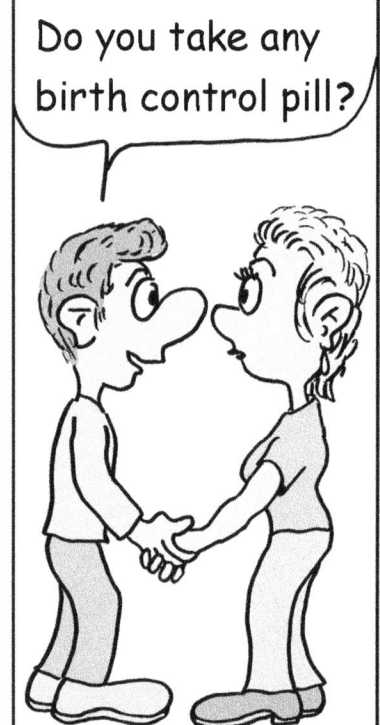
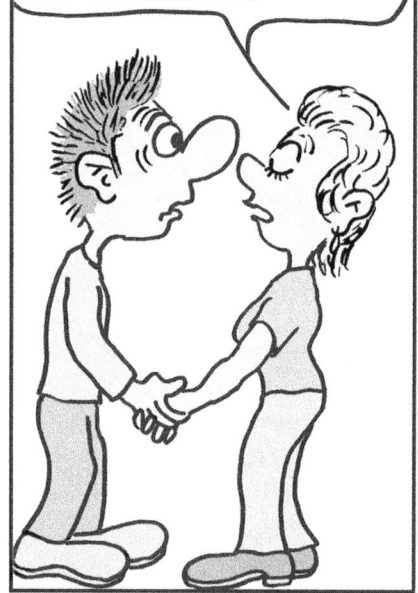
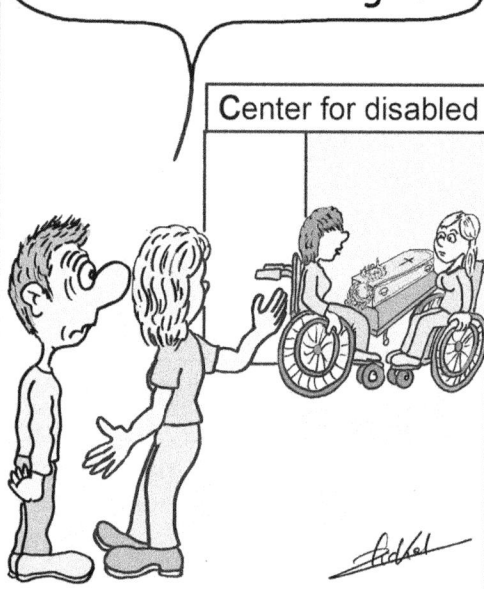

The first problem is that there are over 100 strains of HPV, only 30 of which are even theoretically linked with cervical cancer. In addition, HPV is present in at least half the normal population, almost never causing any disease or problems whatsoever. Indeed, HPV has never been proven as a pathogen for any disease.

... All that has ever been shown is that HPV is sometimes present in cervical cancer tissue, but as we know it's also present in half the normal population. There is a total lack of evidence that cervical cancer appears in women with HPV more often than in women without it. And yet this will be the focus of the vaccine: to pretend to eliminate this ubiquitous virus from the body.

The second enormous impediment to credibility is that the average age for cervical cancer is 50 years. But the plan is to mandate Gardasil to 12 years olds. And the manufacturer is only claiming efficacy for 5 years. So using their own statistics, this makes the vaccine worthless in the long run, because by the time most females need immunity, it will have worn off long ago.

...The original phrase used by Merck to link HPV with cervical cancer was "there is a strong connection." How that phrase got transformed to 'is the cause of' in the past two years is more a matter of marketing than of science.

Gardasil has not been evaluated for carcinogenicity or impairment of fertility. That's great. They want to vaccinate all American 12 year olds with a vaccine for cancer and they don't even know for sure whether or not it causes cancer, or makes the recipients infertile.

Dr. Tim O'Shea, DC
Leading Member of the World Association for Vaccine Education (WAVE)

Shaken Baby Syndrome: still another vaccine adverse effect

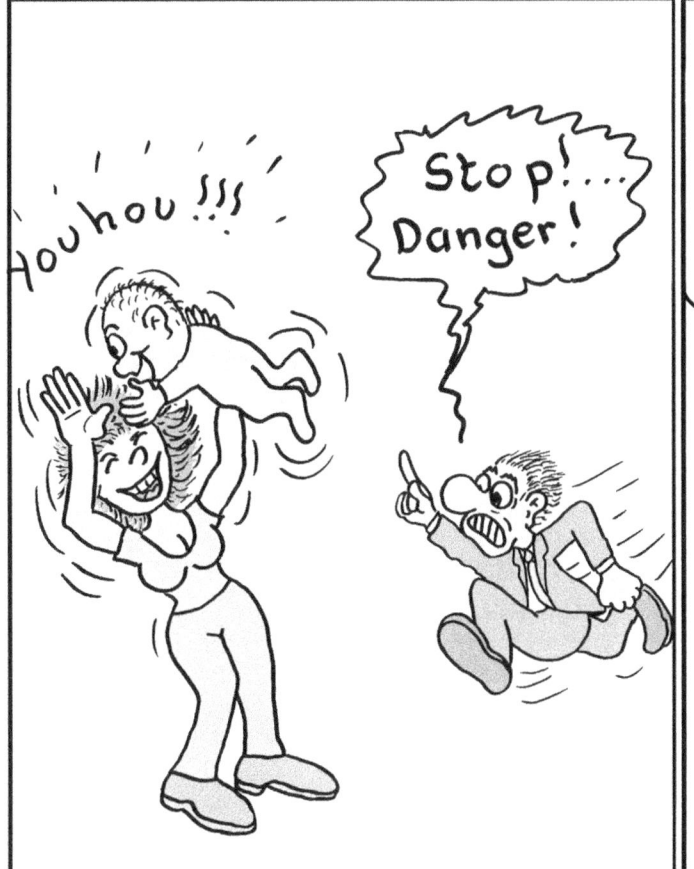
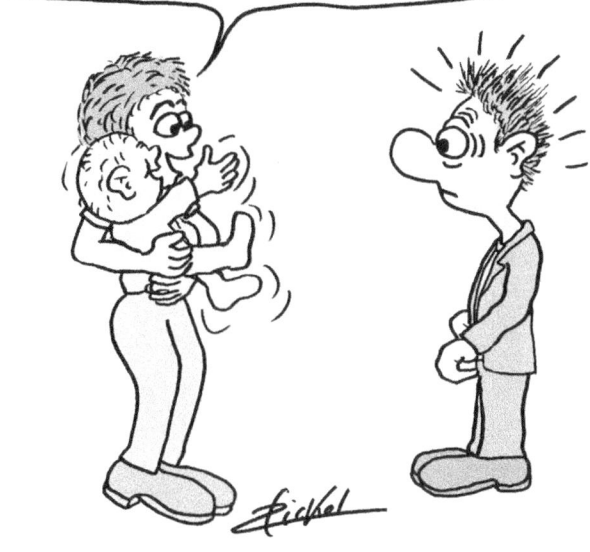

It's estimated that half of infant deaths is attributed to child abuse classified as Shaken Baby Syndrome/Non-Accidental Trauma, for which parents are legally prosecuted ... Subdural hemorrhages can result from brain inflammation due to vaccine adverse events along with other diseases connected with vaccinations ... Gardner noted that there was a distinct age difference between nontraumatic brain hemorrhages in Japan and in America, where most nontraumatic brain hemorrhages tend to occur during the first six months of life. The clear explanation, according to Dr. Gardner, was that Japanese do not begin their vaccines until seven months, whereas in the United States they are administered during the first six months, starting within 24 hours of birth with the Hepatitis B vaccine ... Vaccines can and do cause a significant percentage of subdural brain hemorrhages which, tragically, are being falsely and unjustly misdiagnosed as inflicted abuse by parent or caretaker.

Dr. Harold E Buttram, MD, and Catherine J. Frompovich

Do Childhood Vaccines Cause Subdural (Brain) Hemorrhages, Currently Diagnosed as Shaken Baby Syndrome and Other Health Anomalies?

Cattle Sick of Humans

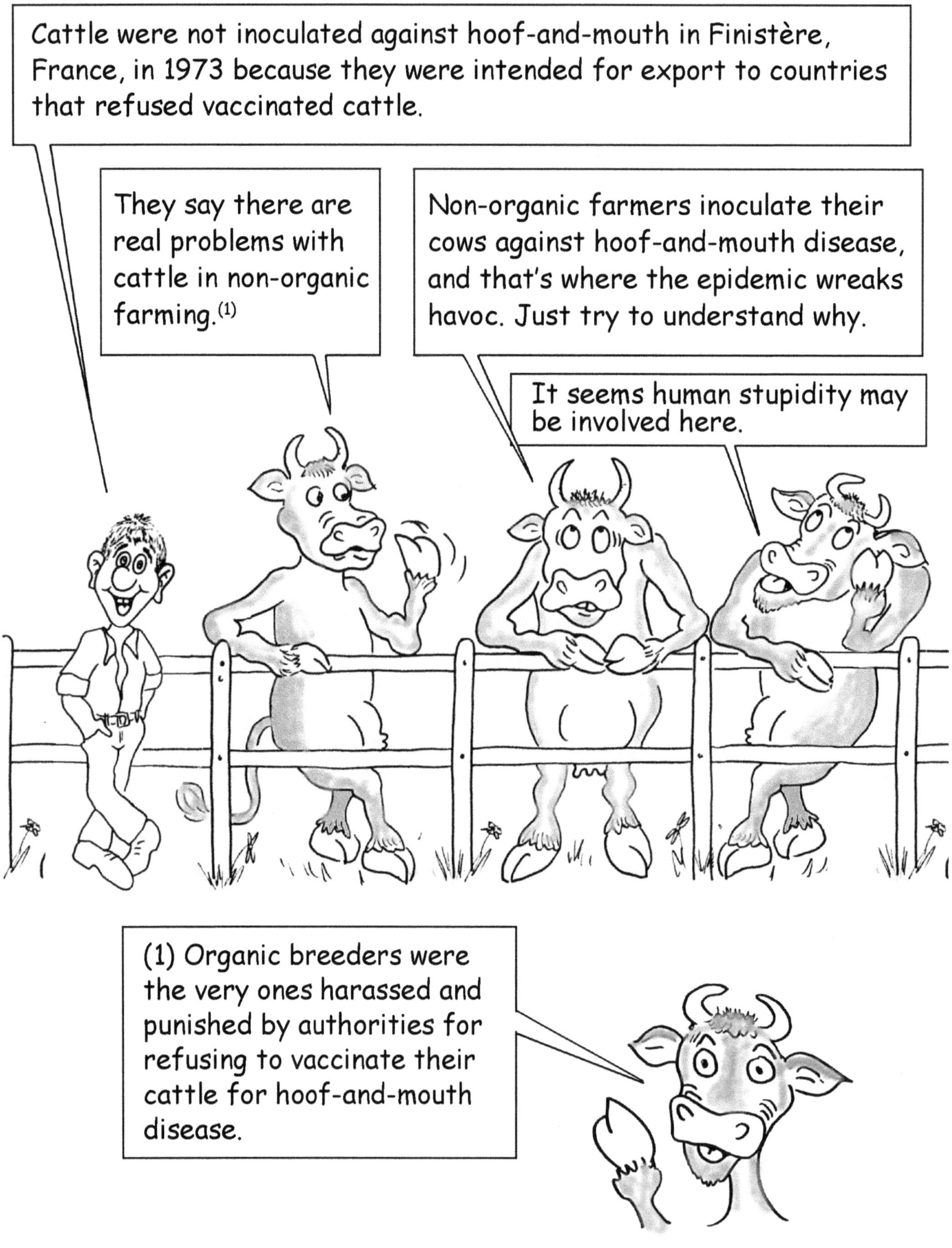

Cattle were not inoculated against hoof-and-mouth in Finistère, France, in 1973 because they were intended for export to countries that refused vaccinated cattle.

They say there are real problems with cattle in non-organic farming.[1]

Non-organic farmers inoculate their cows against hoof-and-mouth disease, and that's where the epidemic wreaks havoc. Just try to understand why.

It seems human stupidity may be involved here.

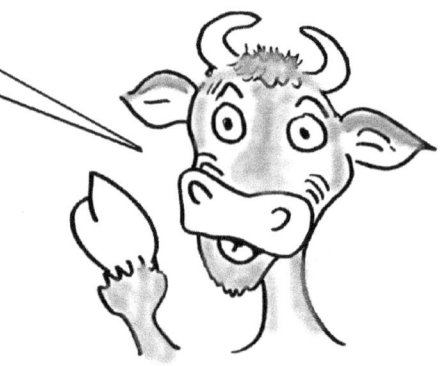

[1] Organic breeders were the very ones harassed and punished by authorities for refusing to vaccinate their cattle for hoof-and-mouth disease.

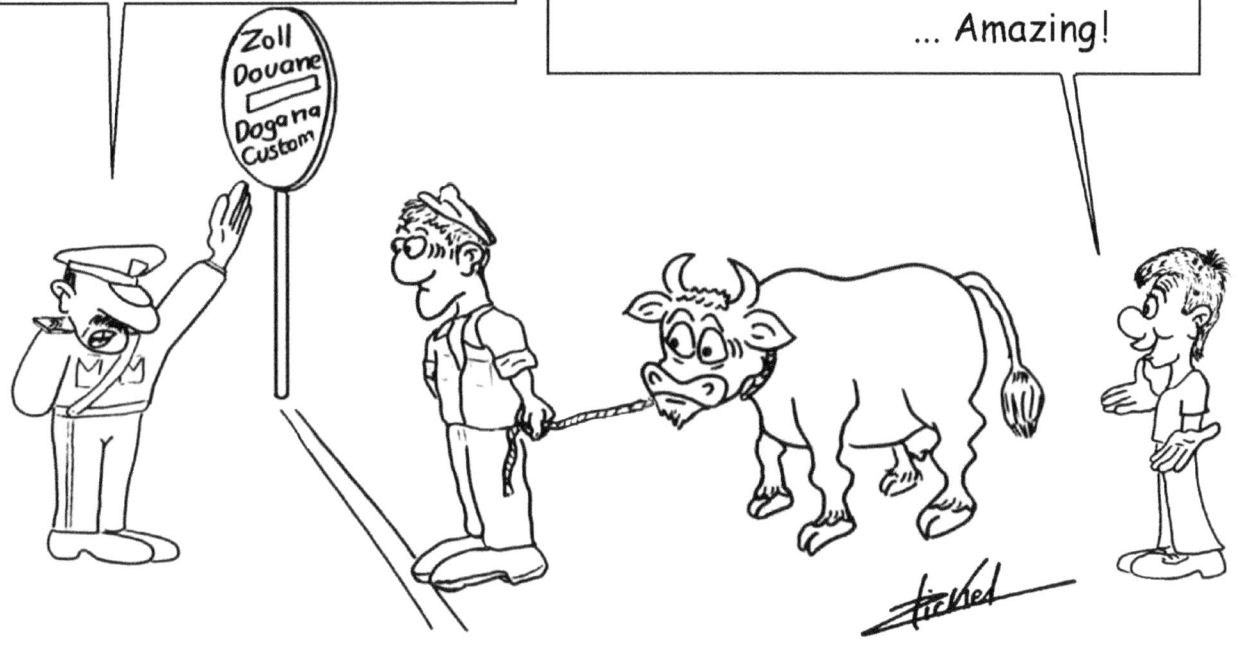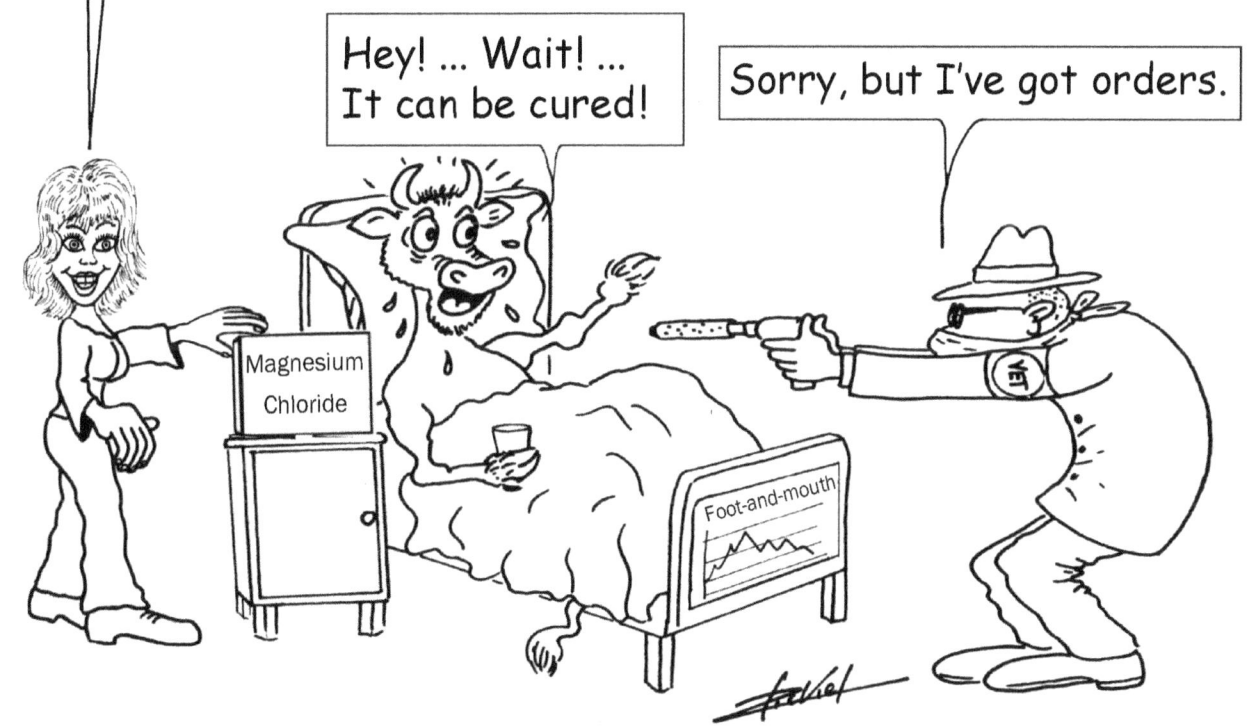

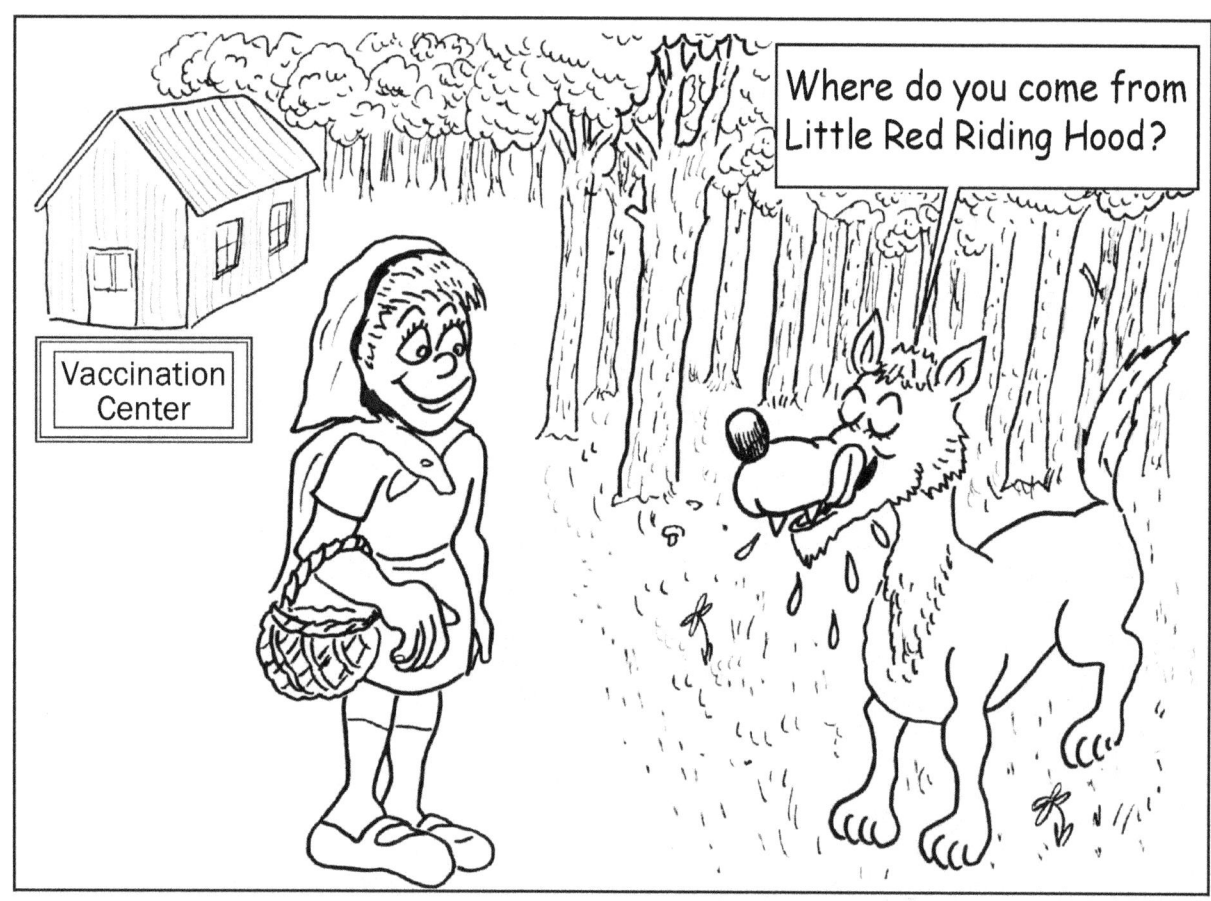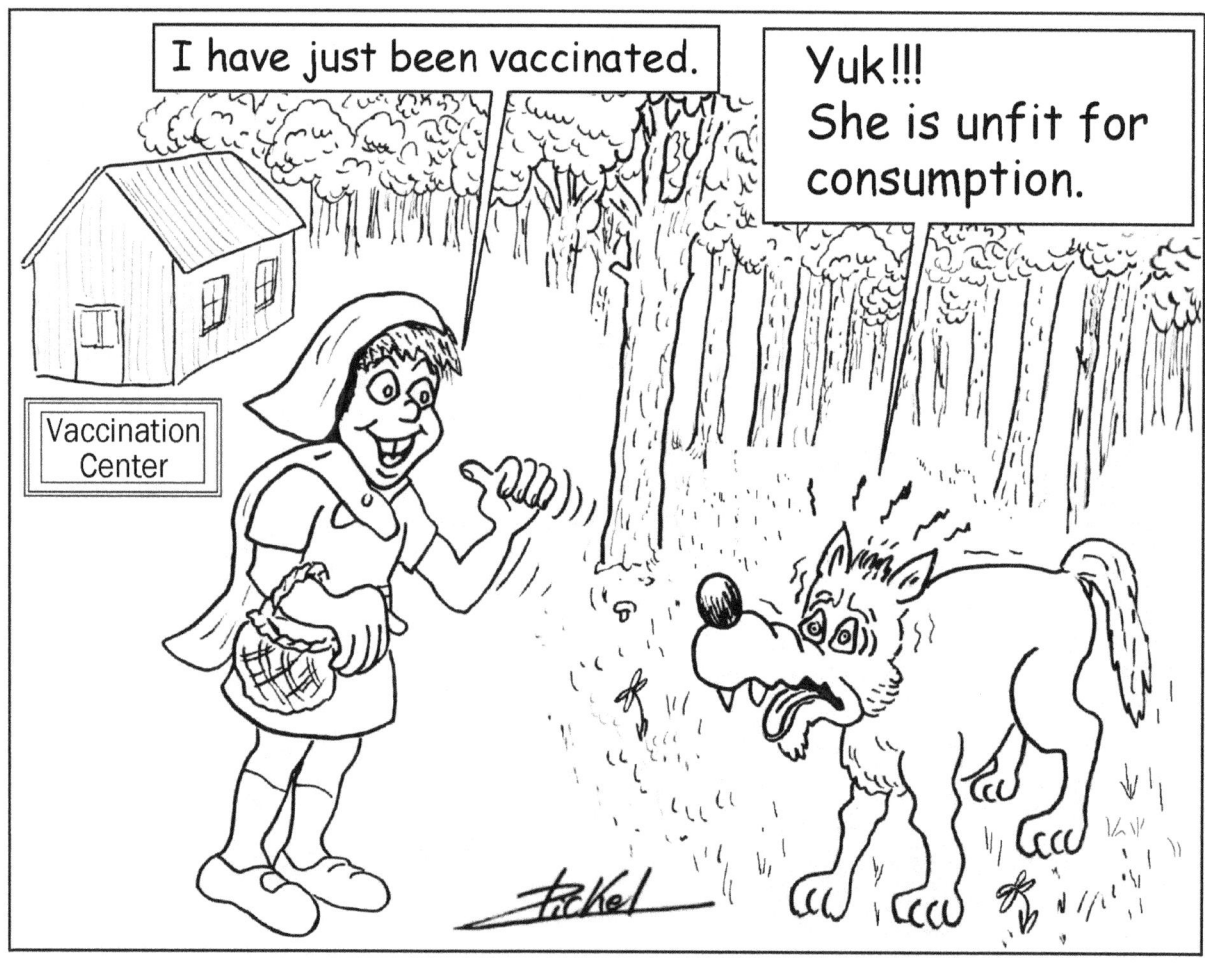

Acquired Immuno-Deficiency Syndrome

If we continue to spread and increase the use of vaccines, we can expect that within a few decades, a new pathology will emerge, that of vaccinated societies.

Professor P. DELOGE
(Trends of Contemporary Medicine, 1962)

According to many researchers, AIDS is a collapse of the immune system. Among others factors is the repetition of vaccinations.[1]

Areas in Africa where AIDS explodes as a pandemic match zones subjected to various vaccination campaigns.[2]

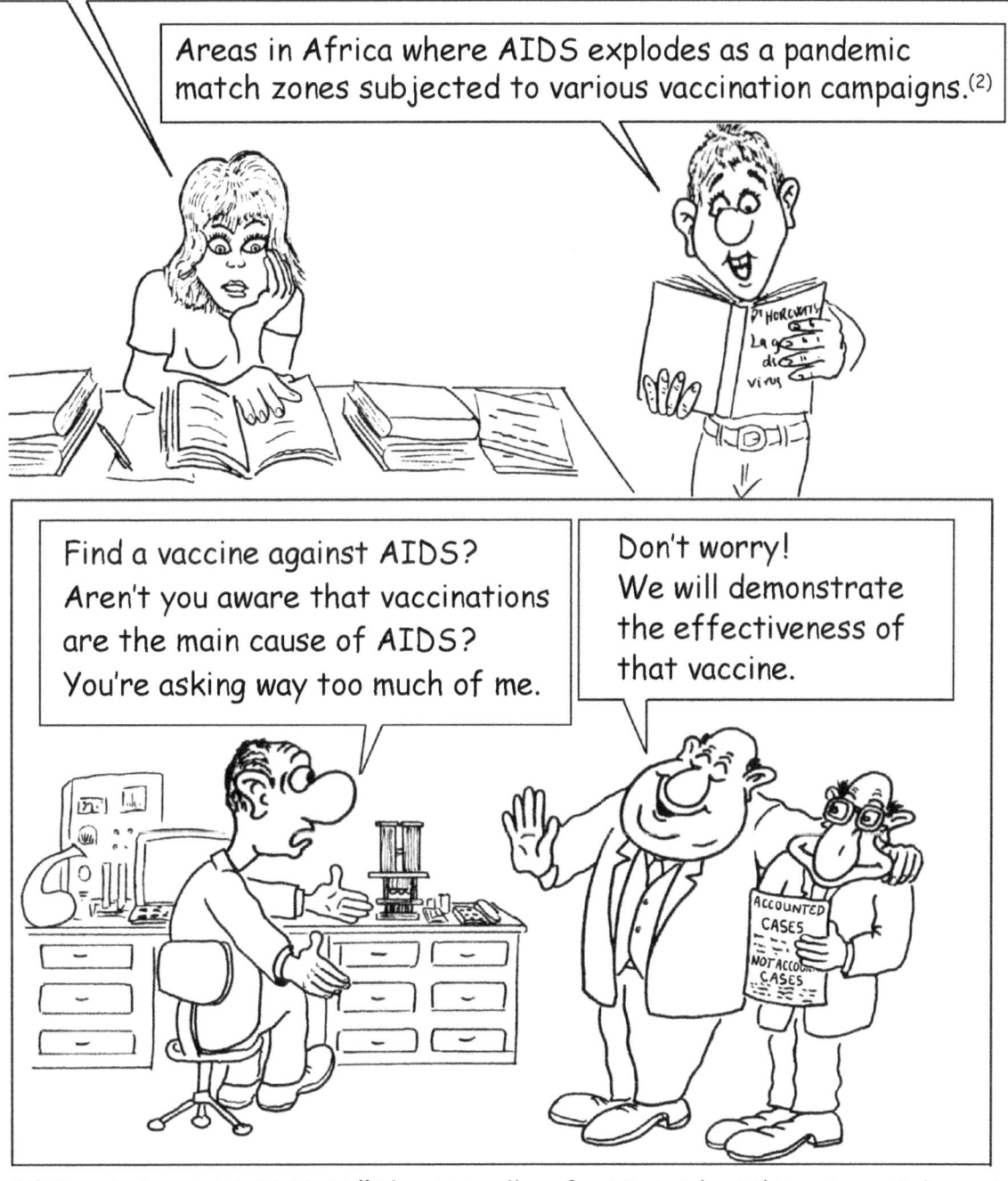

Find a vaccine against AIDS? Aren't you aware that vaccinations are the main cause of AIDS? You're asking way too much of me.

Don't worry! We will demonstrate the effectiveness of that vaccine.

(1) Dr. Robert WILLNER, "The Swindle of AIDS. The Ultimate Trickery"
(2) Dr. Louis de BROUWER, "AIDS Vertigo"

> *Vaccinations, at least as they are presented, relate more to magic than to immunology.*
> — Dr. Jacques KALMAR

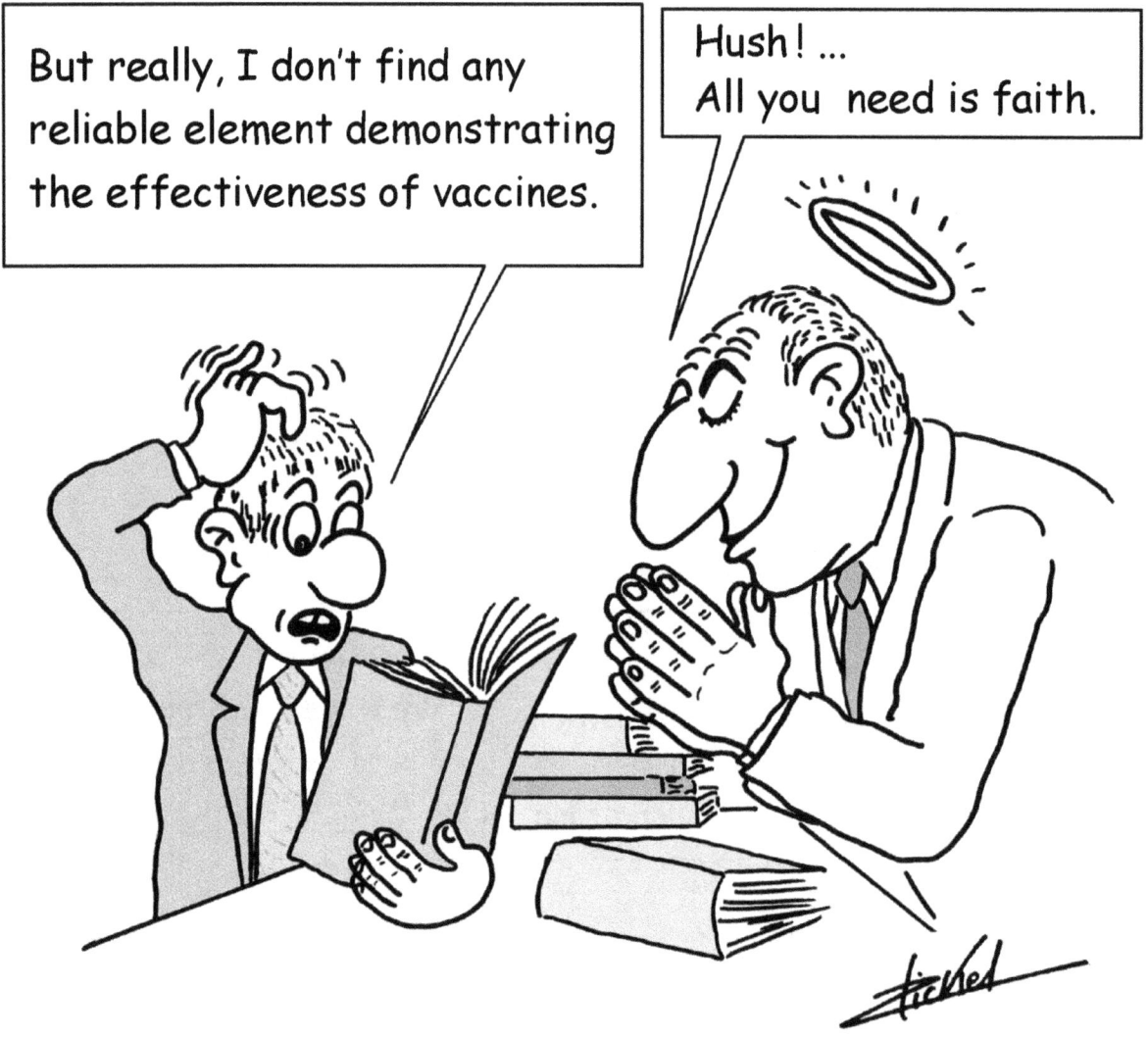

> *As in the holy scriptures, the dogma is unfailingly settled. All one needs to do is follow the ritual in the bliss of great revelations.*
> — Dr. Jacques KALMAR

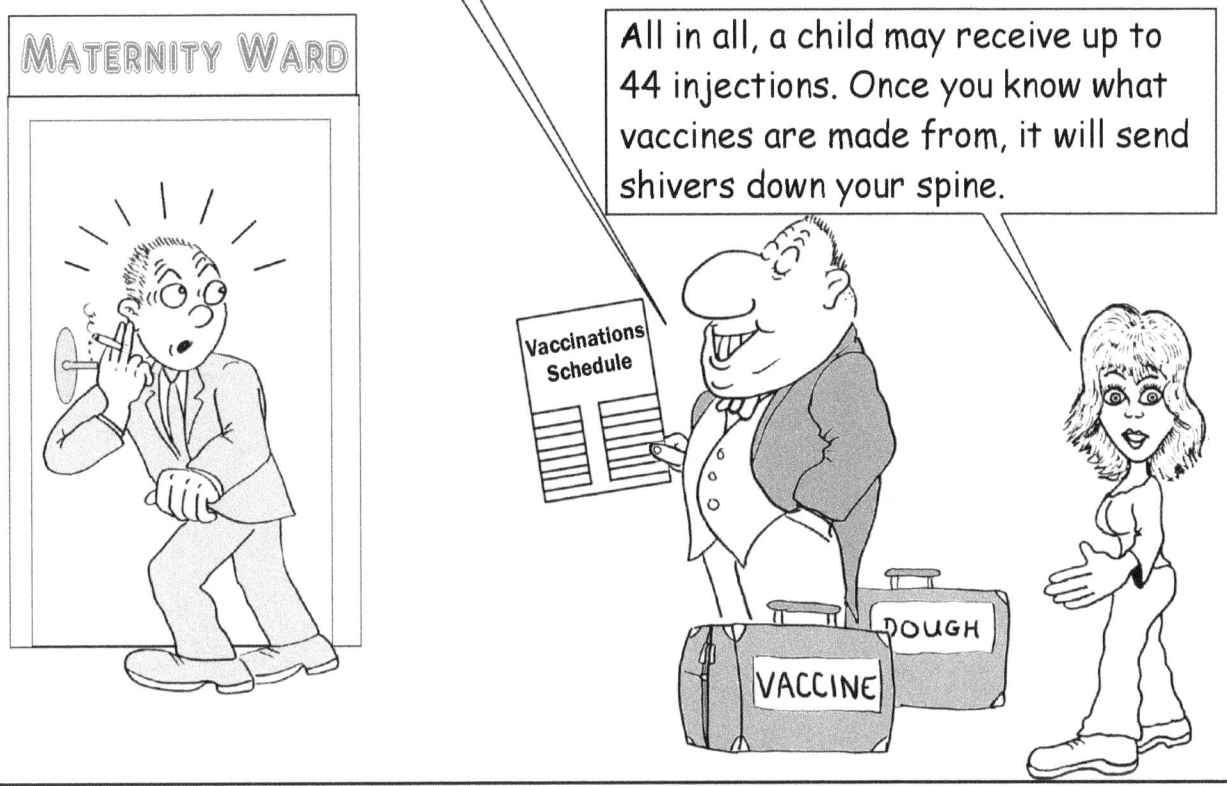
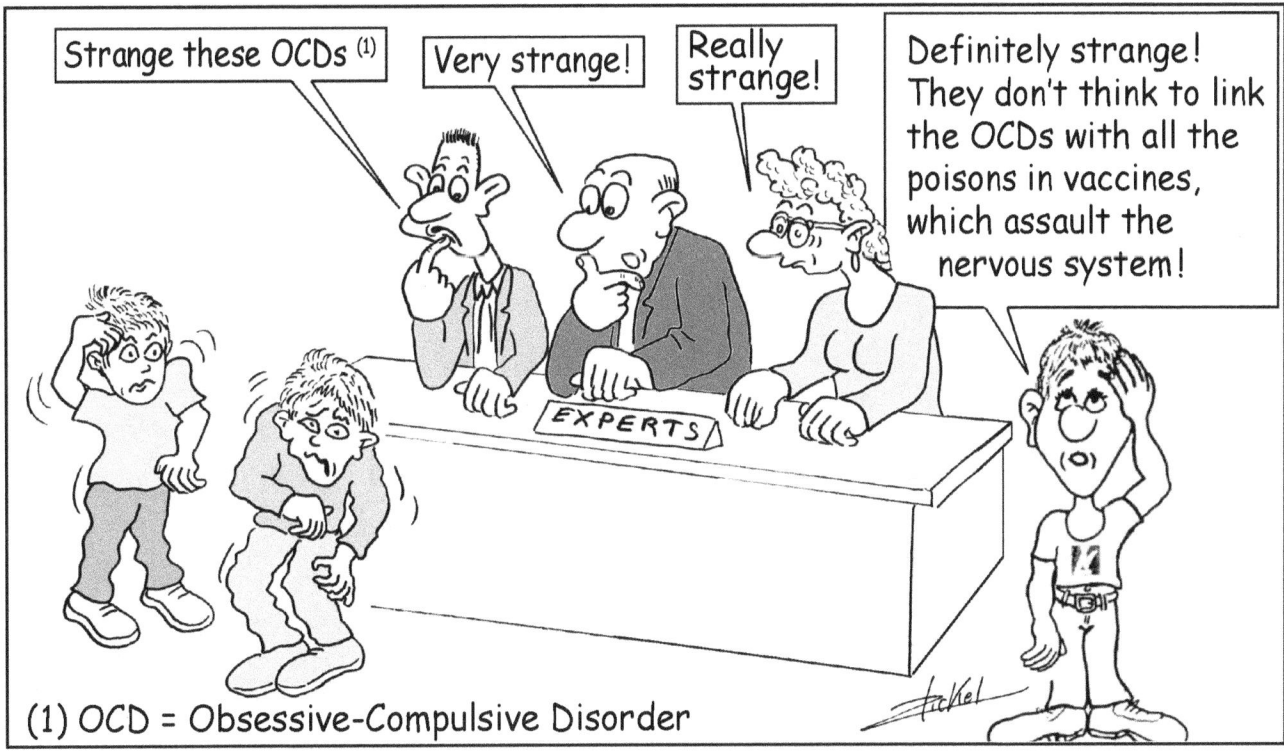

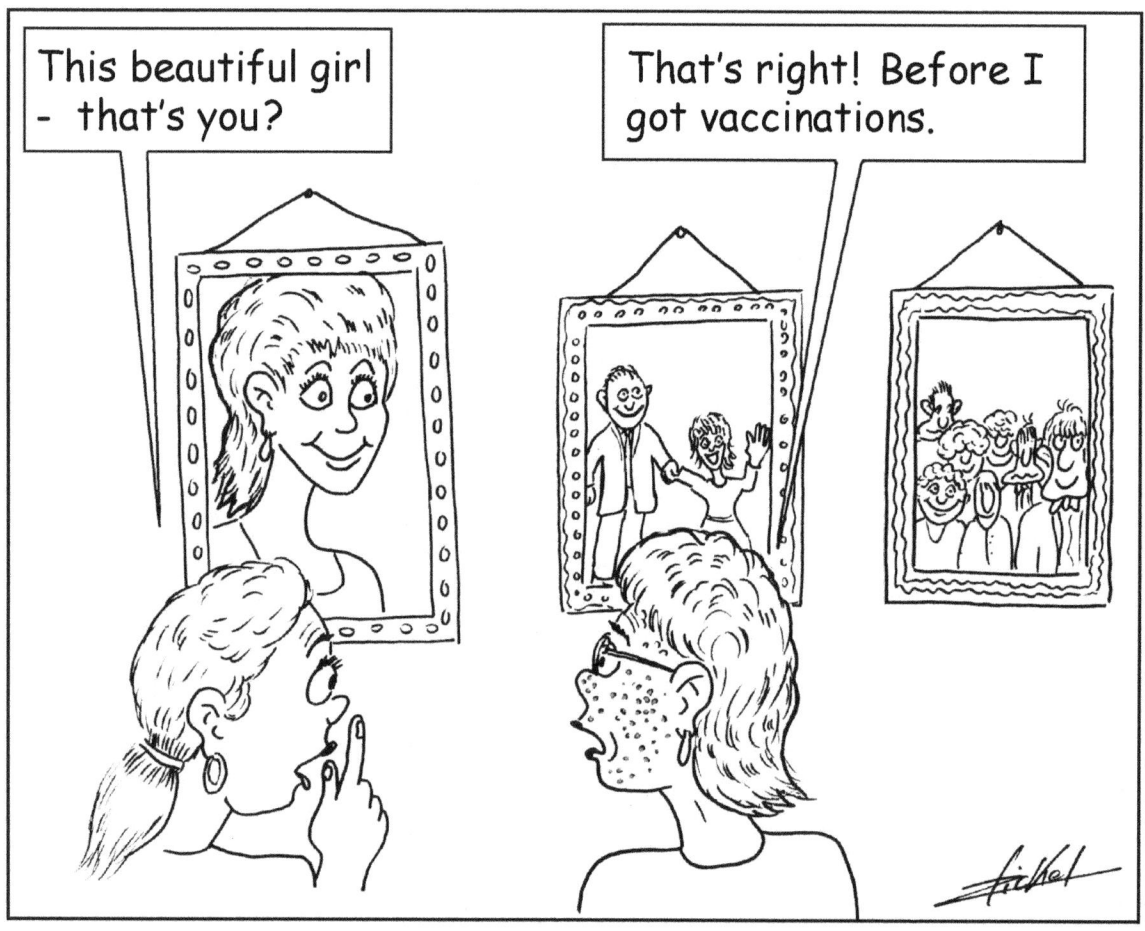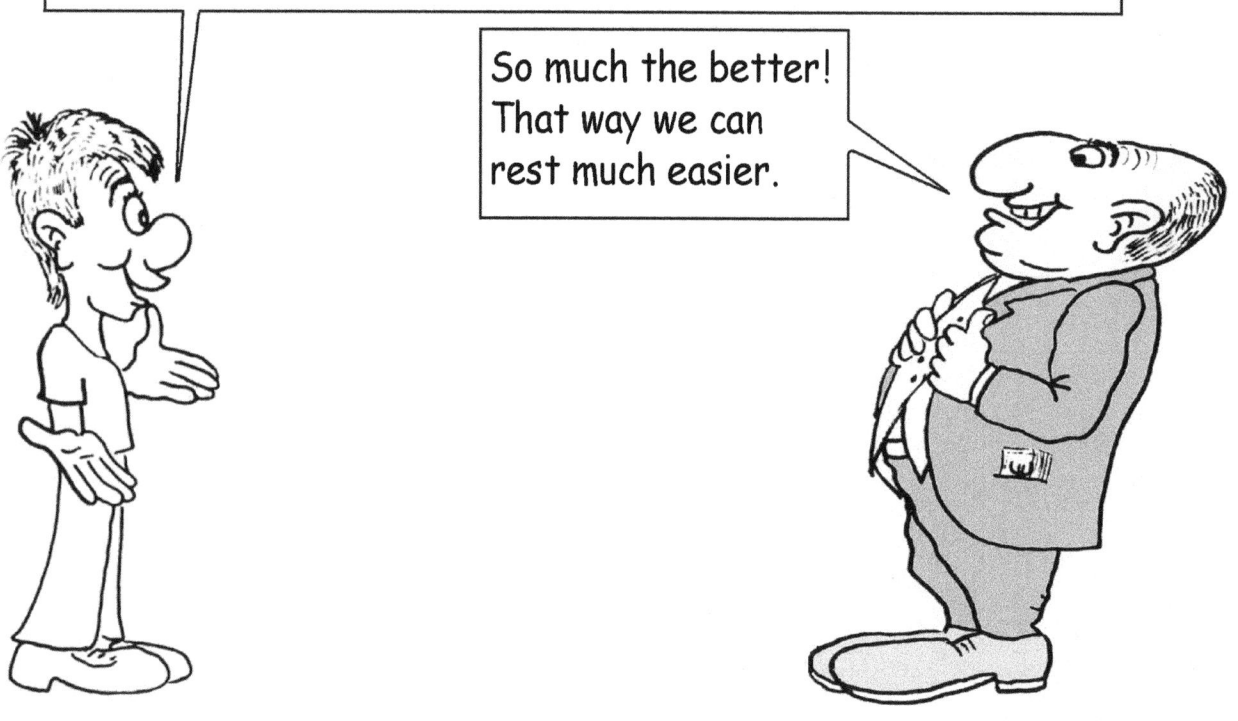

Vaccines bring diseases, create new ones and spread death. The scientific proof that artificially causing a disease prevents the natural appearance of that disease has never been established. As a doctor, I stand against these vaccinations and protest against the myth of Pasteur.

Dr. Paul-Emile CHEVREFILS

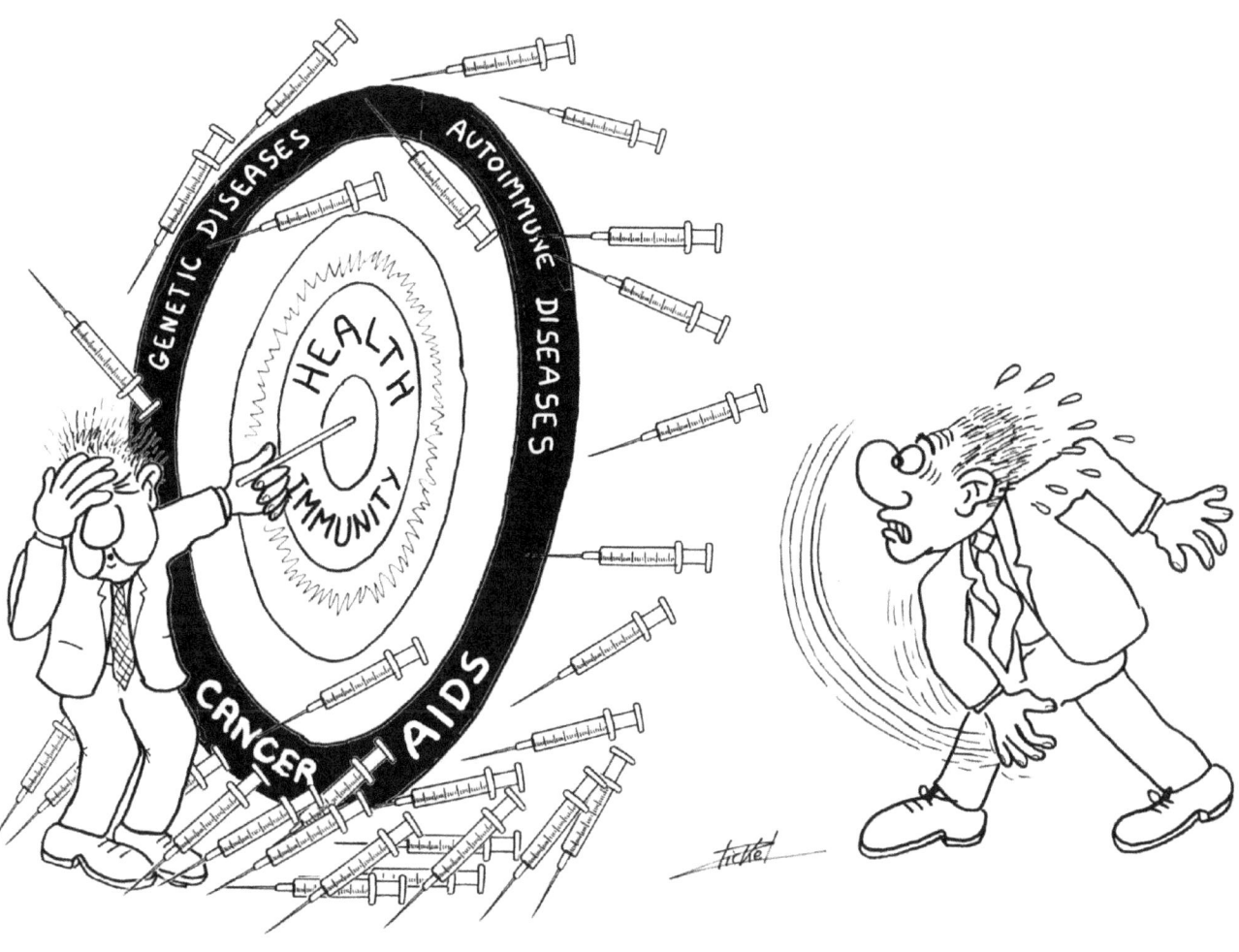

"Beware of false knowledge; it is more dangerous than ignorance."
"If history repeats itself, and the unexpected always happens, how incapable must Man be of learning from experience."

George Bernard SHAW

> *Vaccines can cause progressive chronic arthritis, multiple sclerosis, systemic lupus erythematosus, Parkinson's disease and cancer.*
> *Professor R. SIMPSON of the American Cancer Society*

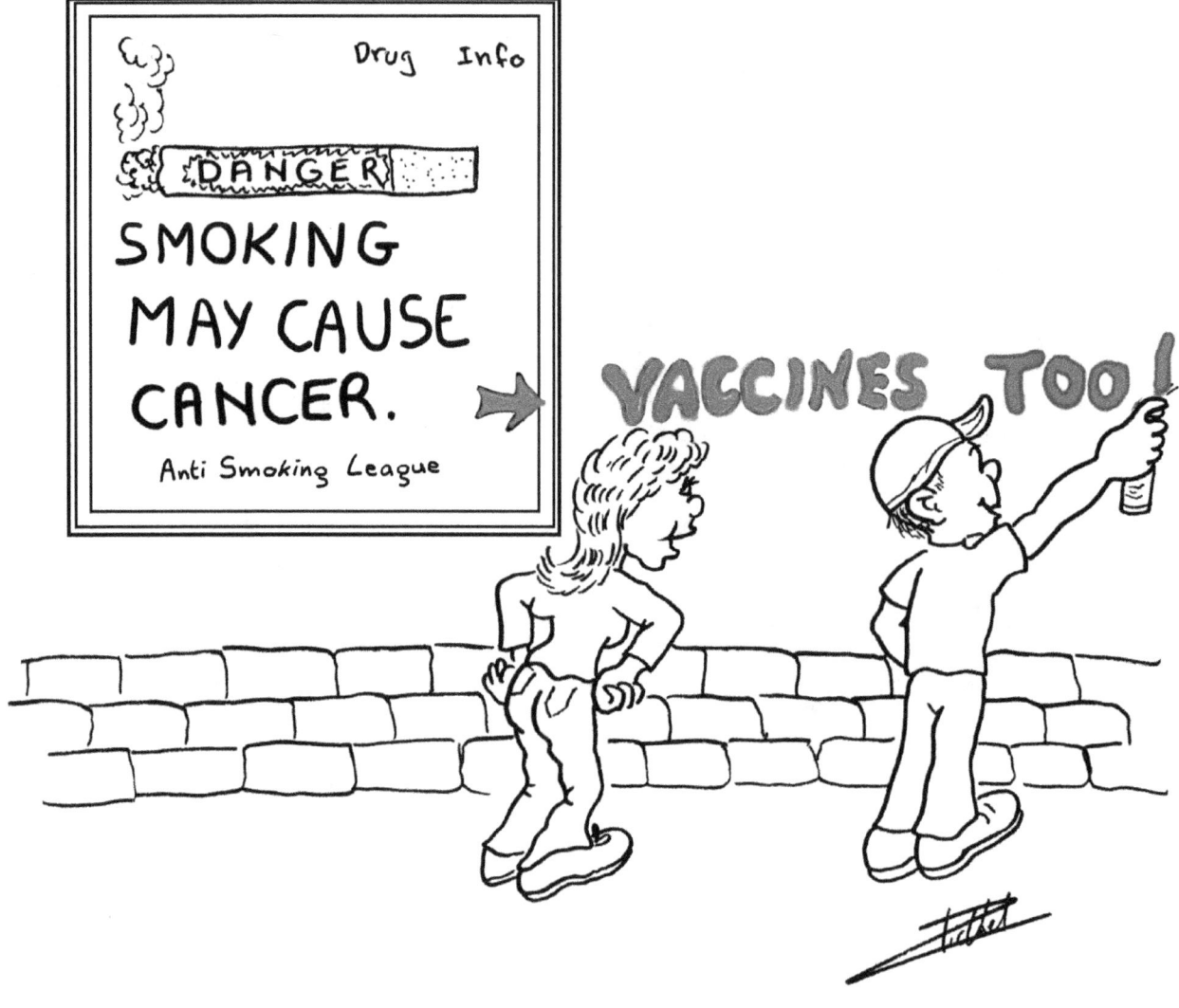

> *Have we traded mumps and measles for cancer and leukaemia?*
> *Dr. Robert S MENDELSOHN*

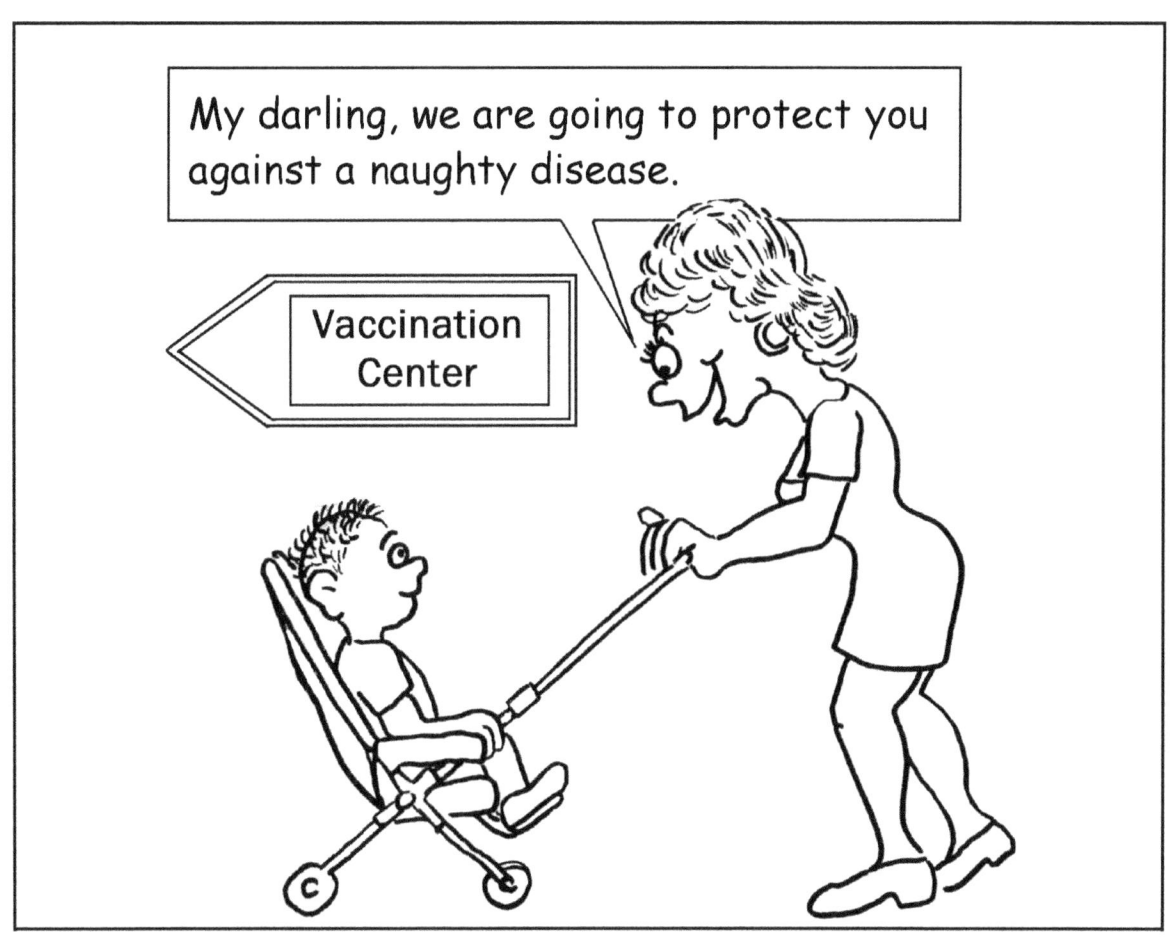
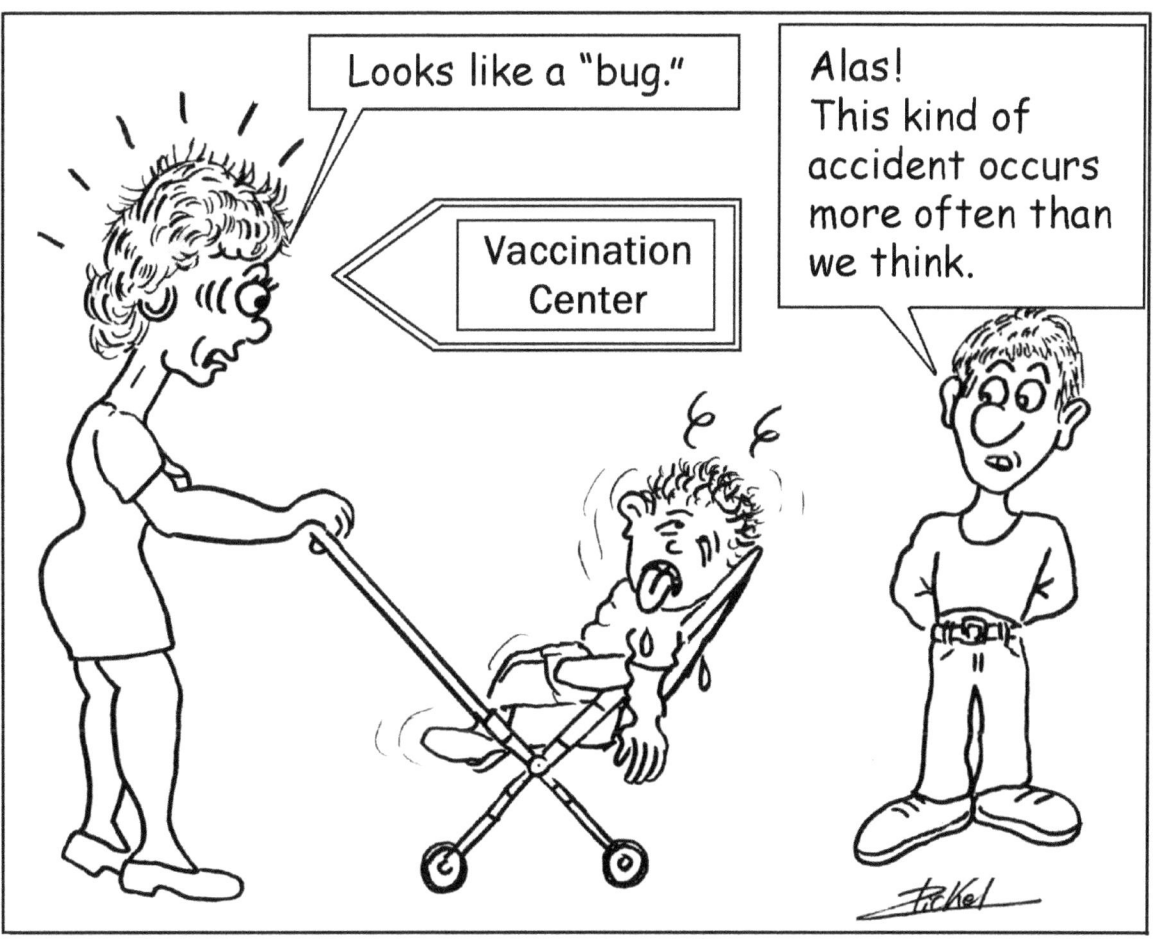

Several German authors have described the link between multiple sclerosis and the vaccinations against smallpox, typhoid, tetanus, poliomyelitis and the tuberculosis.
                              British Medical Journal, 1967

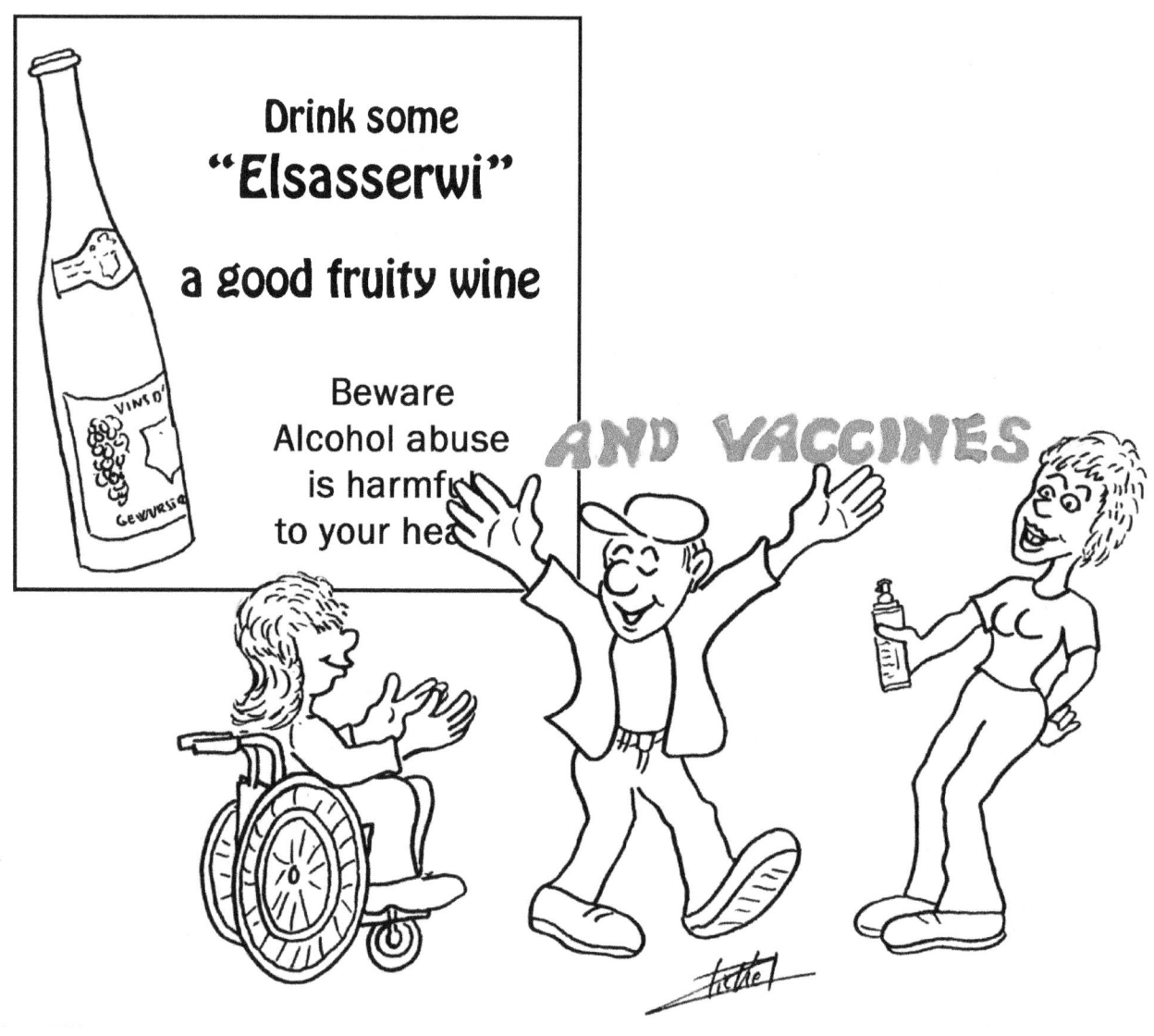

Certain strains of vaccines can be involved in degenerative diseases such as rheumatoid arthritis, leukemia, diabetes and multiple sclerosis.
                              Dr. G. DETTMAN (Australian Nurses Journal)

> *Any vaccination may cause a light or serious encephalitis.*
>
> Harris COULTER, PhD
>
> (Vaccination Social Violence and Criminality: The Medical Assault on the American Brain)

> *Every vaccination causes at least a minor encephalopathy, which destroys brain cells.*
>
> Dr. Gerhard BUCHWALD
>
> (Vaccination: A Business Based on Fear)

The consequences of vaccinating are not always immediately visible. Neurological and mental disorders such as ADHD, autism, dyslexia, bi-polar and even mental retardation can be attributed to early childhood vaccinations.

Adult and vaccinated!

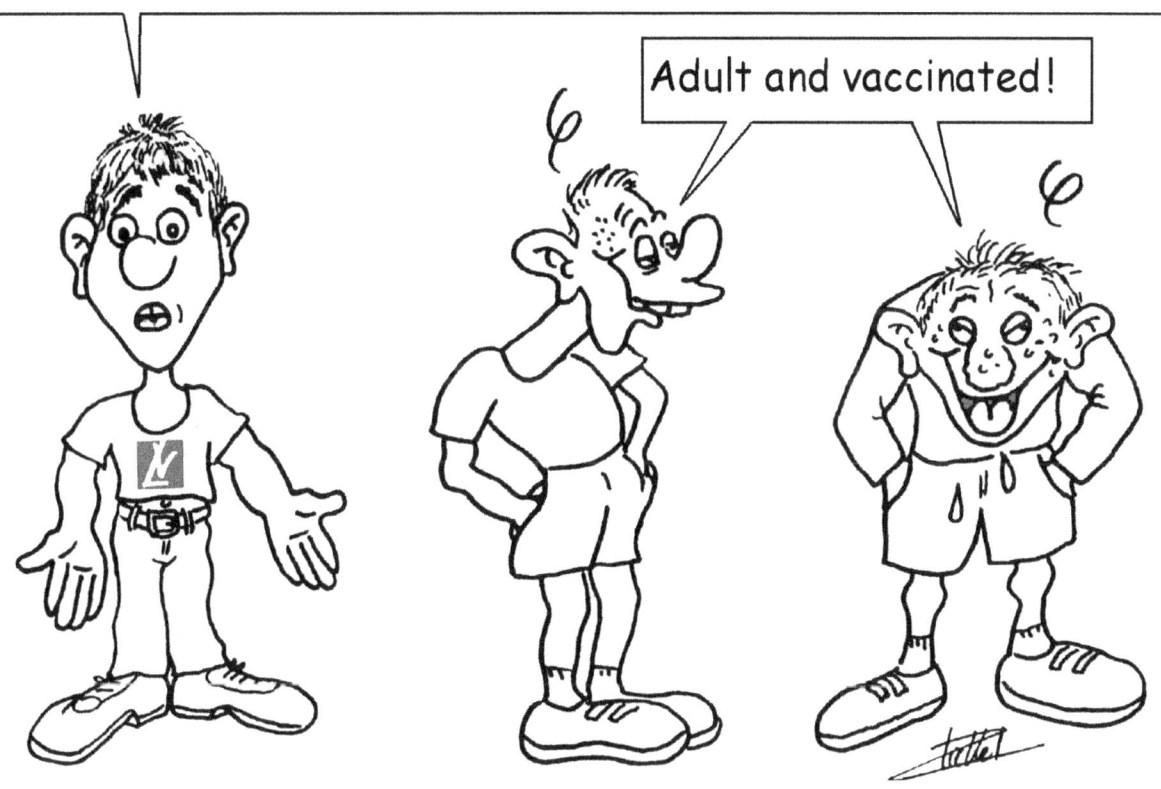

> *It is a real epidemic ... It is ridiculous to claim that there is no link between autism and vaccination except coincidences. The truth is that children are hurt by vaccinations.*
>
> Bernard RIMLAND, PhD,
> Director and Founder of the Autism Research Institute of San Diego, California

> Among the 3.3 million children annually inoculated in the United States with the DPT, 16,038 demonstrated acute crises and persistent tears, which is considered by several neurologists as revealing an irritation of the central nervous system; 8,484 had convulsions within 48 hours following the injection of the DPT. [1]
>
> Dr. Allan HINMAN and Jeffrey COPELAN
> (Newspaper of the American Medical Association)

(1) DPT = Diphtheria, Pertussis, Tetanus.

Parents frequently observe emotional disorders after vaccinations.

Neurological after-effects may arise even in the absence of extreme reactions.

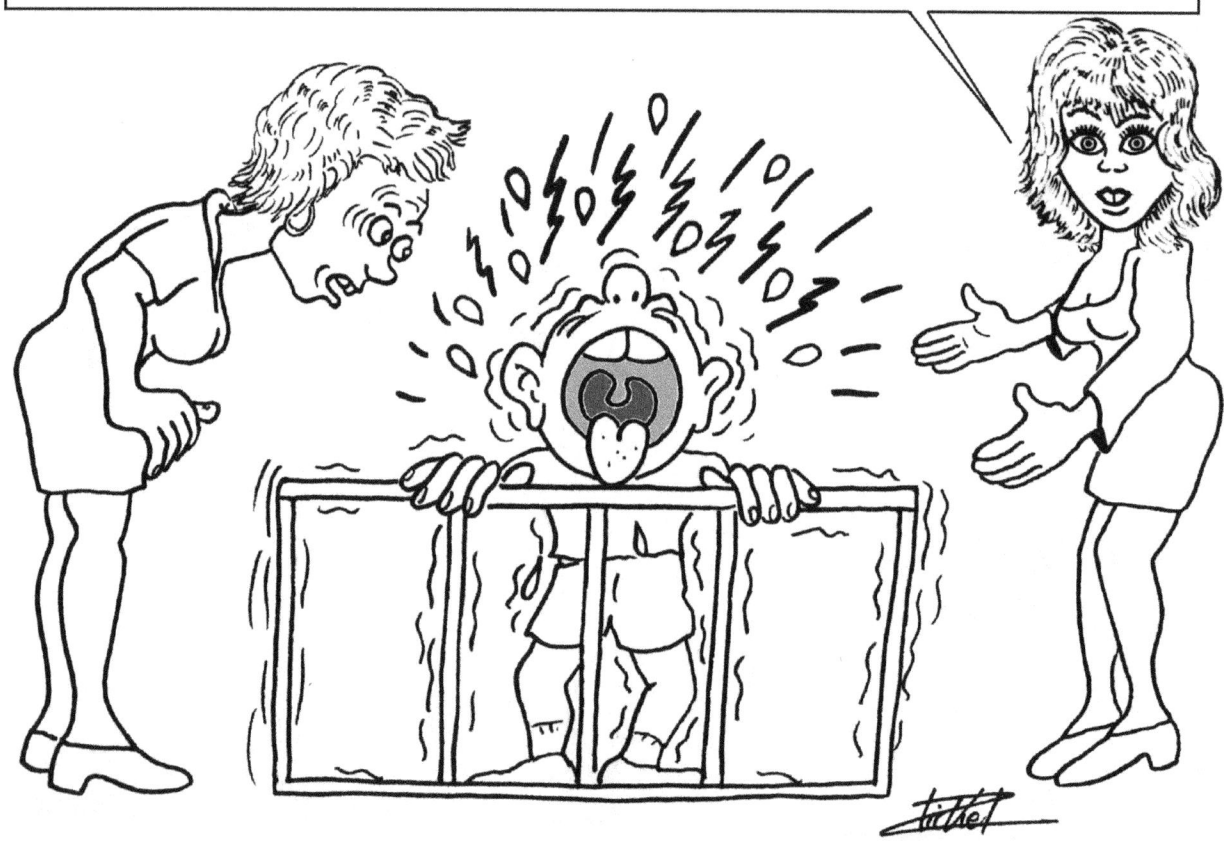

> For 23 years, I have been observing that unvaccinated children were healthier and stronger than the vaccinated ones. Allergies, asthma and behavioral disturbances clearly occurred more frequently in my young vaccinated patients. Besides, the former suffered more often or more severely from infectious diseases than the latter.
>
> Dr. Philip INCAO

> *If we could uncover all the cases of death by vaccination in the world, these figures would make Herod himself shudder.*
> George Bernard SHAW

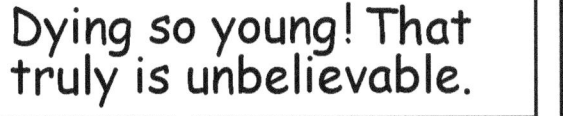

> *These are the Mass vaccinations with live viruses, both useless and dangerous, are the cause of the spread of AIDS.*
> Professor Richard DELONG (Live Viral Vaccines)

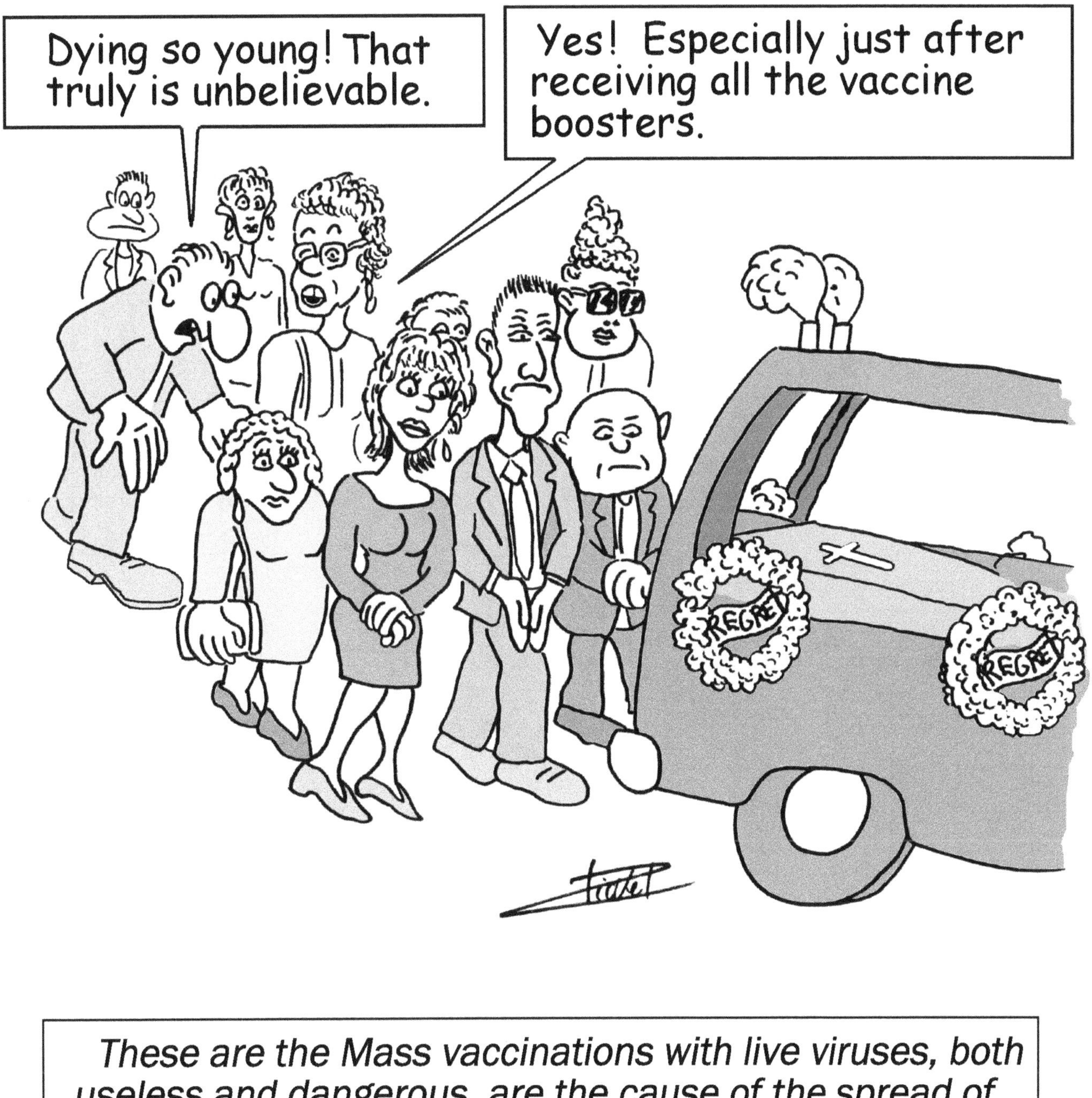

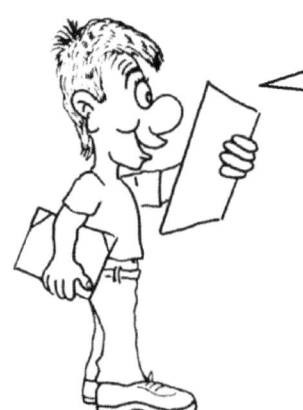

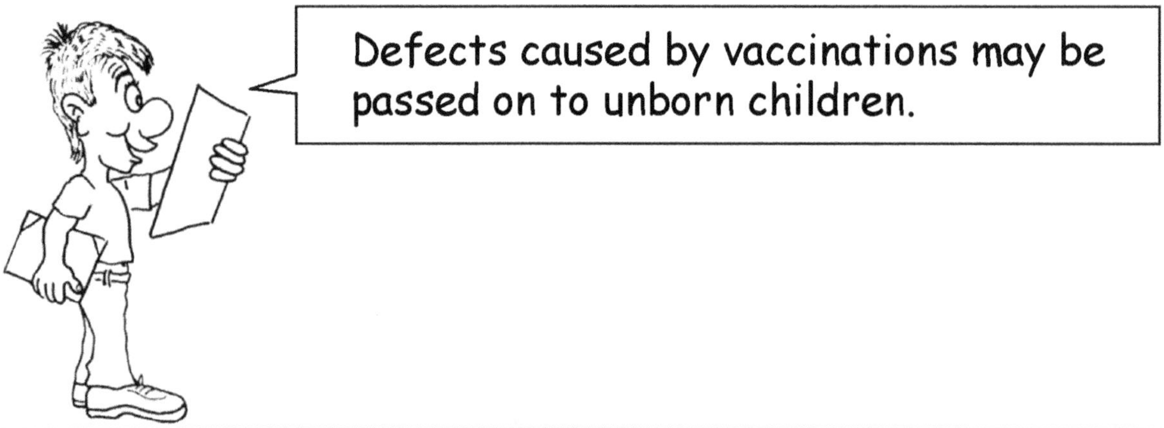

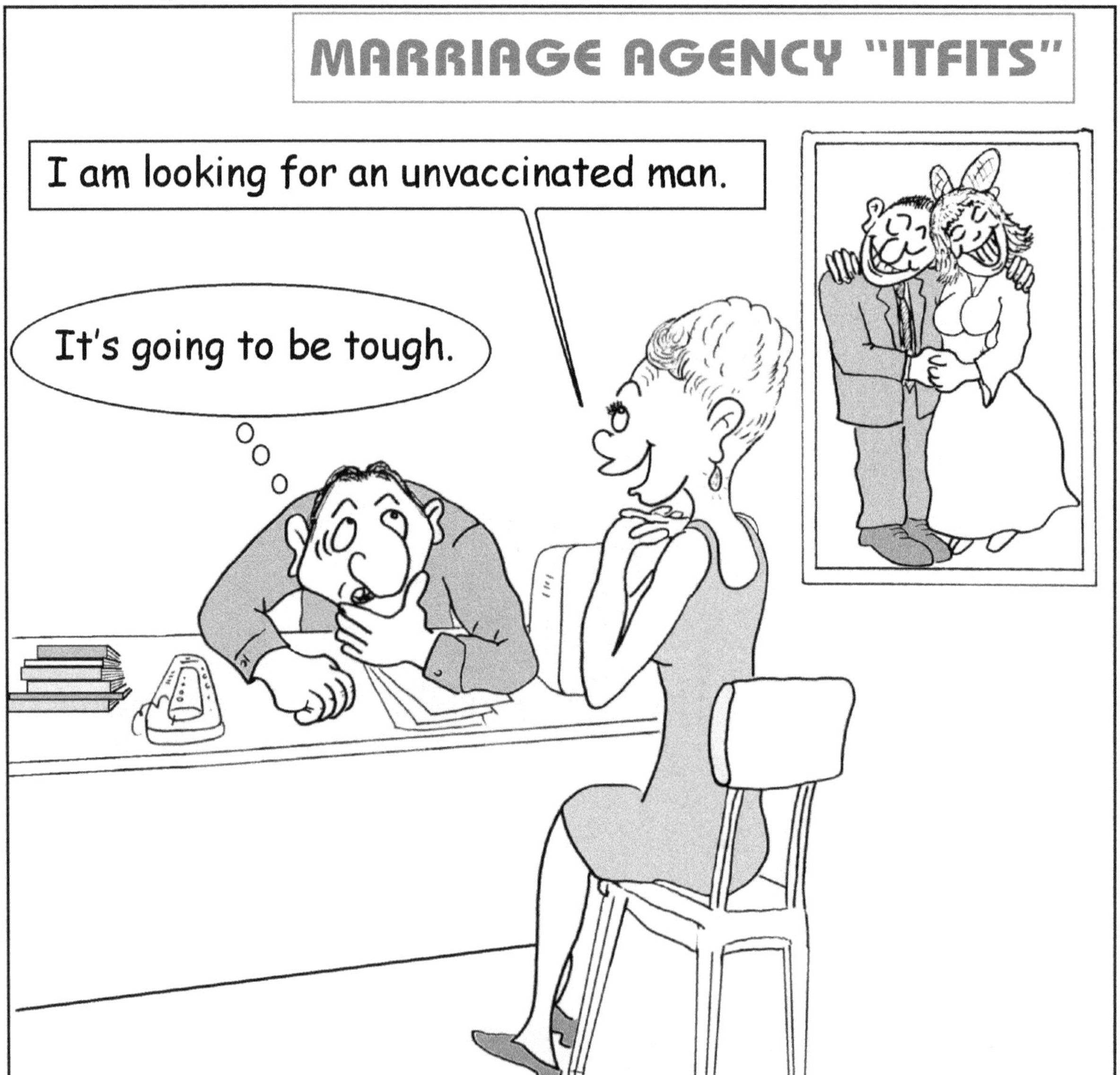

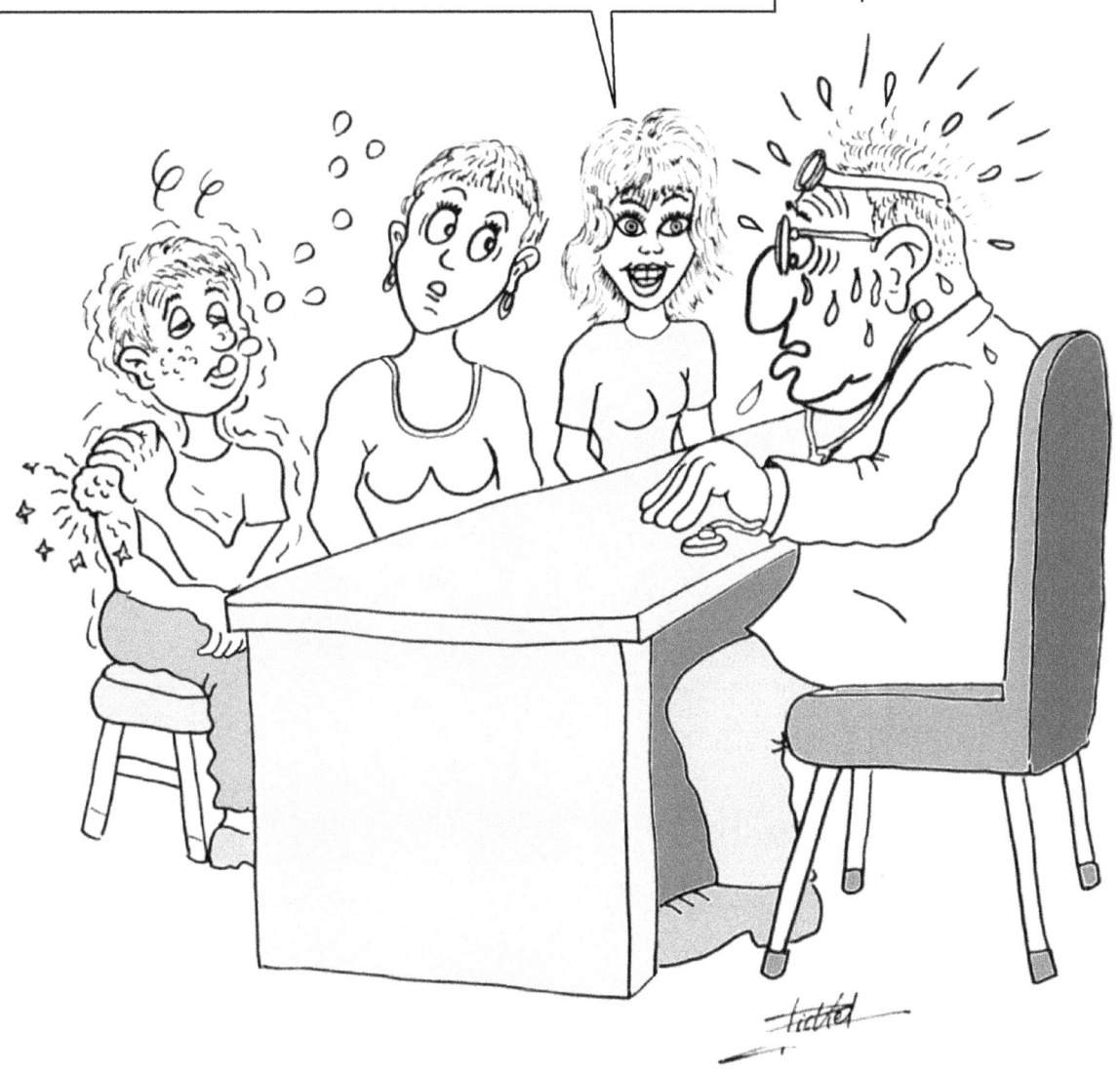

> Few doctors are willing to attribute a death or a complication to a method which they recommended and believe in.
>
> Professor Georges DICK
> (British Medical Journal, July, 1971)

> Medical authorities are very reluctant to recognize and admit post-vaccination adverse events.
>
> In France, thanks to the intervention of the LNPLV [1], a 1956 law was passed to compensate victims of compulsory vaccinations.

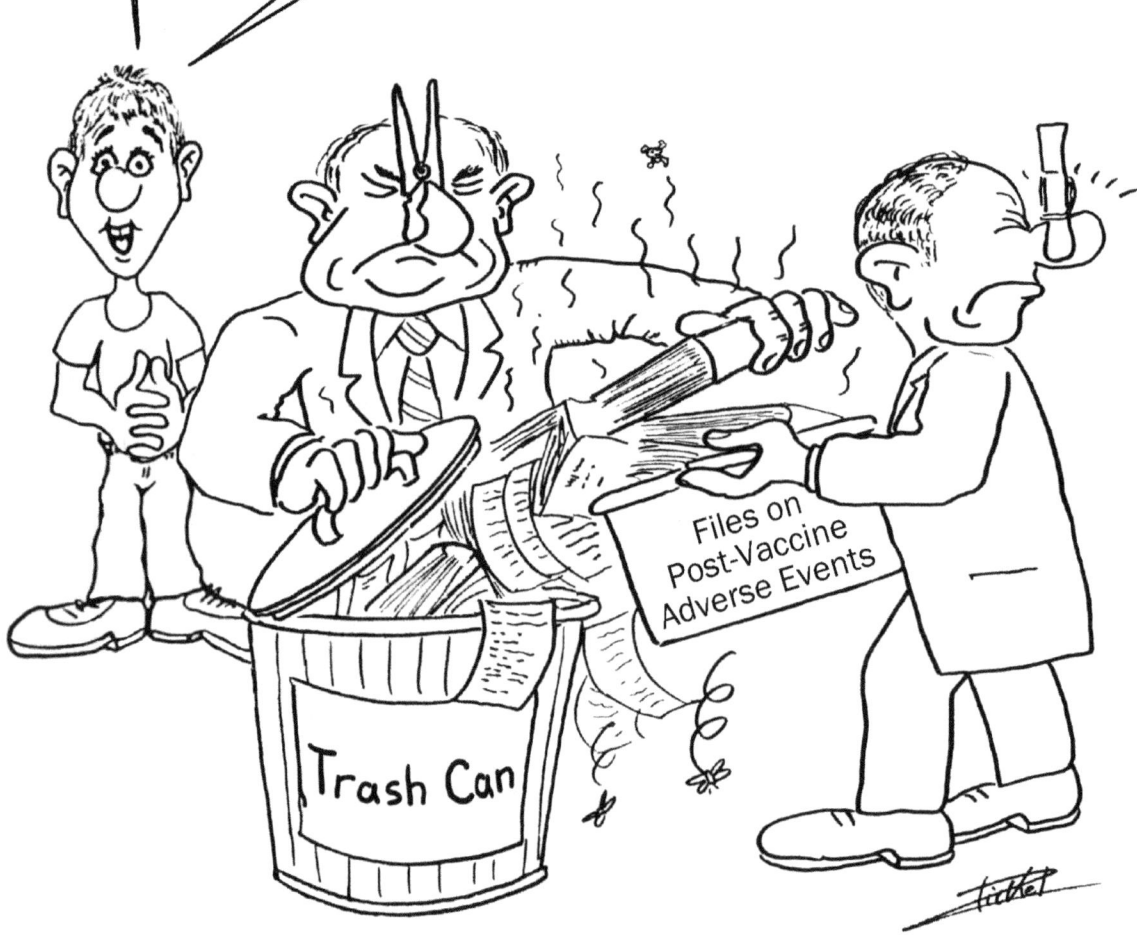

(1) Ligue Nationale Pour la Liberté des Vaccinations
(National League for Freedom in Vaccinations)

> *Vaccinations often result in complications which are never mentioned, but are still numerous and sometimes fatal.*
>
> *Dr. Jacques KALMAR*

« .In May of 1960, Dr. Ratner chaired a panel discussion, at the 120th Annual Meeting of the Illinois Medical Society to review the increasing rise in paralytic polio in the U.S. The proceedings were reprinted in the August, 1960, Illinois Medical Journal which exposed the Salk vaccine as a frank and ineptly disguised fraud. One of the experts on the panel, statistician Dr. Bernard Greenberg, who went on to testify at Congressional hearings, revealed how data had been manipulated to hide the dangers and ineffectiveness of the vaccine from the pubic. Dr. Greenberg explained that the perceived overall reduction in polio cases was achieved by changing the criteria by which polio was diagnosed. »

J.I. Rodale, The Encyclopedia of Common Diseases (1962 edition)

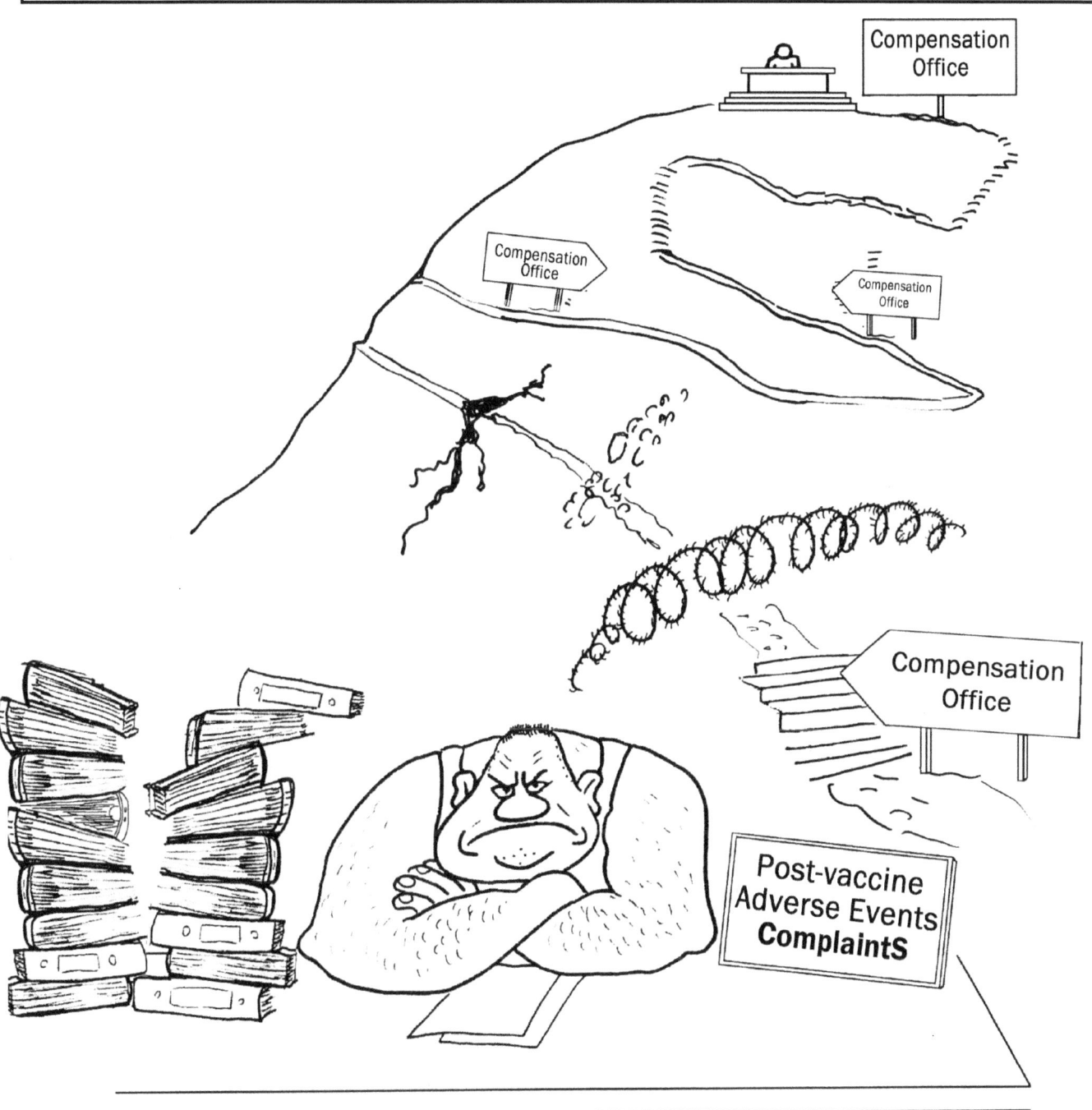

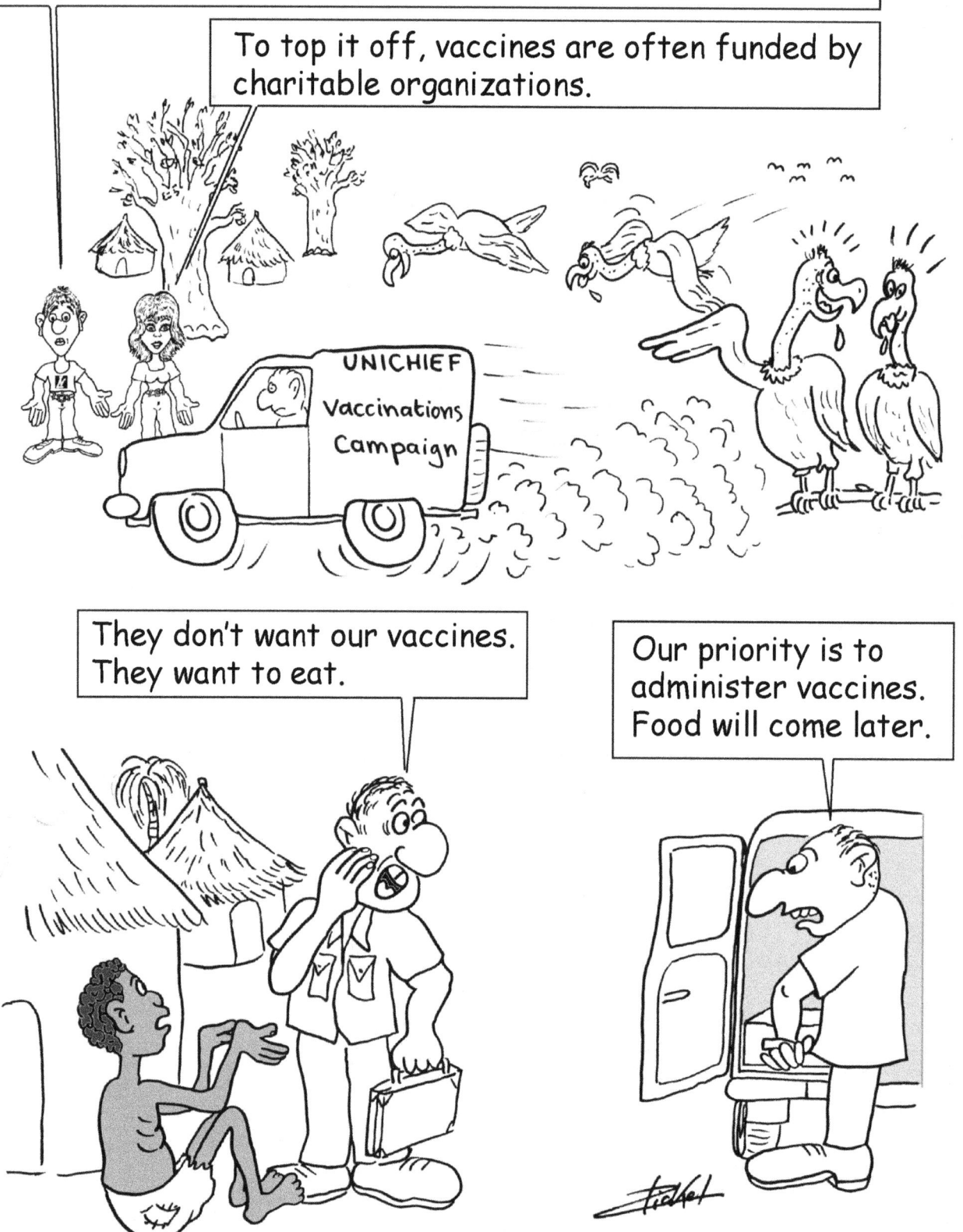

Vaccines: The Great Illusion

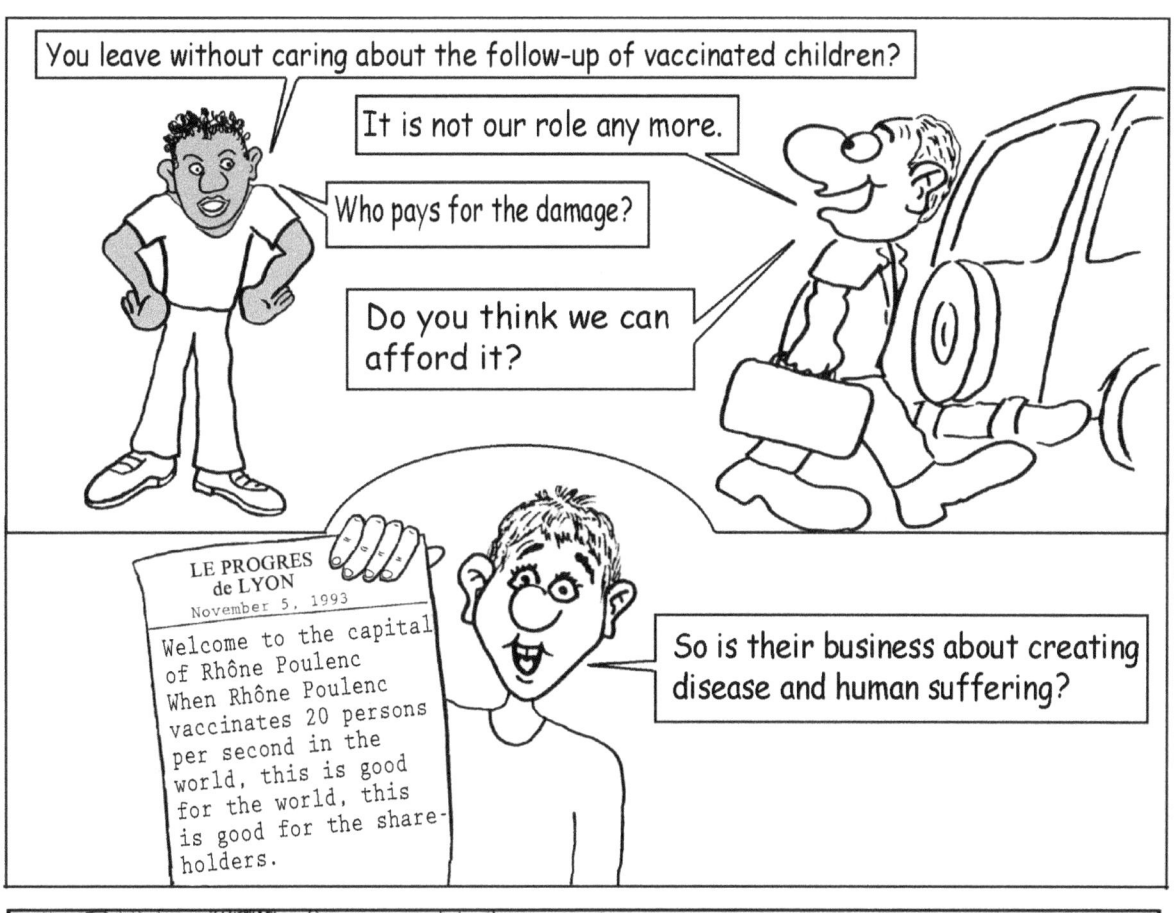
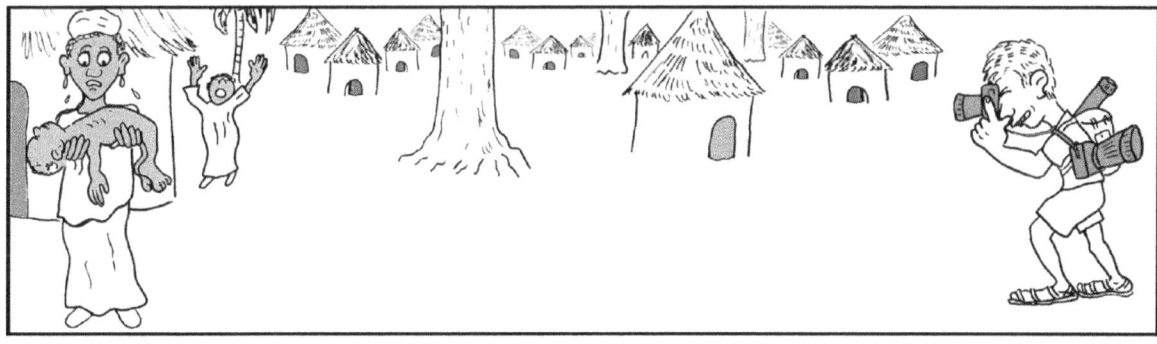
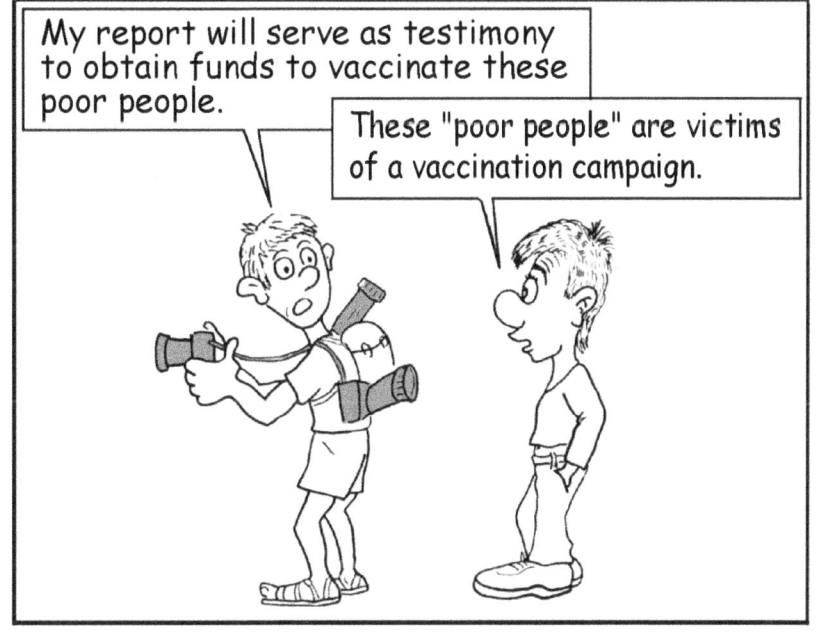
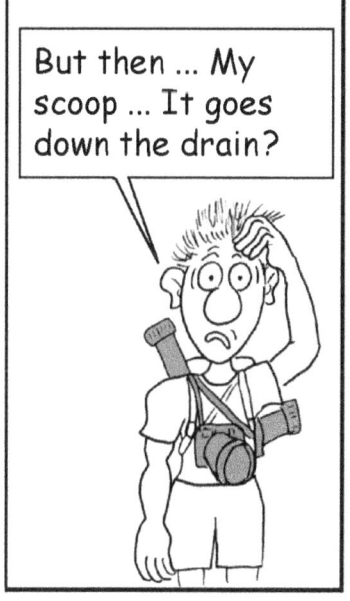

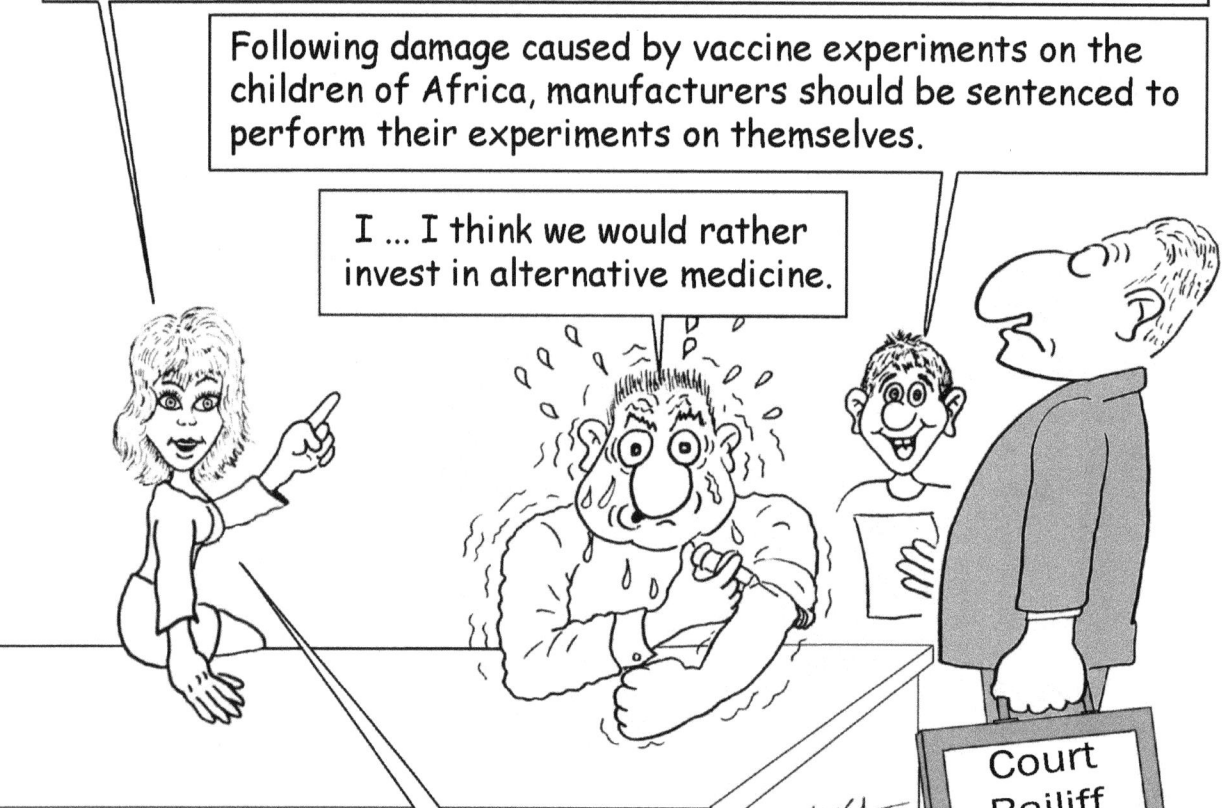

(1) in secession war with Nigeria (1967/1970)
(2) 2 million doses of oral polio vaccine and 800,000 doses of measles (MMR) vaccine.

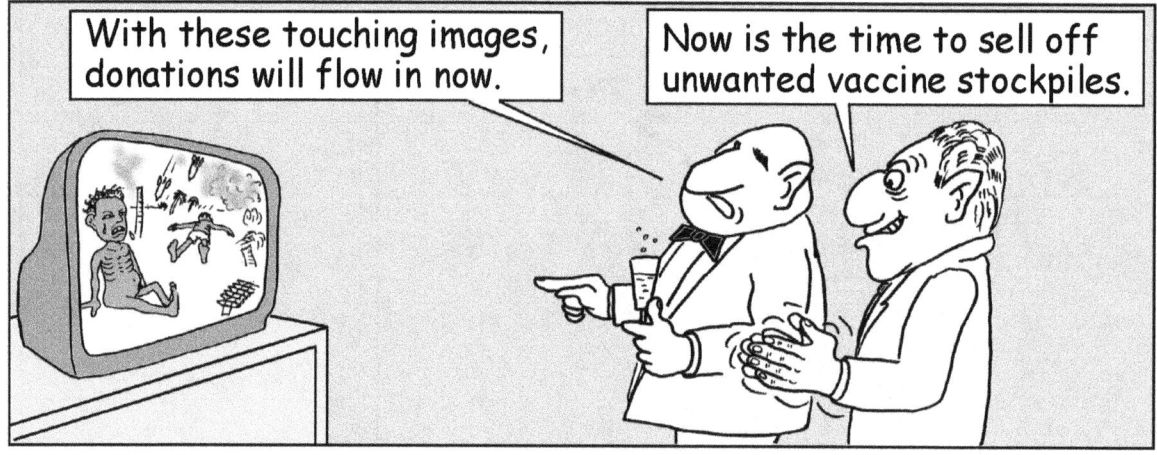

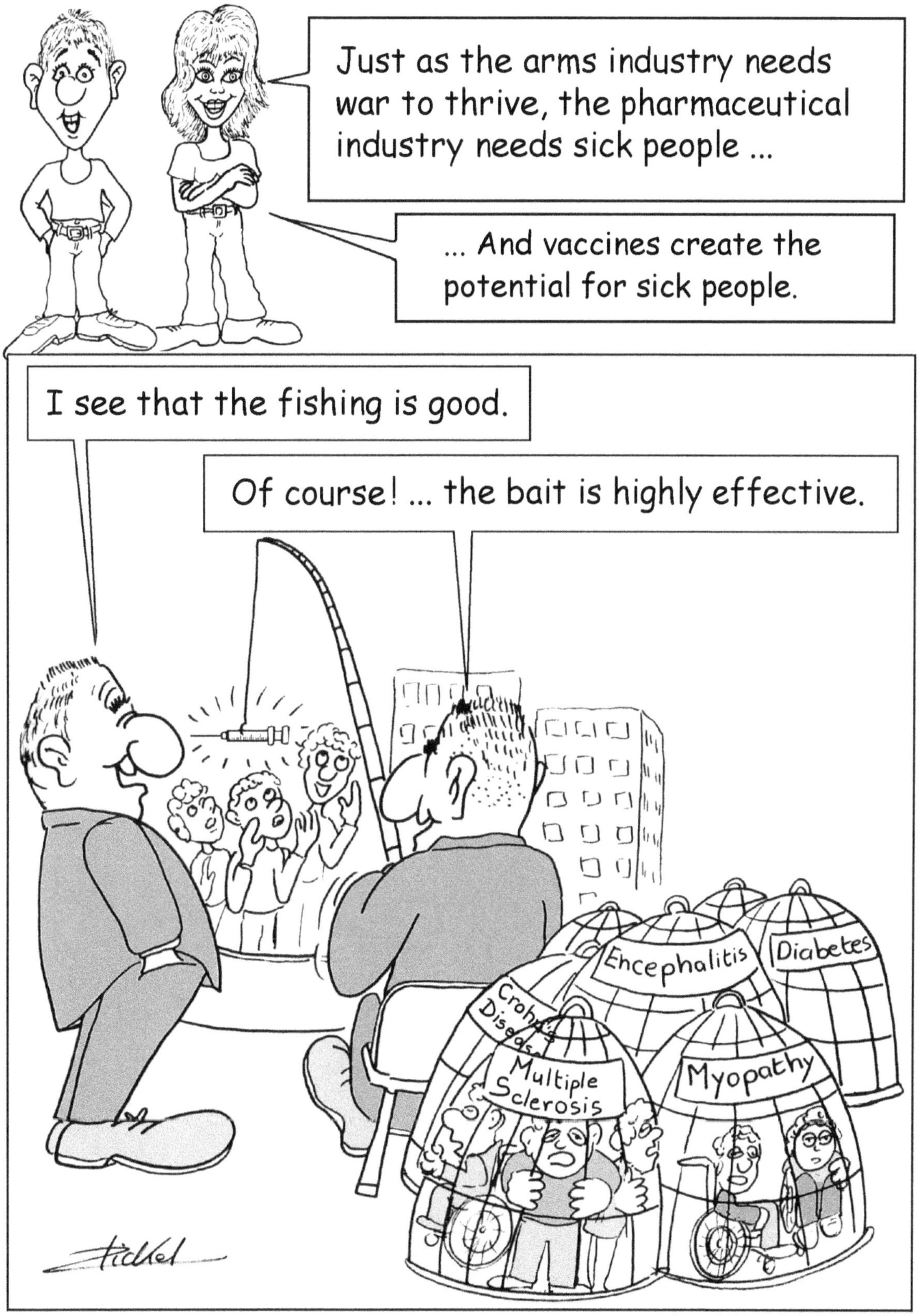

Vaccines: The Great Illusion

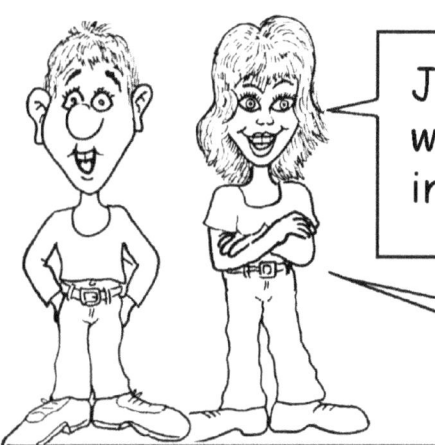

Medicine creates its own customers and keeps them for life.

Professor PEQUIGNOT (World Conference of Doctors)

Two thirds of the 103 children who died of sudden infant death had received the D. T. P. vaccine within the 3 weeks preceding death. Some were even dead the next day.
　　　　　　　　　Dr. TORCH ("Neurology 1982")

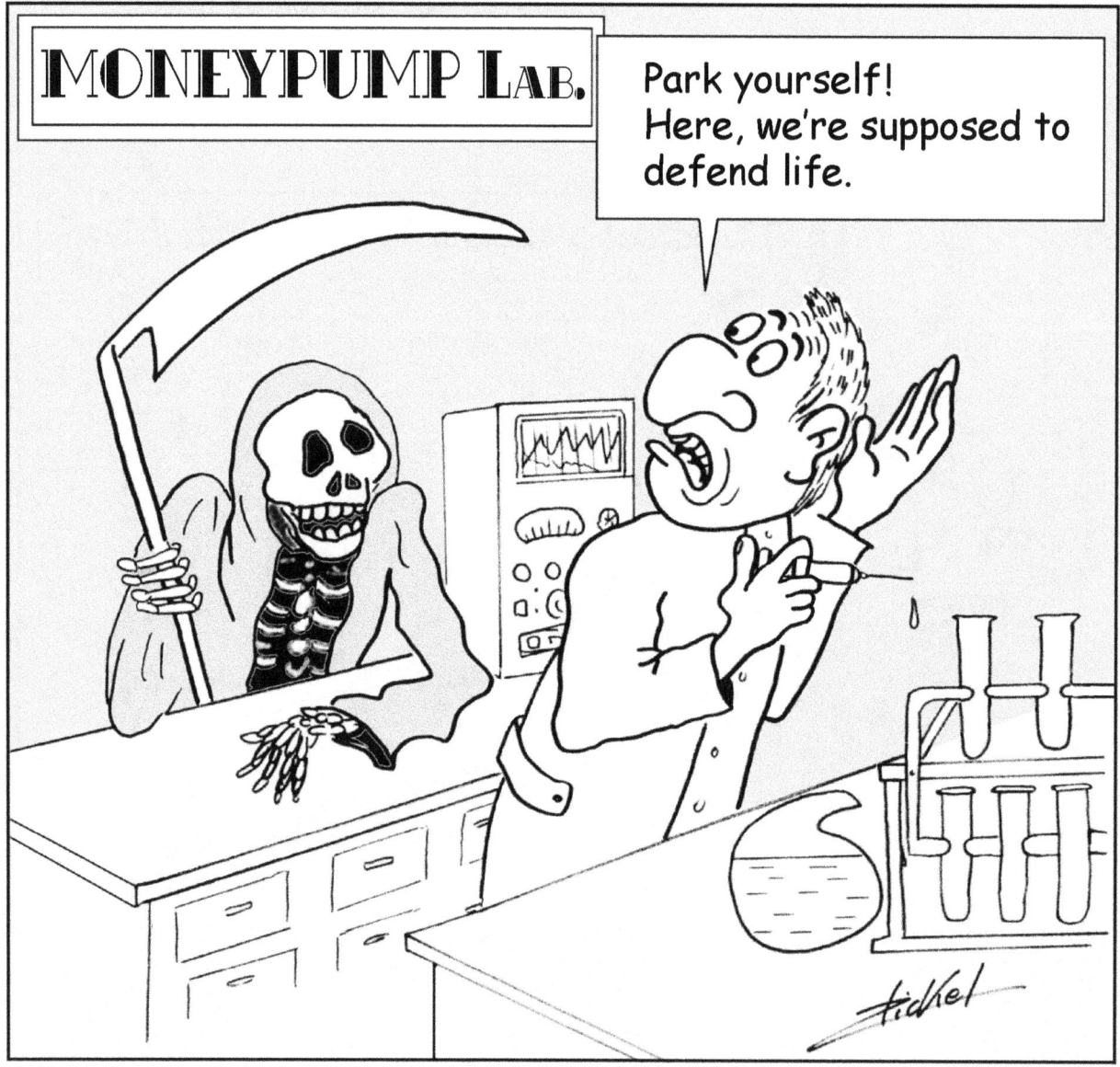

In 1992, a study published in "The American Journal of Epidemiology" showed that a child is 8 times more likely to die three days after having received the DPT vaccine (Diphtheria, Pertussis and Tetanus) than a non-vaccinated child.

> We will always get the same remarks concerning the adverse effects of vaccinations. Considered from a biological or immunological standpoint, every vaccination is an offense to the body.
>
> Professor R. BASTIN (Medical Assistance. 1 February 1986)

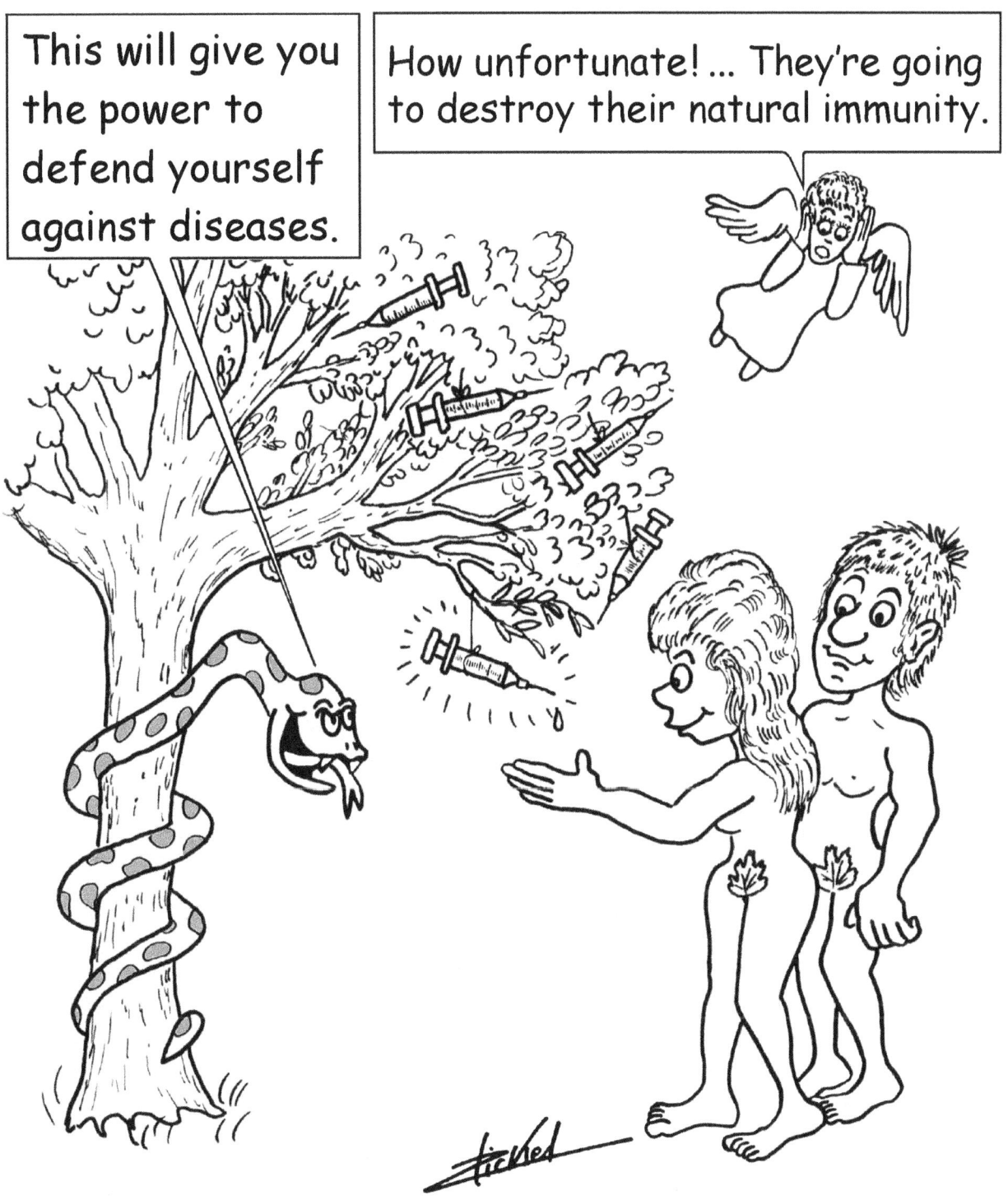

> *Vaccines are useless,*
> *vaccines do not protect,*
> *vaccines are harmful.*
> Dr. Gerhard BUCHWALD
> (Impfen.Das Geschäft mit der Angst)

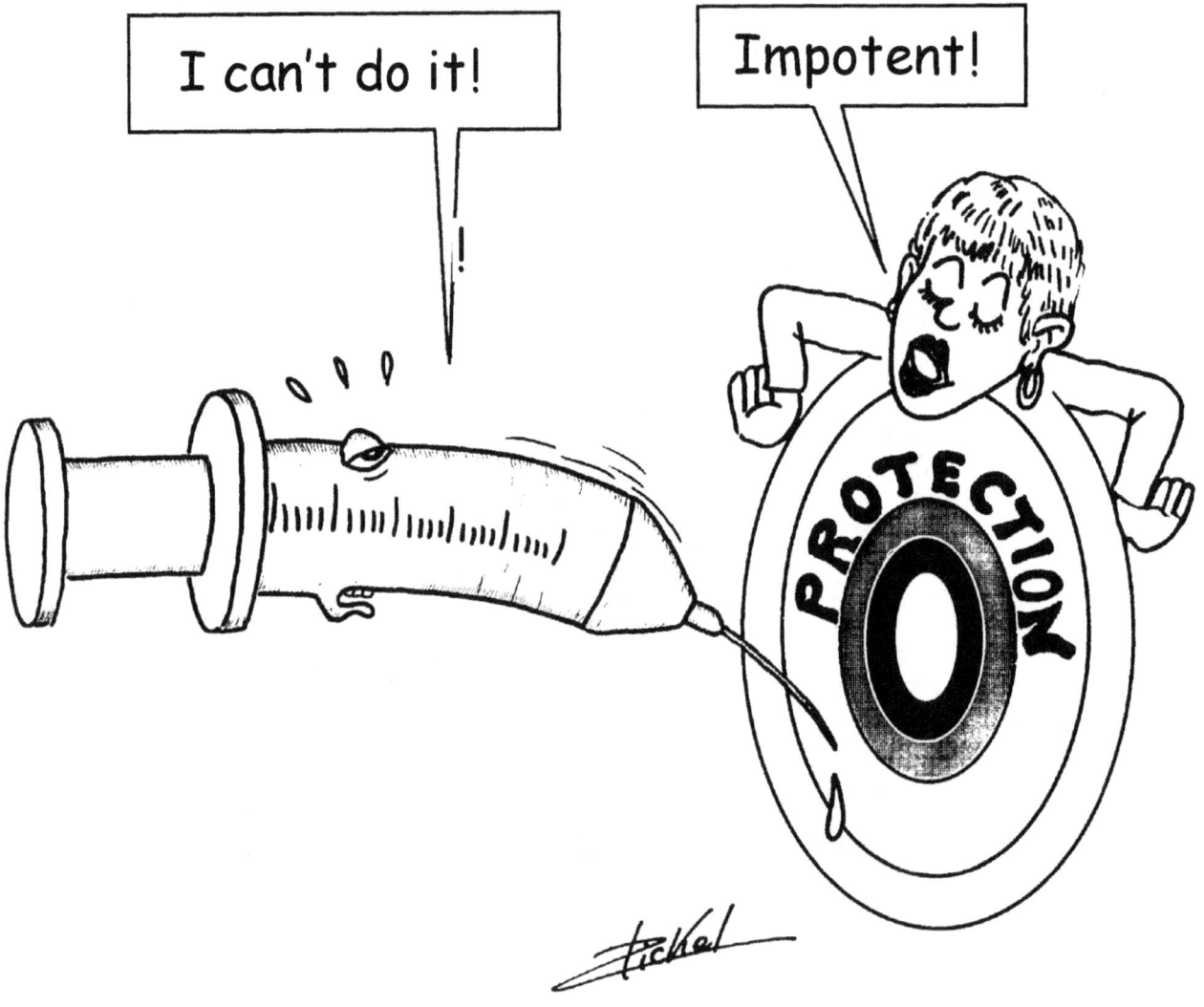

> Claiming to establish a collective immunizing barrier with vaccinations, and blindly applied in an anti-hygienic context, reaches the highest level of idiocy.
> Dr. Jacques KALMAR

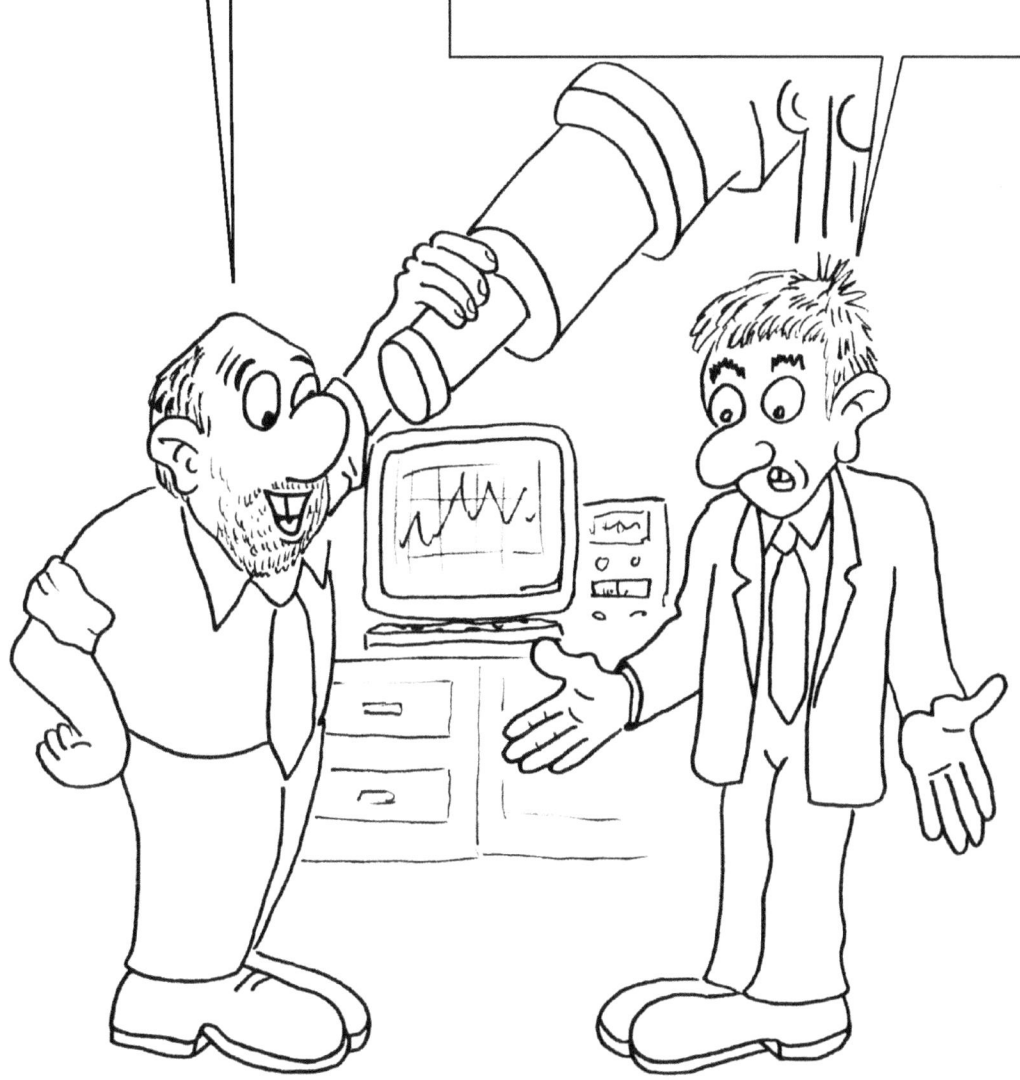

"The more we discover about the universe, the more we raise questions about it."

"In immunology, the more we know, the more we question the benefit of vaccinations.
This has been lasting for a century."

> If the principle of vaccination was conceivable at the beginning of the 20th century when medical and scientific experts ignored virtually everything about molecular biology, endogenous as well as exogenous viruses, retroviruses and their recombination, this became quite different a few decades ago.
> Continuing to inoculate whole populations, hundreds of millions since 1978, is not only a mistake, but a criminal act, a real genocide, on a global scale.
>
> Dr. Louis de BROUWER (AIDS Vertigo)

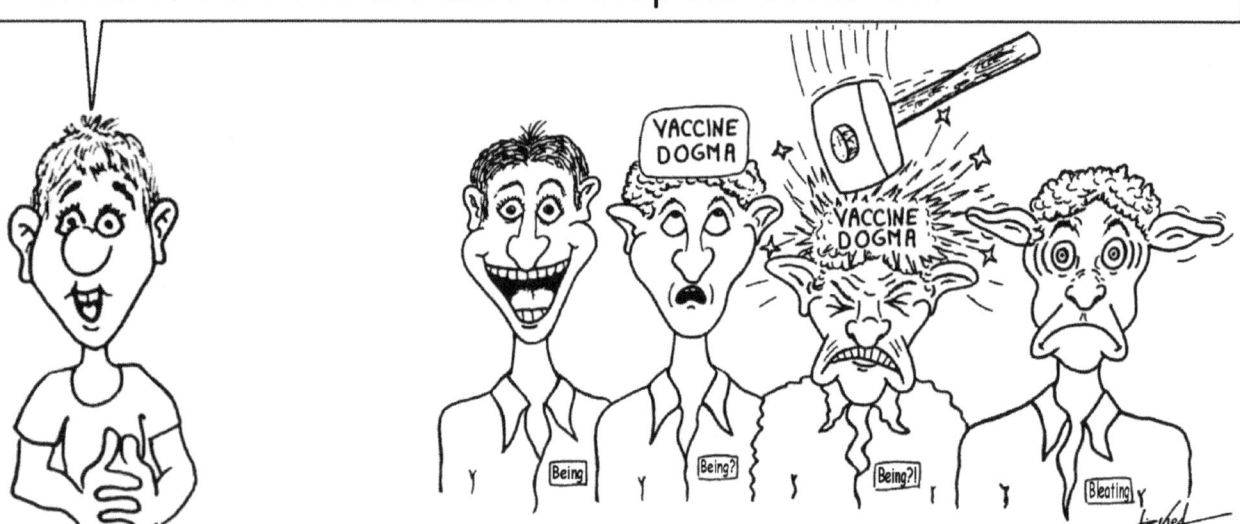

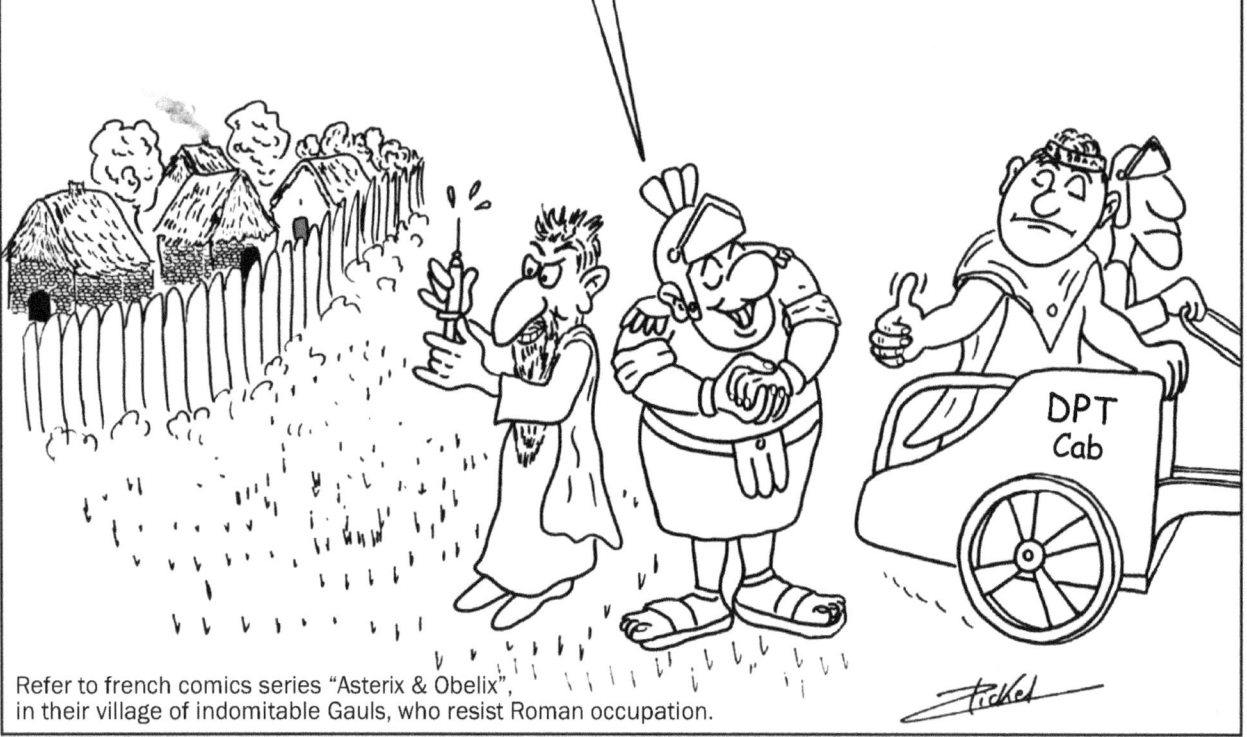

Refer to french comics series "Asterix & Obelix", in their village of indomitable Gauls, who resist Roman occupation.

The Composition of Vaccines

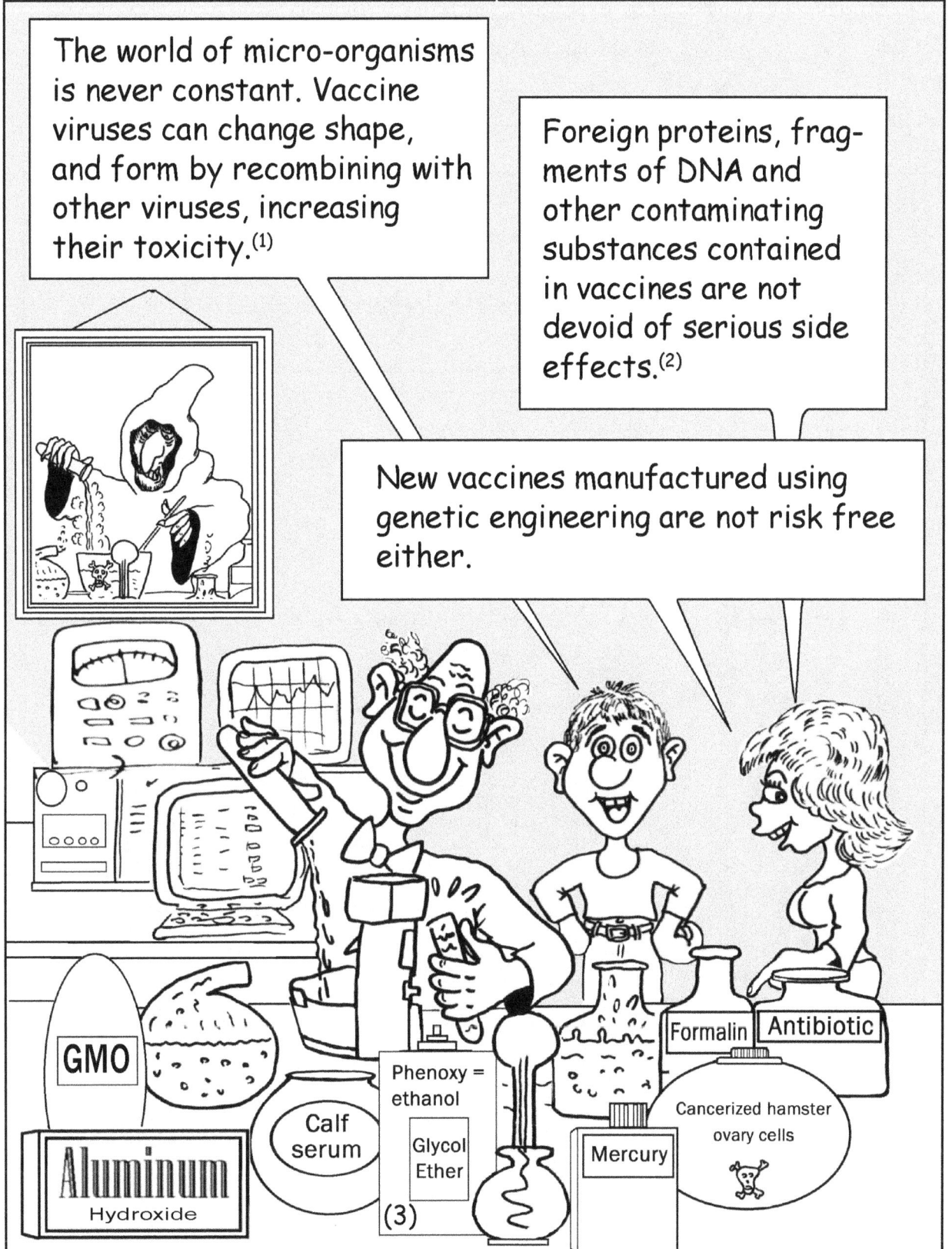

Michel GEORGET: Vaccinations – Les vérités indésirables
(1) Pages 73 – 78 (with numerous scientific references)
(2) Pages 91 to 124 ("   "   "   ")
(3) Collective Expertise of the INSERM on 1999 (Med. Research)

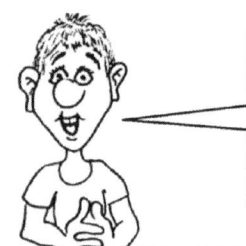

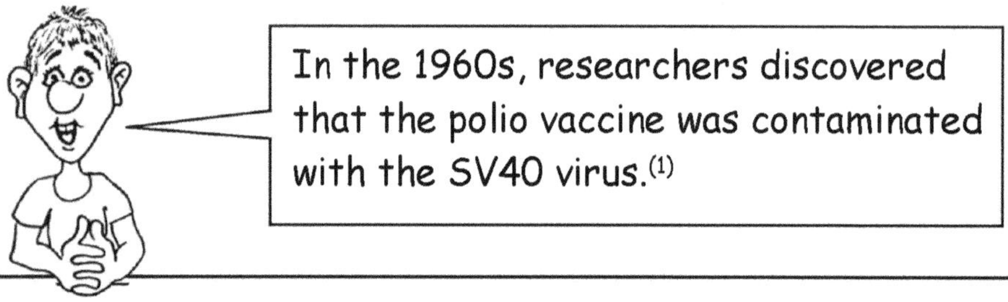

In the 1960s, researchers discovered that the polio vaccine was contaminated with the SV40 virus.[1]

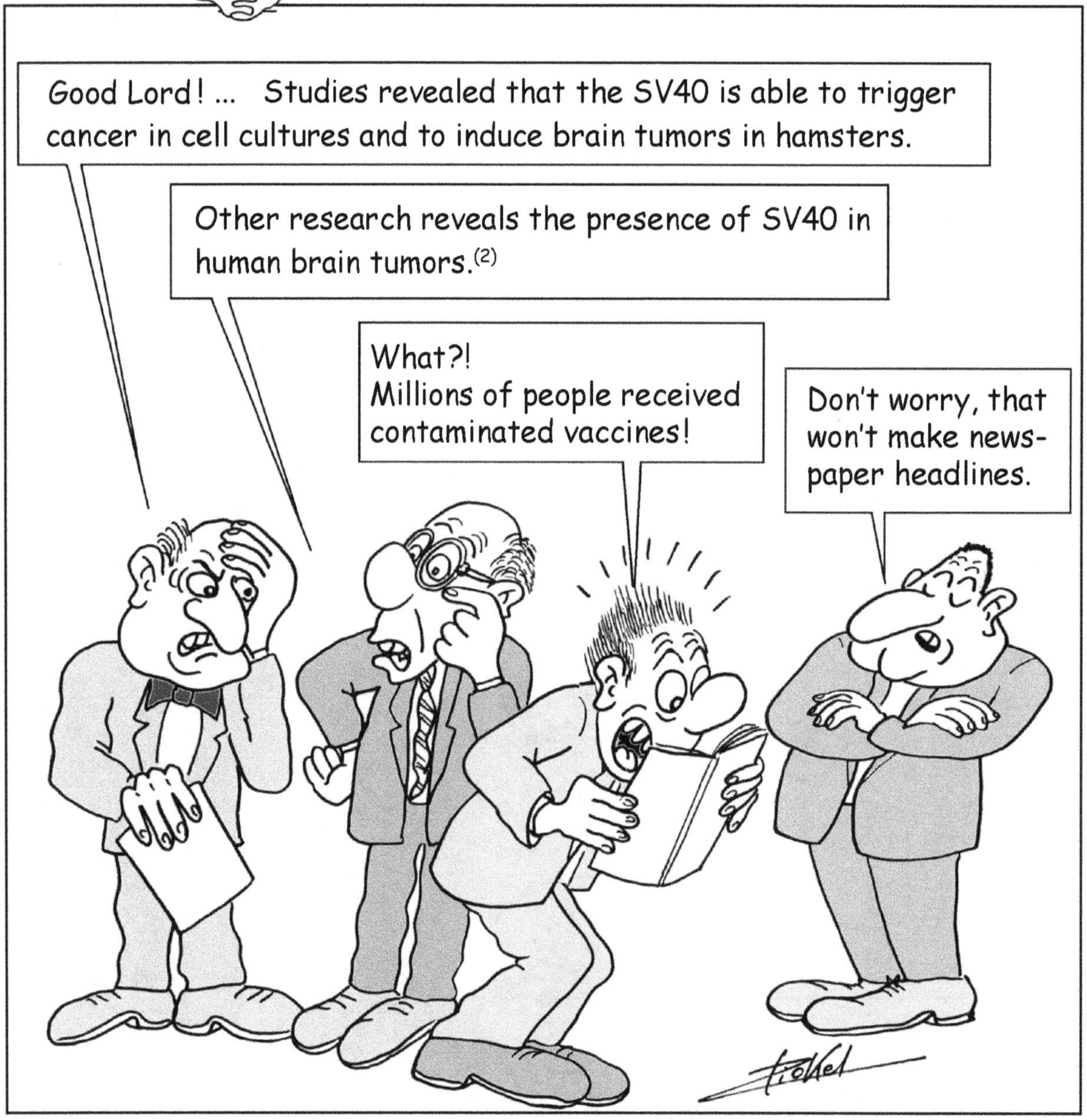

Good Lord! ... Studies revealed that the SV40 is able to trigger cancer in cell cultures and to induce brain tumors in hamsters.

Other research reveals the presence of SV40 in human brain tumors.[2]

What?! Millions of people received contaminated vaccines!

Don't worry, that won't make newspaper headlines.

(1) The 40th simian virus discovered in cultures of monkey kidney cells.
(2) As well as in various types of cancers.

A medical team from Baylor College in Houston found the virus SV40 in tissues of patients suffering from brain tumors and mesothelioma. This virus, recognized as a carcinogen, has been injected into 600 million people throughout the world through the polio vaccine ...
Michel THIBON-CORNILLOD   *(technical adviser for the Ministry of Health in France)*
(Sciences-Actualités - May, 1998)

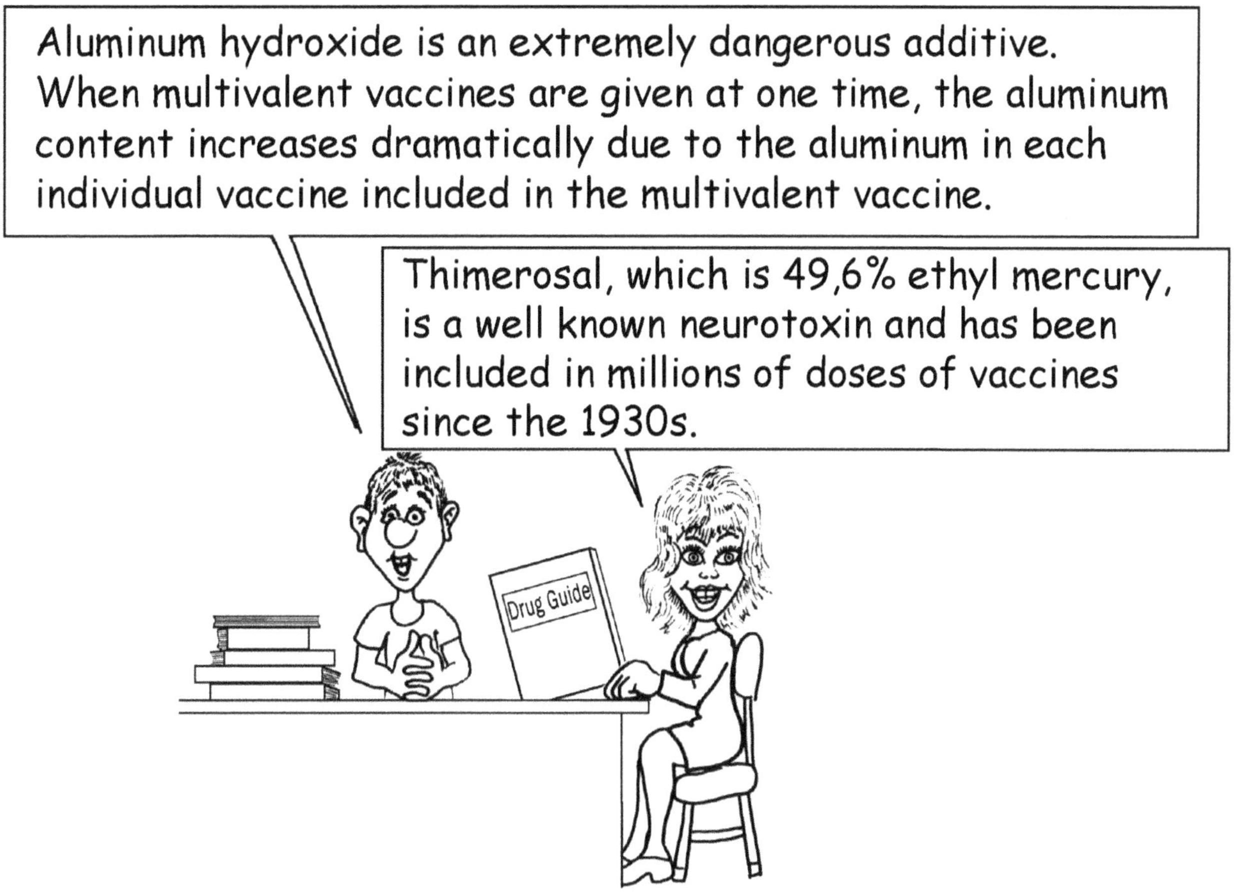

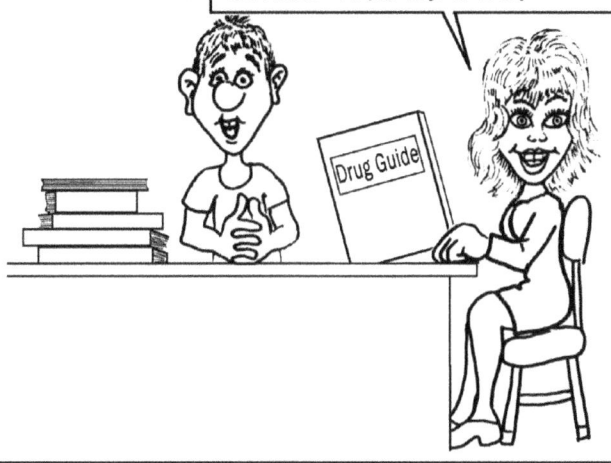

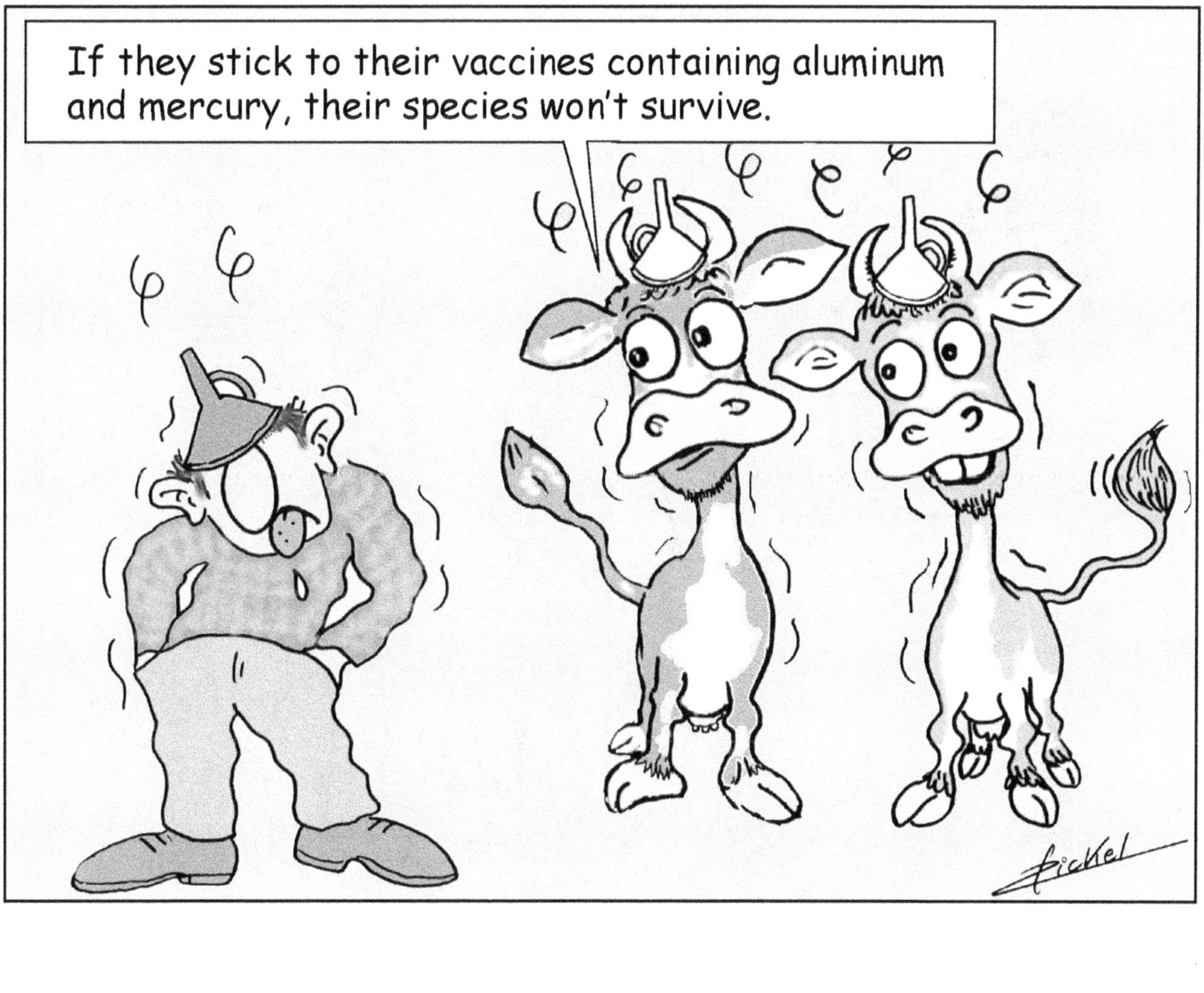

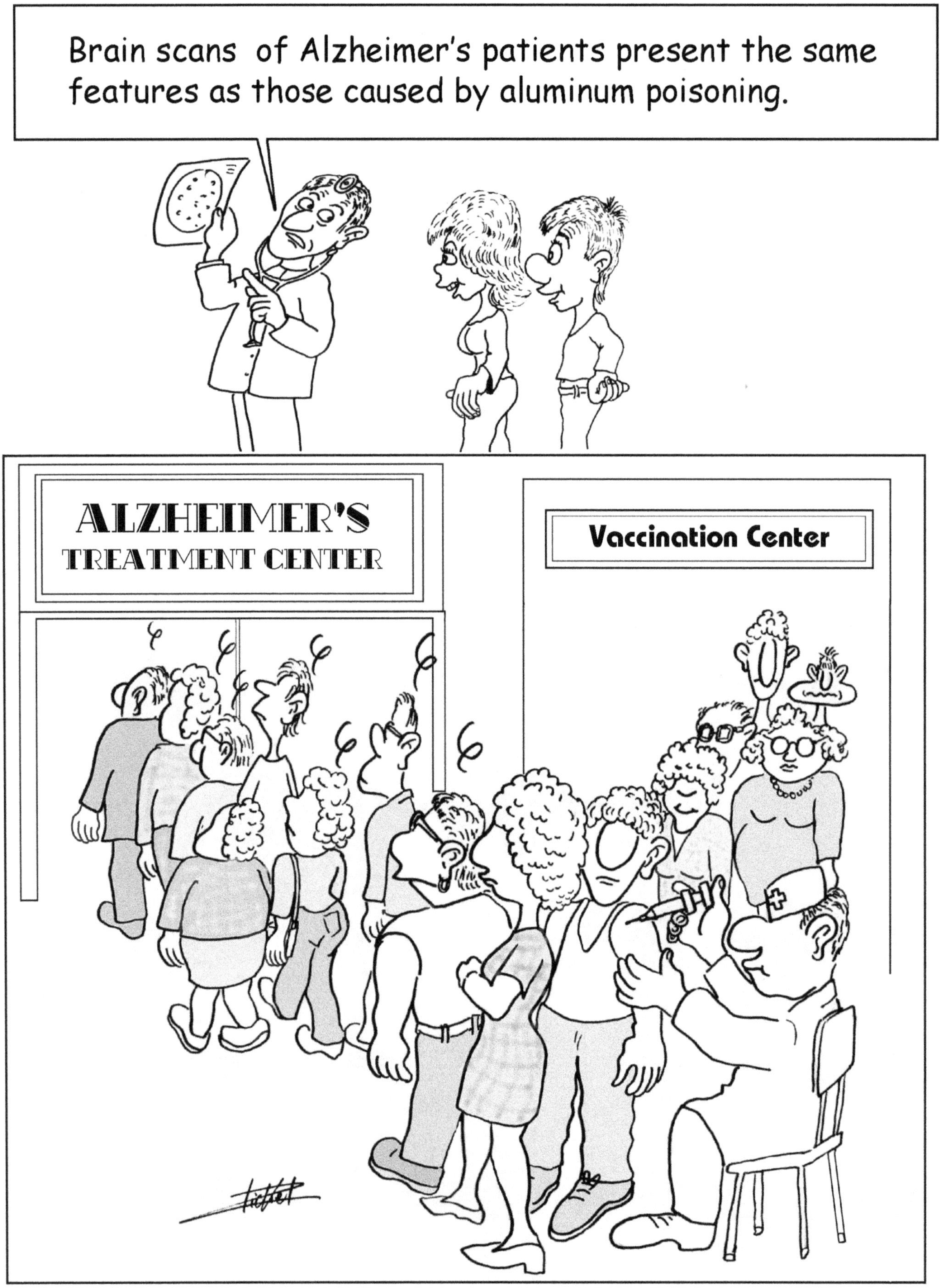

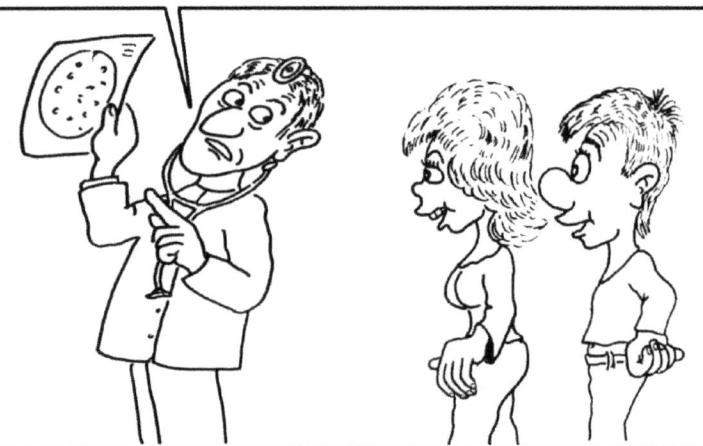

Vaccines: The Great Illusion

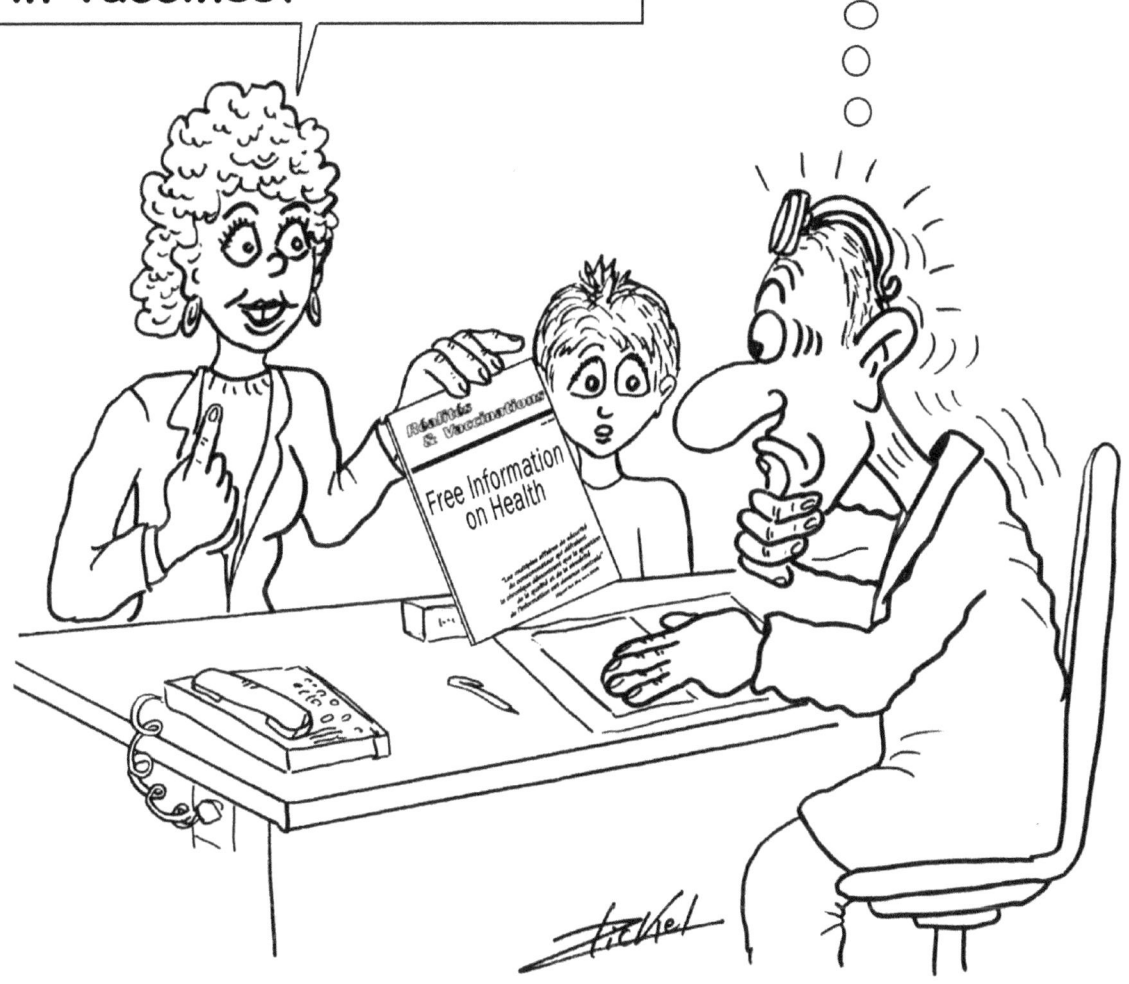

We are besieged by our fears. We will fight germs until death with methods that will horrify generations to come.

Dr. Jacques KALMAR

> *The deliberate and unnecessary introduction of infectious viruses into a human body is an insane act which must be dictated by a deep ignorance of virology and of the processes of infection. [...] The harm caused is incalculable.*
>
> Pr. R. DELONG, Virologist and Immunologist, University of Toledo, United States

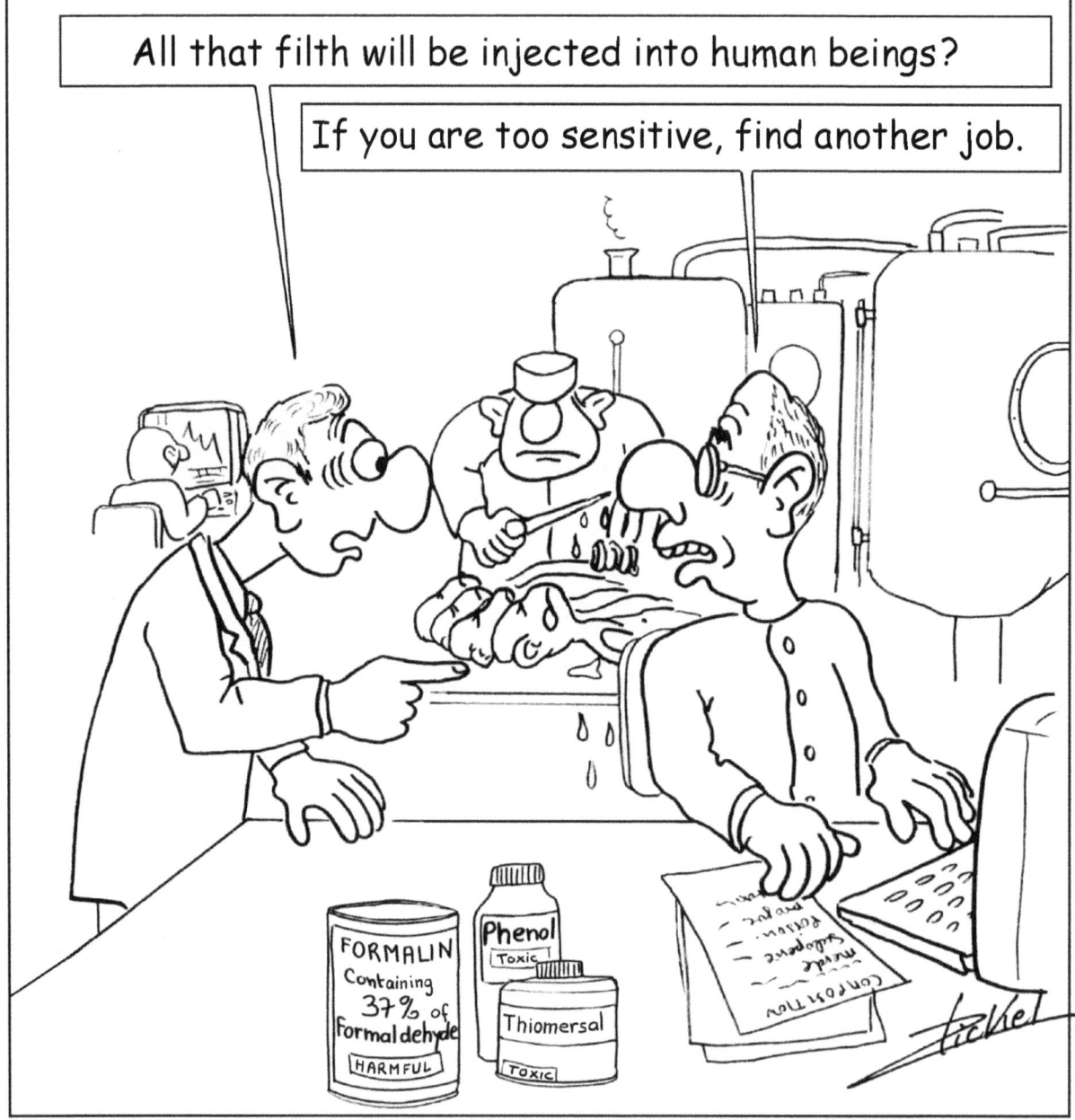

> *The microorganisms inoculated bypassing all the natural barriers have been tinkered in such a way that the majority of the people develop chronic pathologies, the symptoms of which are not easy to connect with their initial cause.*
>
> Dr. Jacqueline BOUSQUET (Doctor of Science and honorary researcher at the CNRS (NATIONAL CENTER FOR SCIENTIFIC RESEARCH, France)

> Most infants have been receiving up to 15 doses of mercury-containing vaccines by the time they are 6 months old. It is almost inconceivable that these heavy burdens of foreign immunologic materials, introduced into the immature systems of children, could fail to bring about disruptions and adverse reactions in these in systems.
>
> Dr. Harold E BUTTRAM, MD

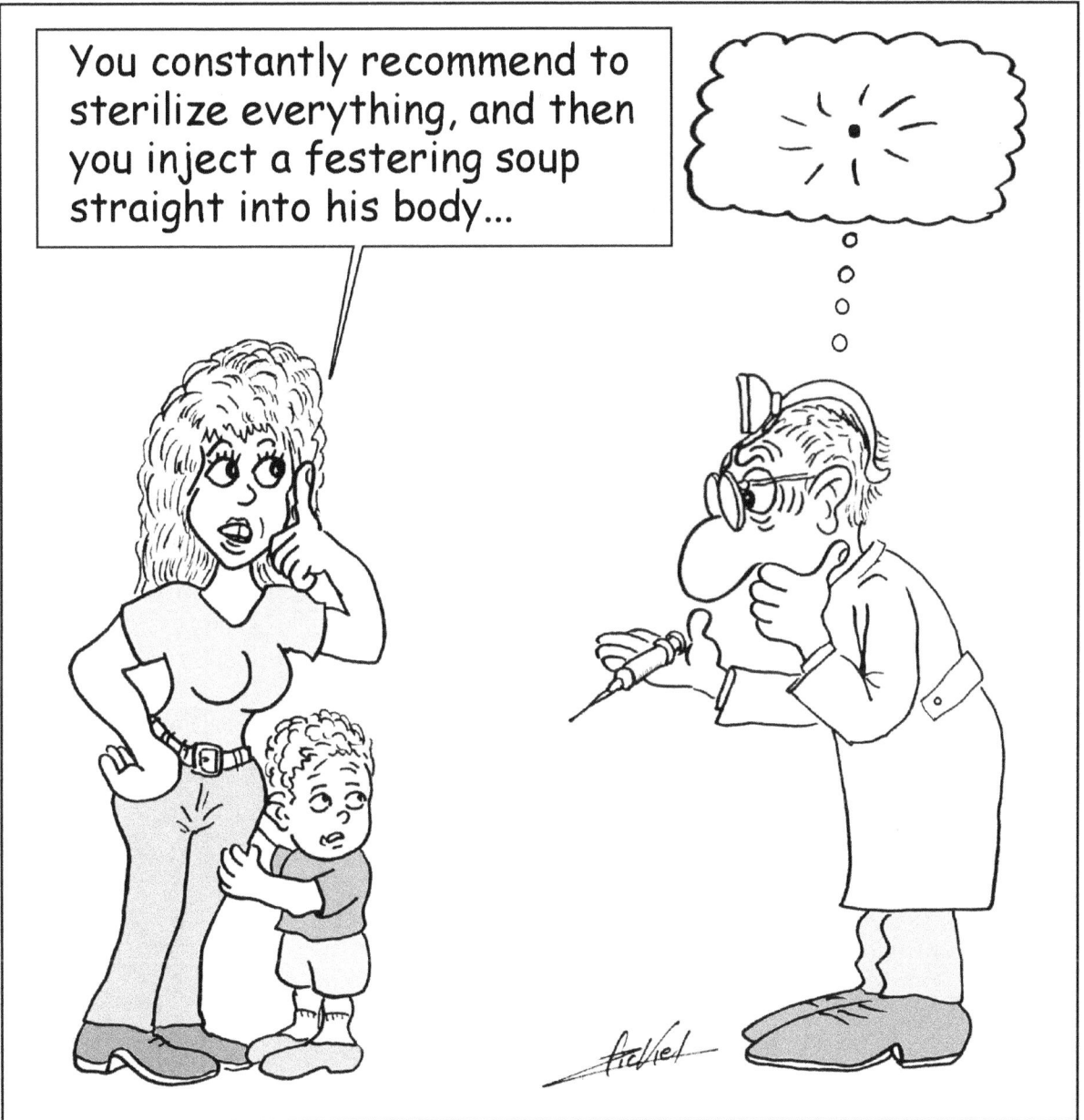

> The intjection of foreign proteins and even live viruses (contained in "modern" vaccines) into the bloodstream of a child is a great offense committed against his/her immune system.
>
> Dr. Richard MOSKOWITZ

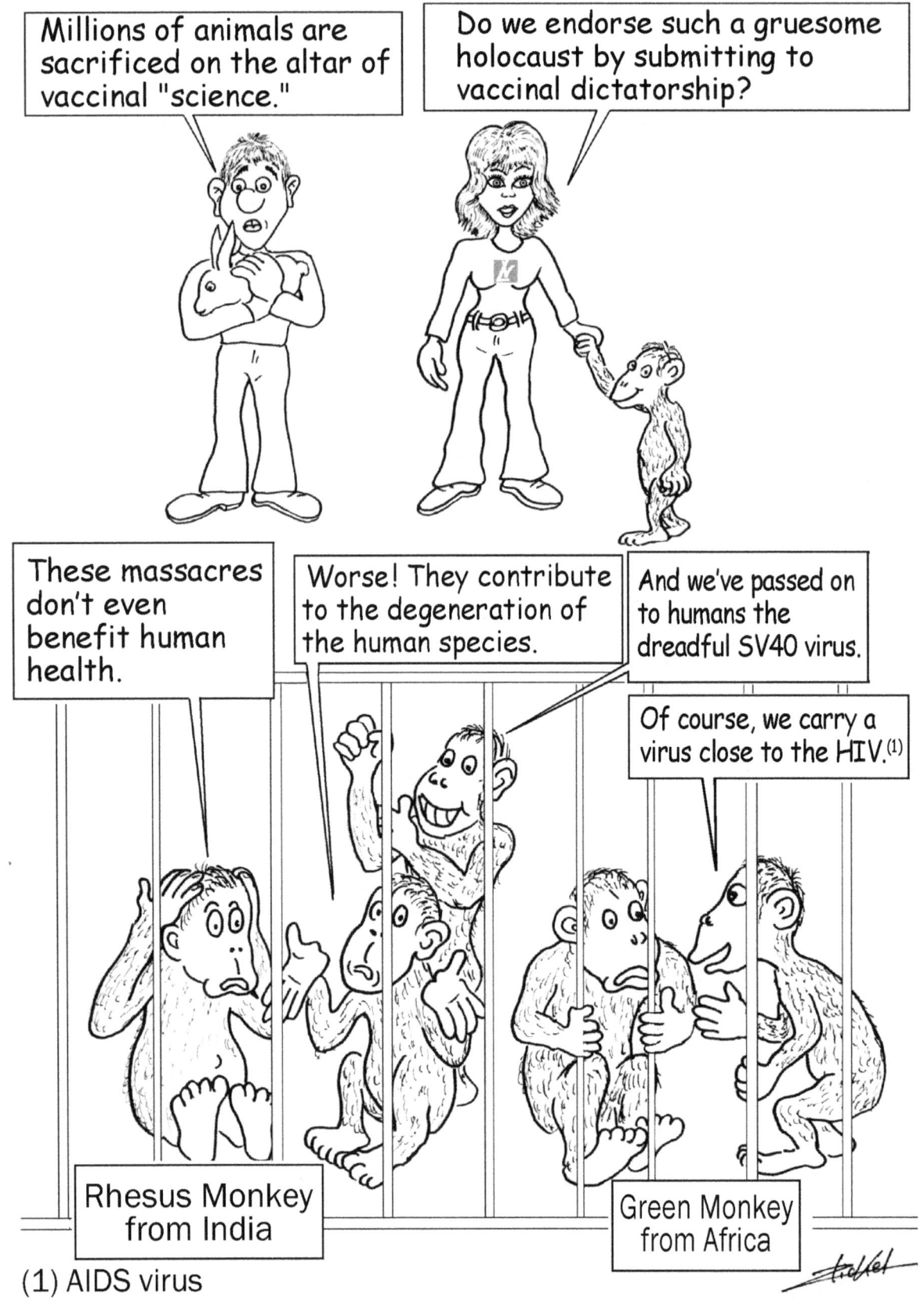

(1) AIDS virus

None of the vaccine strains taken from monkeys is devoid of neurological toxicity.
   Dr. Garcia SILVA ("Le Maroc Médical," No. 43)

Vaccines Are Identical For All Individuals Who Really Are Different.

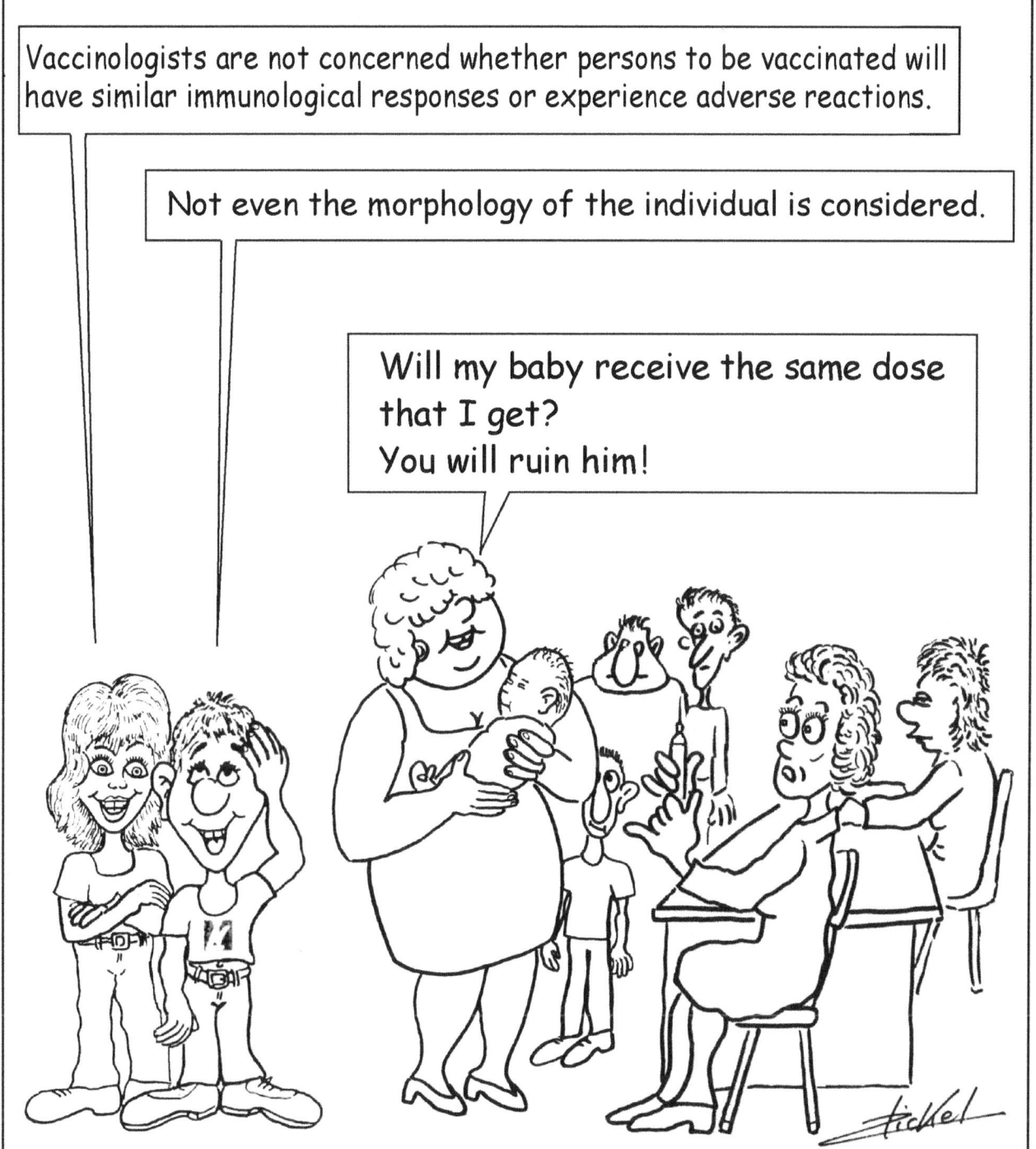

Vaccinologists are not concerned whether persons to be vaccinated will have similar immunological responses or experience adverse reactions.

Not even the morphology of the individual is considered.

Will my baby receive the same dose that I get?
You will ruin him!

> *One can very easily —sadly!— standardize huge crowds on the mental level but, as far as I know, no one ever managed to standardize them on the immunological level.*
>
> Dr. Jacques KALMAR

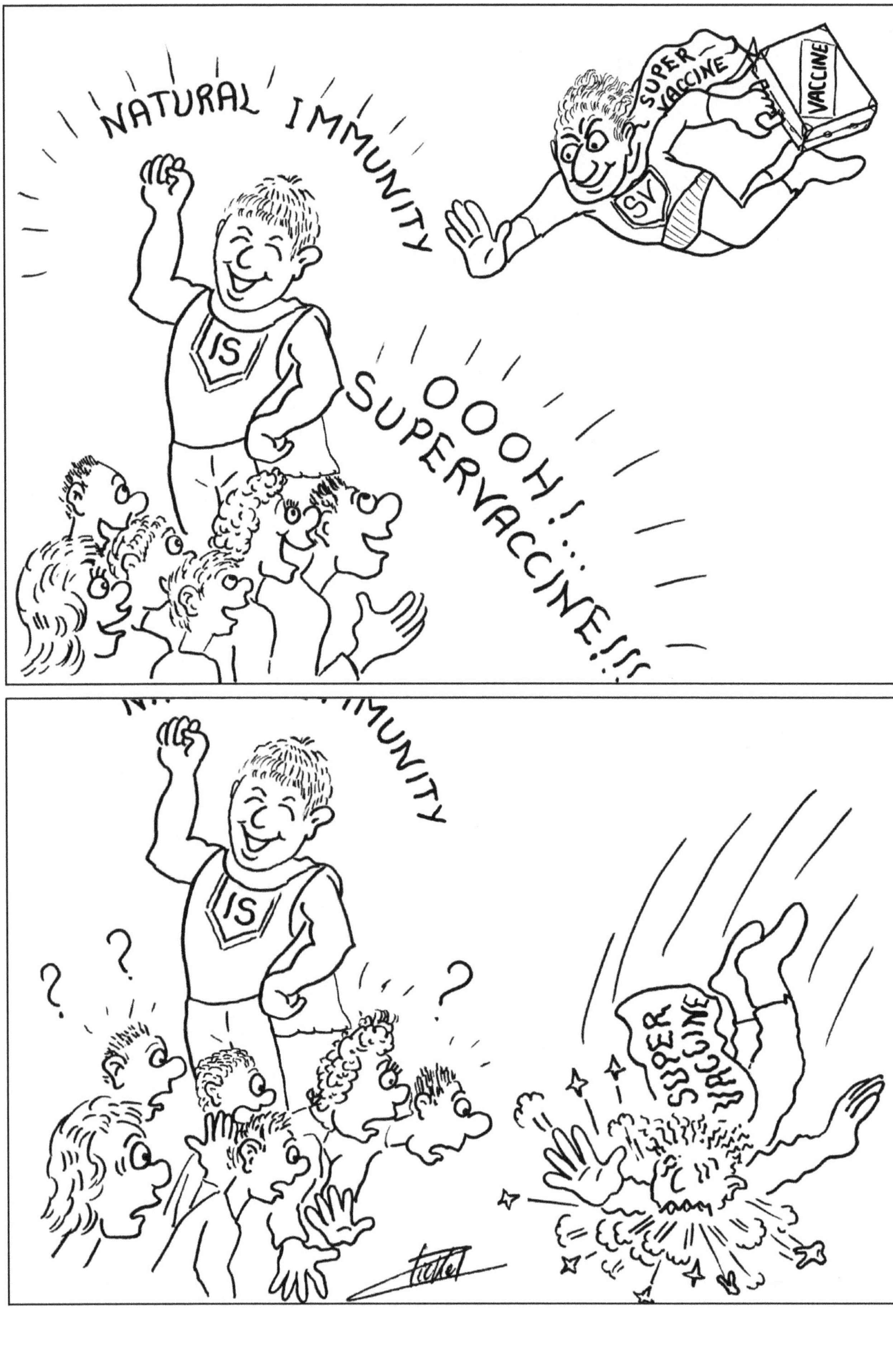

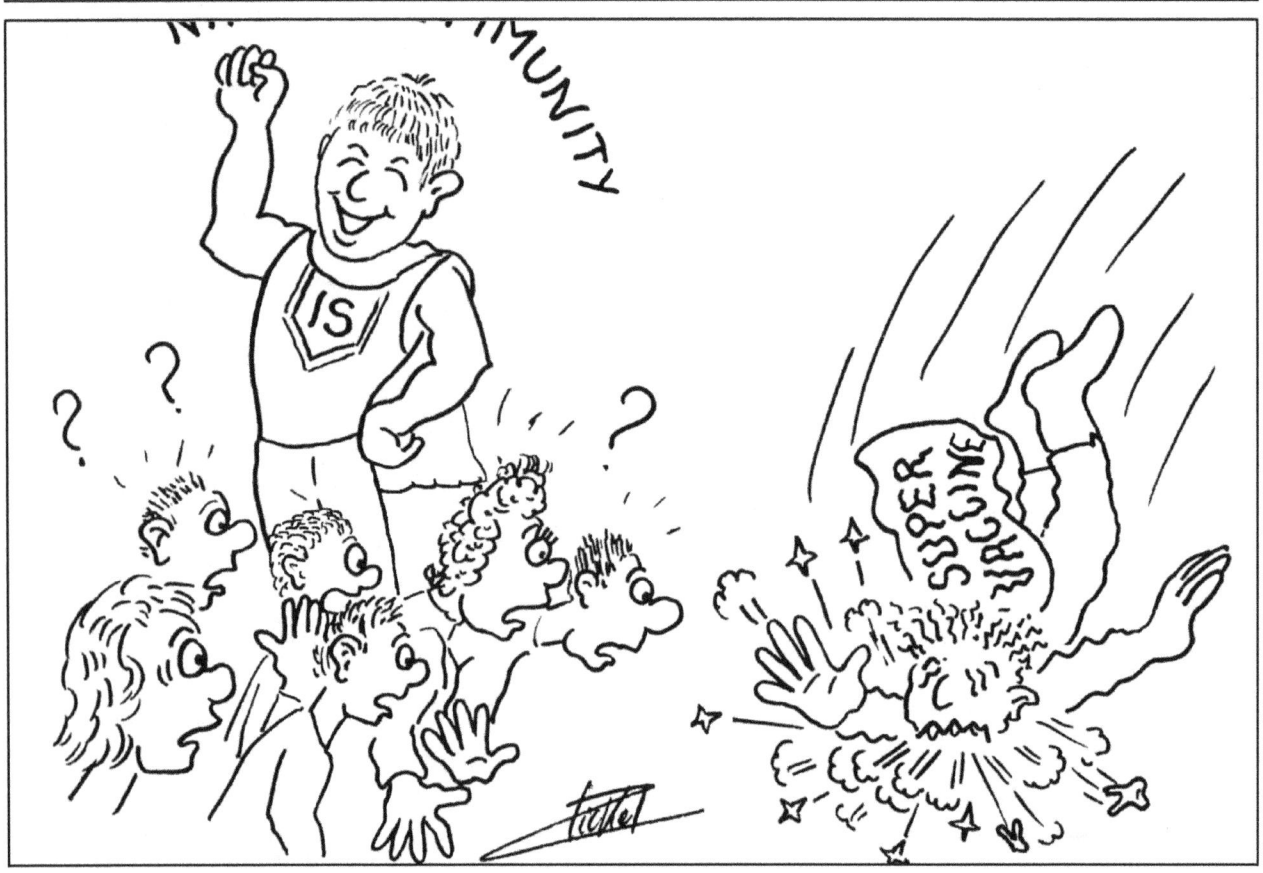

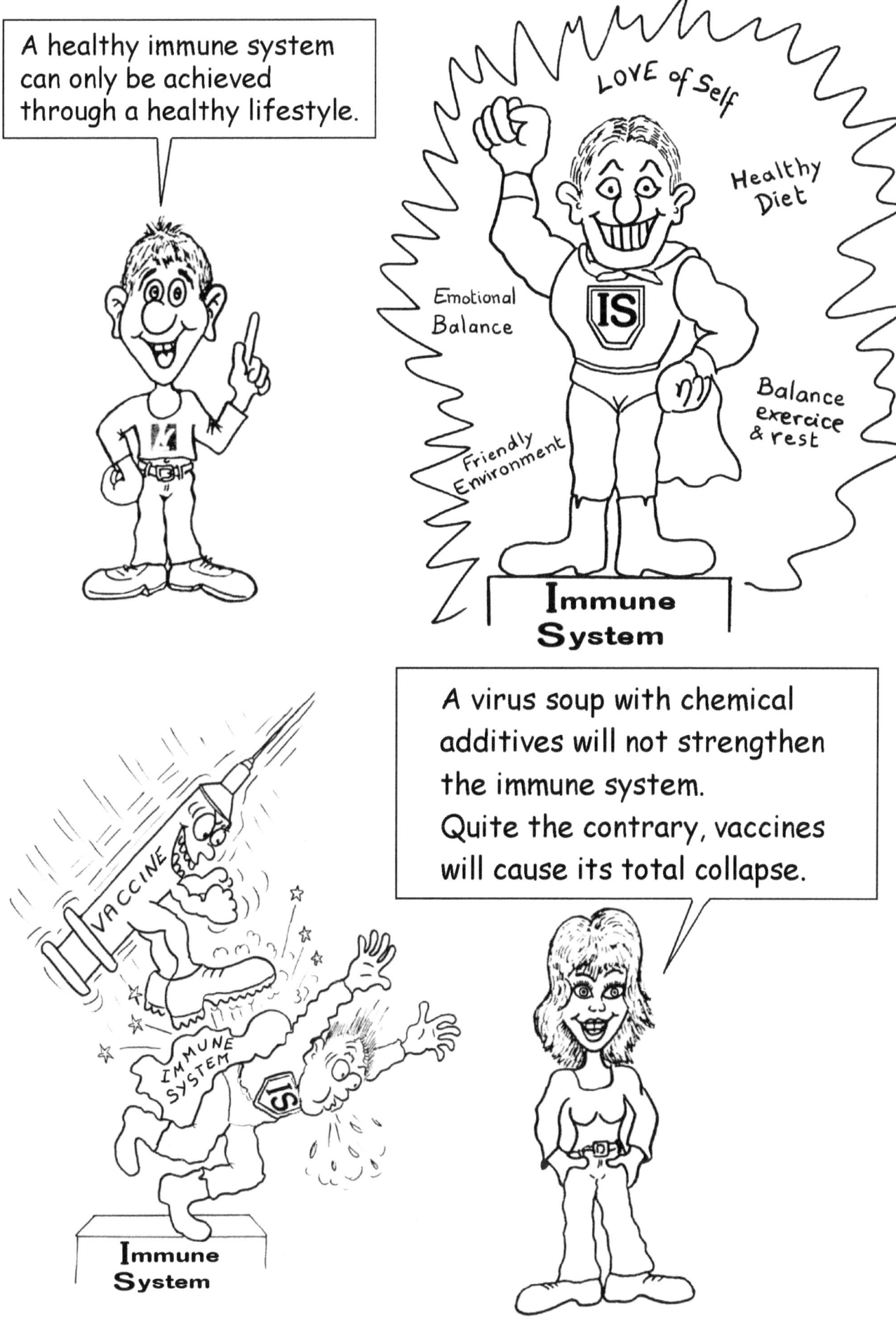

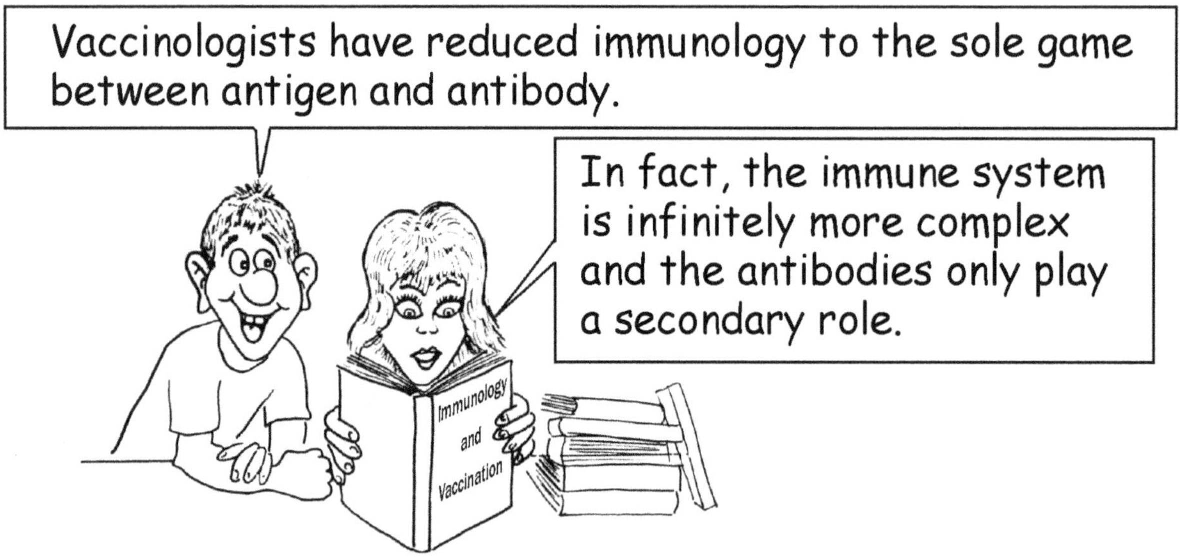

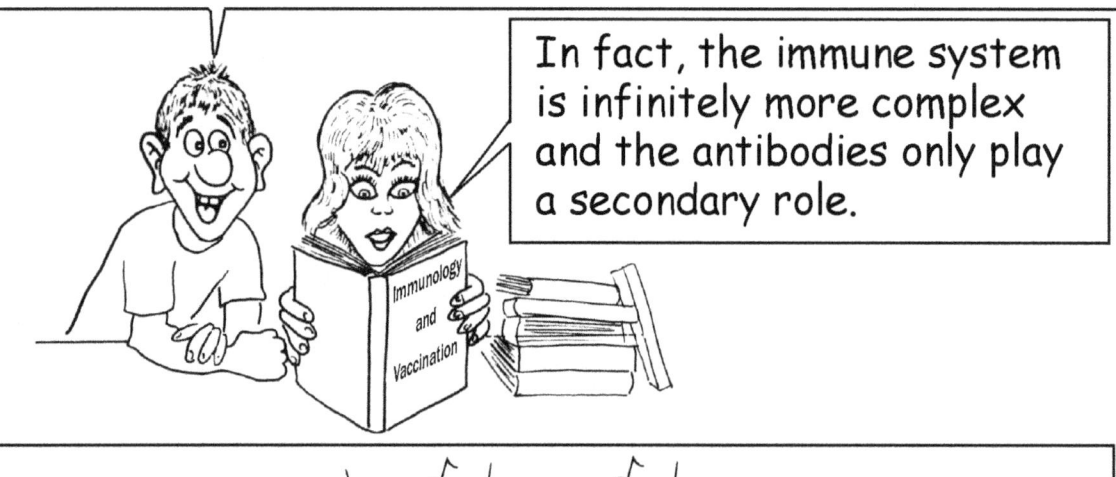

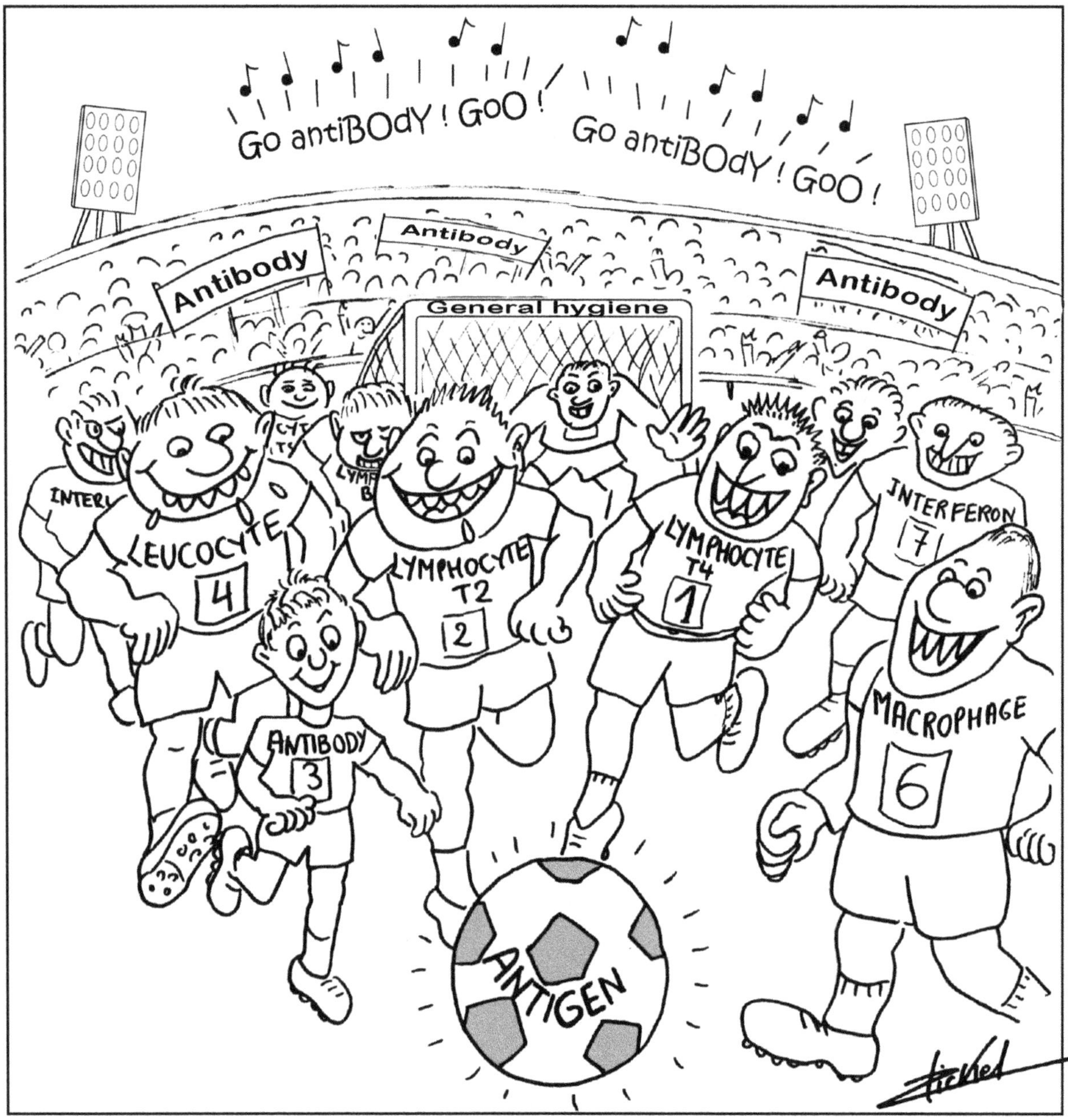

Inspired from "Immunology and vaccination" by Dr. Jacques KALMAR

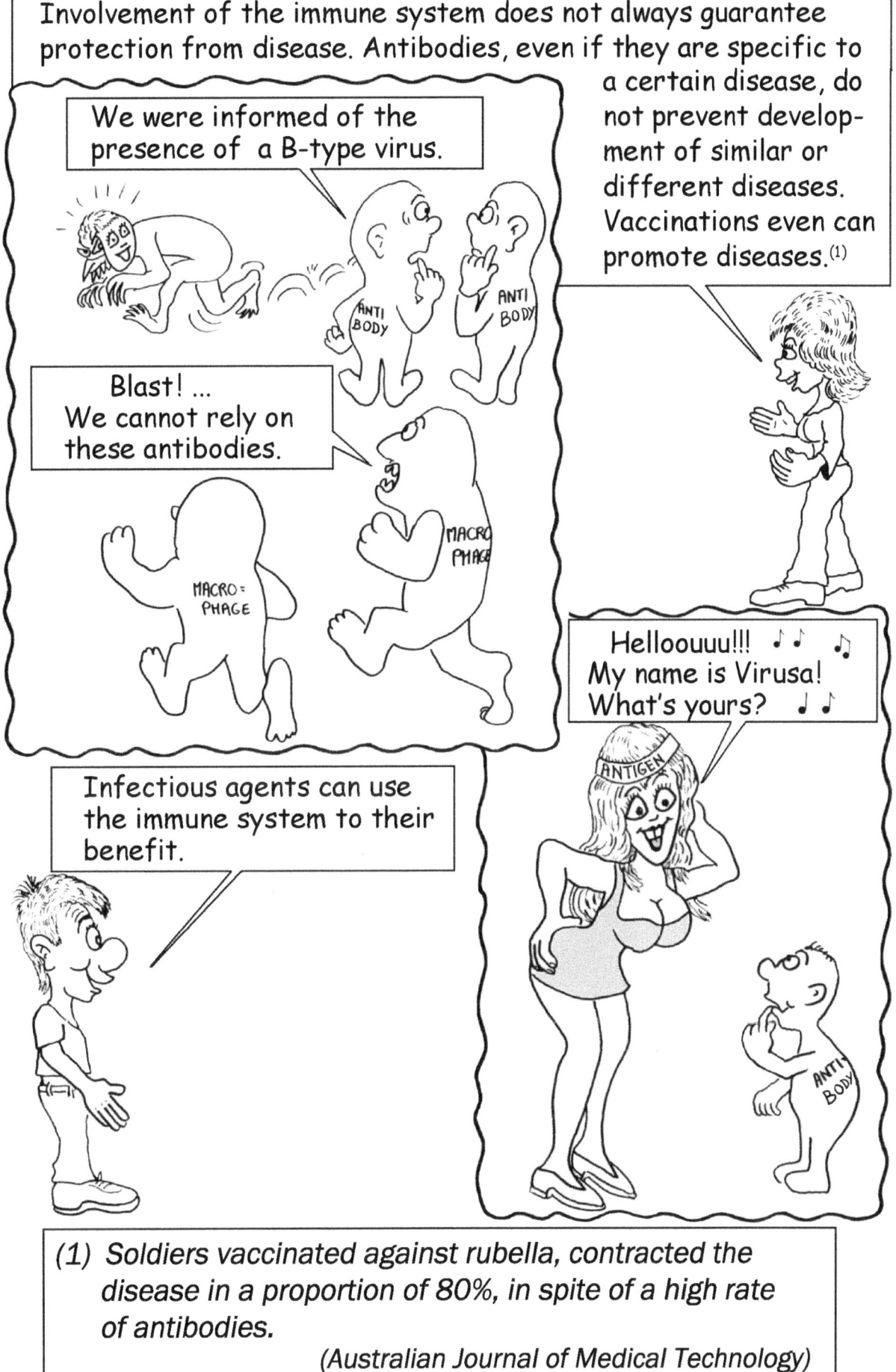

Immuno-Neuro-Hormonal Harmony

The immune system interacts with the nervous and hormonal systems.

Health depends on the proper functioning and interactions of these three systems.

Stress assaulting the nervous system also causes hormonal and immune imbalances.

Vaccinations also cause stress to the immune system. Constantly assaulted by multiple vaccinations, the immune system adversely affects neuro-hormonal balance.[1]

(1) Michel GEORGET: "Vaccination - Les vérités indésirables" (pages 61 to 63)
Harris COULTER, PhD: "Vaccination Social Violence and Criminality: The Medical Assault on the American Brain"

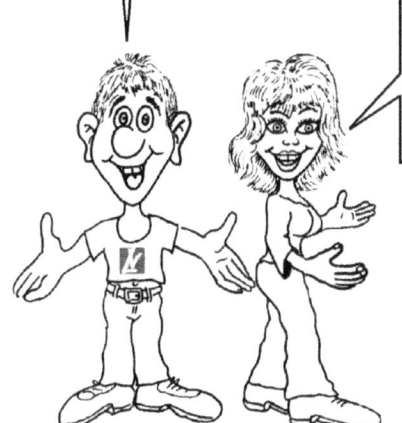

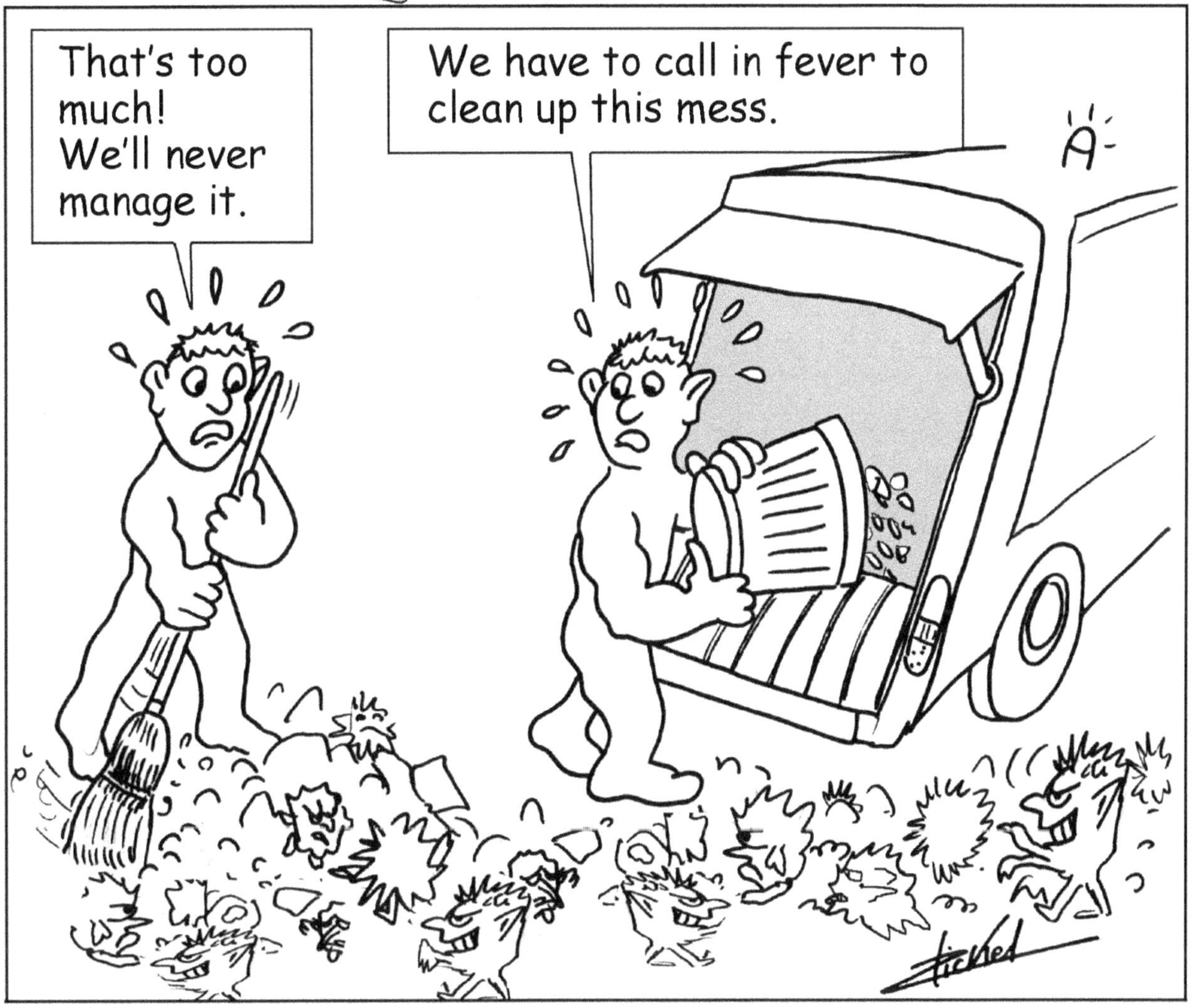

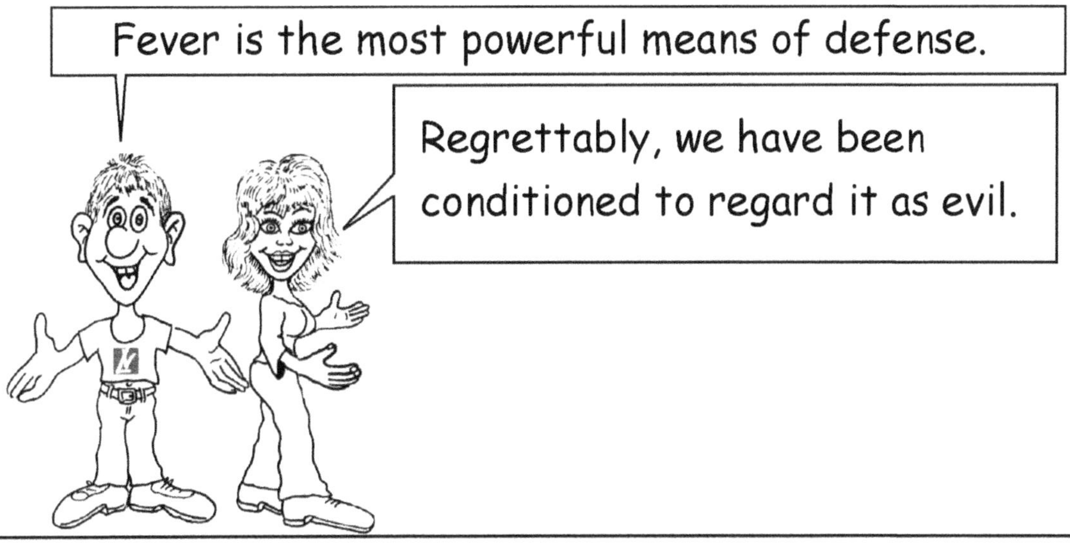

Vaccines: The Great Illusion

The microbe is nothing, the soil is everything.

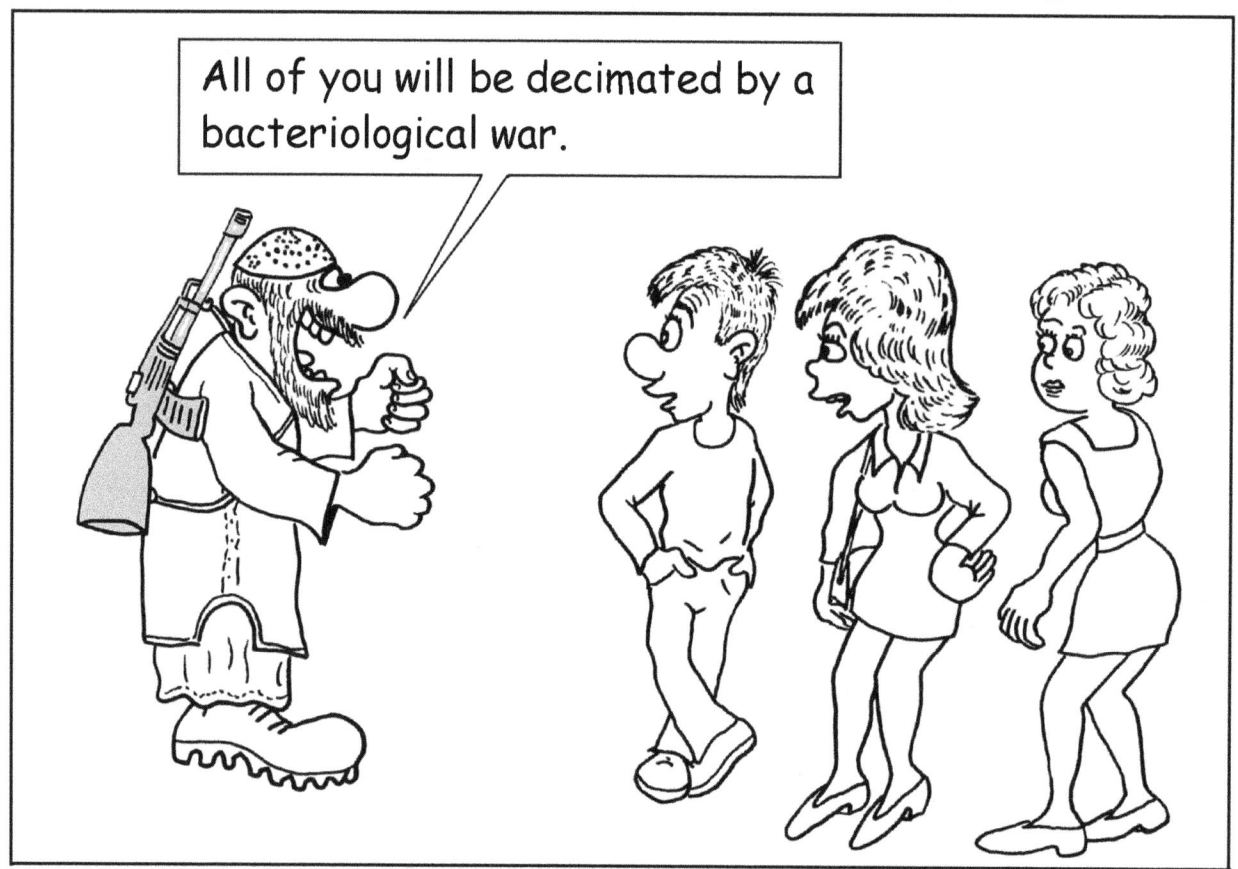

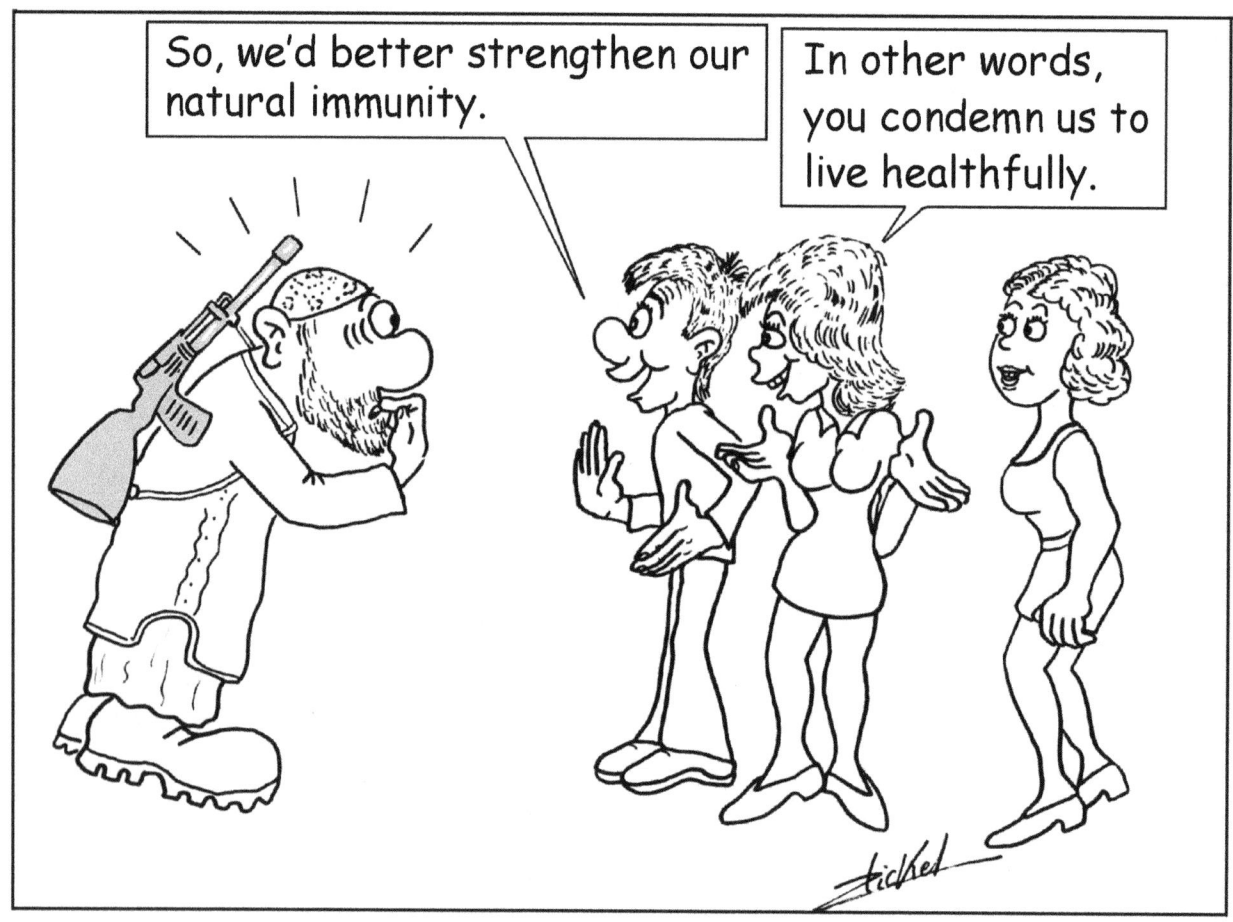

> *I call this vaccinomania. We have reached a point which is no longer scientifically justifiable. Injecting new vaccines into the body, without knowing how they may affect the functions of the immune system over time, verges on criminality.*
>
> Nicholas REGUSH, Medical Journalist

> *Nobody would be foolish enough to argue that vaccines render us "immune" to viruses if in fact they merely weakened our ability to expel them, and forced us to harbor them chronically instead. On the contrary, such a long-term carrier state would also tend to compromise our ability to respond to other infections as well, and would have to be regarded as immunosuppressive to that extent.*
>
> Dr. R. MOSKOWITZ (graduated from Harward)

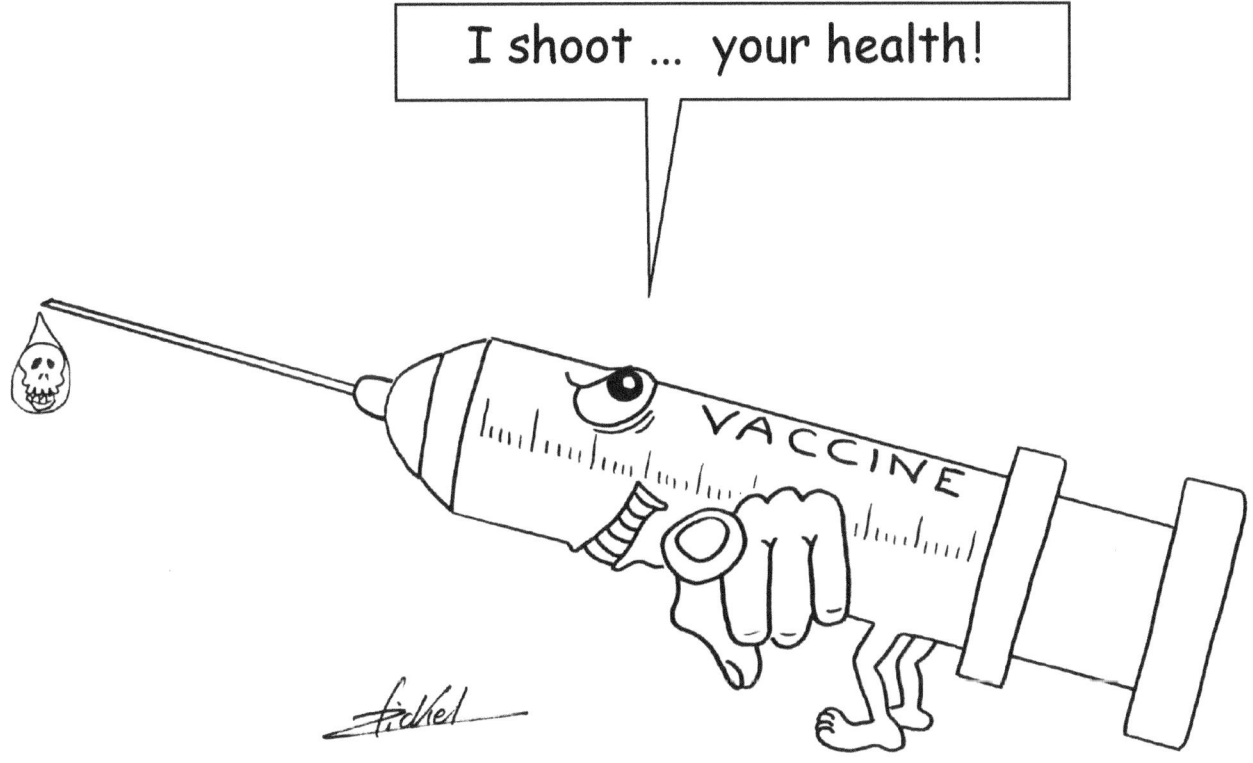

> *"The immune system gets particularly damaged following routine vaccinations."*
>
> *"Immunological resources diminish sustantially among the many children subjected to usual vaccination programs."*
>
> Concours Médical (French publication - January 20, 1974)

> *The vaccinated, far from constituting a protection for the non-vaccinated, are conversely dangerous and may contaminate the rest of the population, since it has been proven that they can carry and transmit polioviruses via the intestinal tract, and maybe other ways.*
>
> Dr. Yves COUZIGOU

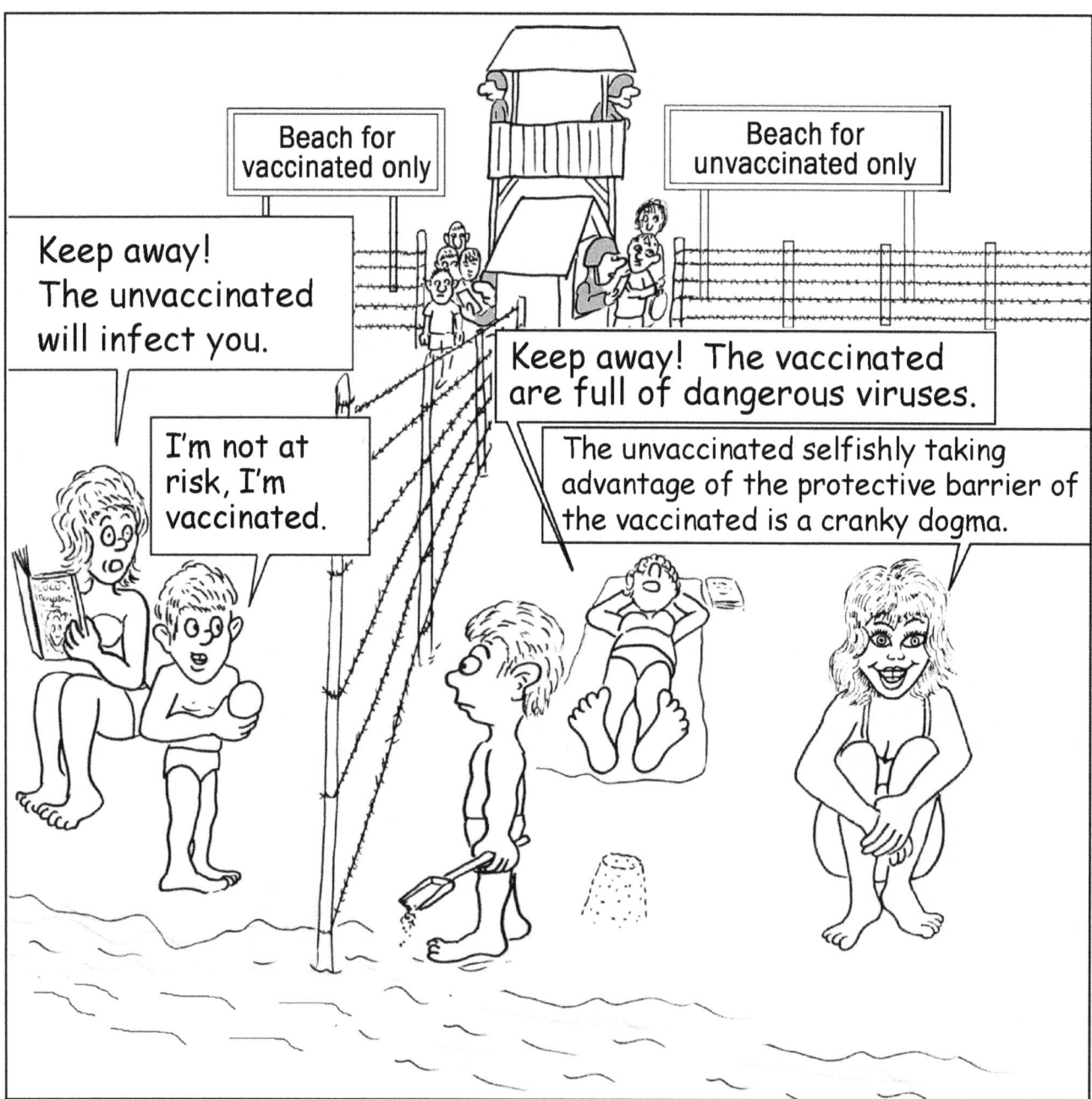

> *The cases of polio from contacts with the inoculated by the oral vaccine are well known.*
>
> (The General Practitioner, February 19, 1985)

Who's really at risk and why?

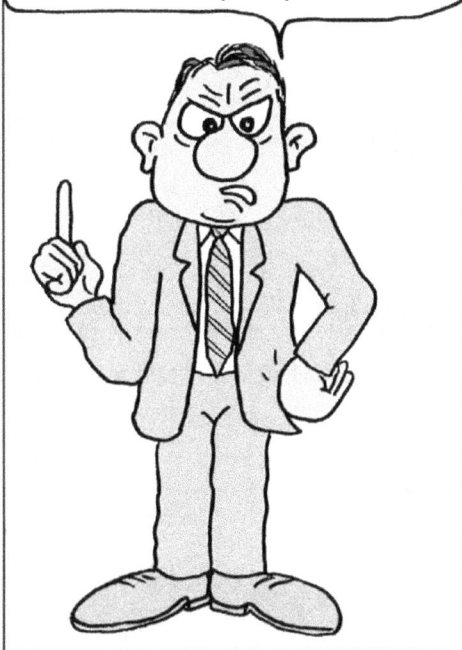

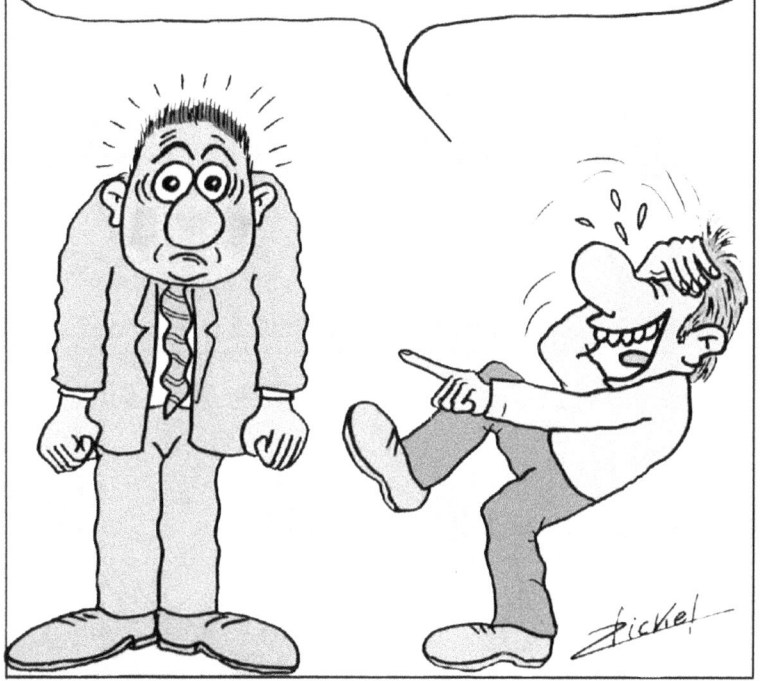

Vaccine pushers often resort to an interesting fear tactic to try to mandate vaccine obedience among the masses: They insist that those who are unvaccinated are a health threat to the rest of the vaccinated population because the vaccinated people might get infected by the unvaccinated disease carriers!

The quack logic of such a claim should be self-evident. If vaccines protect people from infectious disease, then vaccinated people should not be concerned at all about being around unvaccinated people. After all, the vaccine made them all "immune," right?

But of course that's all propaganda. Vaccines don't really work at all. They are marketed under a blanket of disease hysteria and pimped by a cult following of medicalized quacks and needle junkies who abandoned real science long ago.

Mike Adams, aka the Health Ranger
Editor of NaturalNews.com

Vaccination: a kind of magic

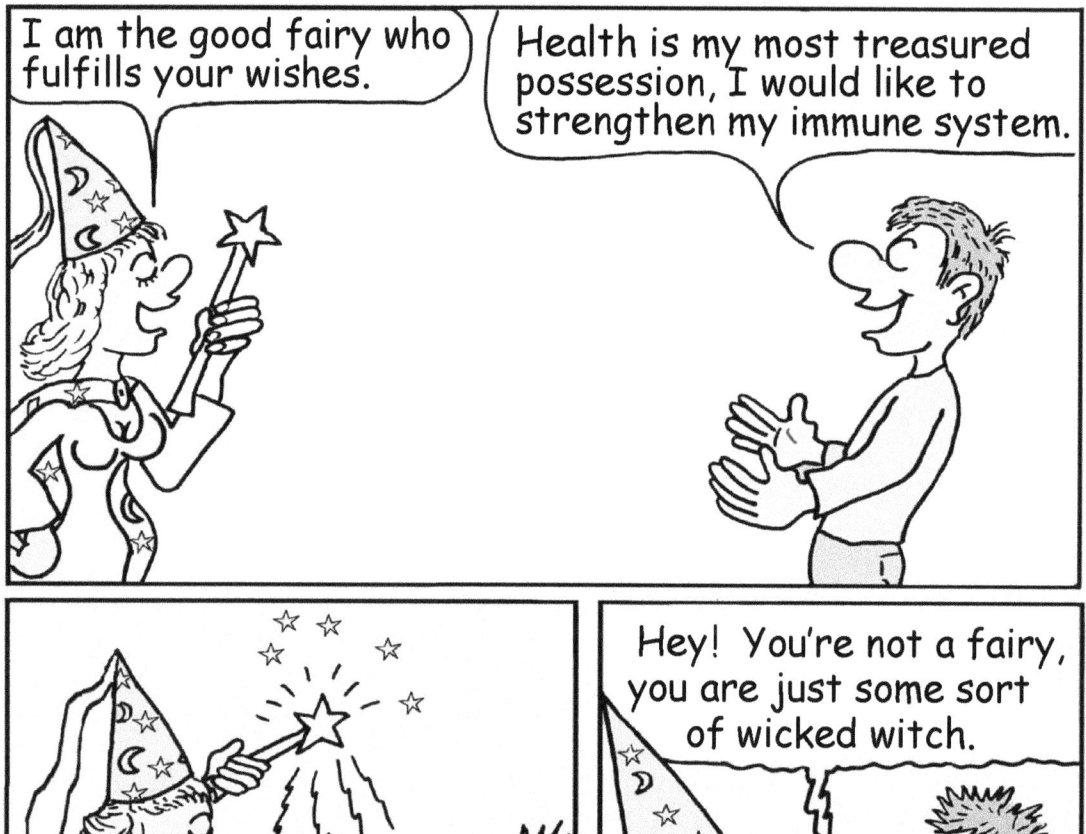

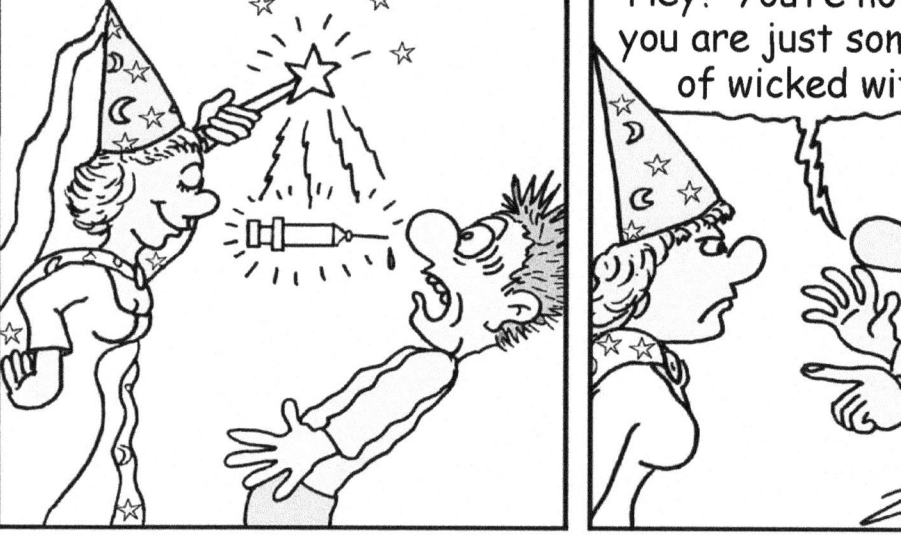

The mechanics of vaccination to build immunity, on the other hand, *is quite unnatural.* Rather than space exposure to a relatively minuscule level of micro-organisms in a gradual manner, massive quantities of antigens are introduced into the body through a series of vaccinations that are given right in a row over a short period of time.

All vaccines, with the exception of the OPV (oral polio vaccination) are injected directly into the bloodstream, by-passing the mucosal immune system known as the secretory IgA*. The secretory IgA is the first in a series of defensive levels within the immune system. It serves as a buffer, filtering microbes so that the impact of these invading organisms is greatly reduced once it reaches the bloodstream. The IgA allows the antigen to be removed in the same manner in which it arrived –through the mucosal barrier– by sneezing, coughing and sweating.

So a vaccine that has been injected "gives the body no warning, no generalised inflammatory response, no chance to recognise, duplicate or defend itself against future challenges from typical antigens.

Dr. Robert Mendelsohn
in "How to Raise a Healthy Child In Spite of Your Doctor."

Vaccines: The Great Illusion

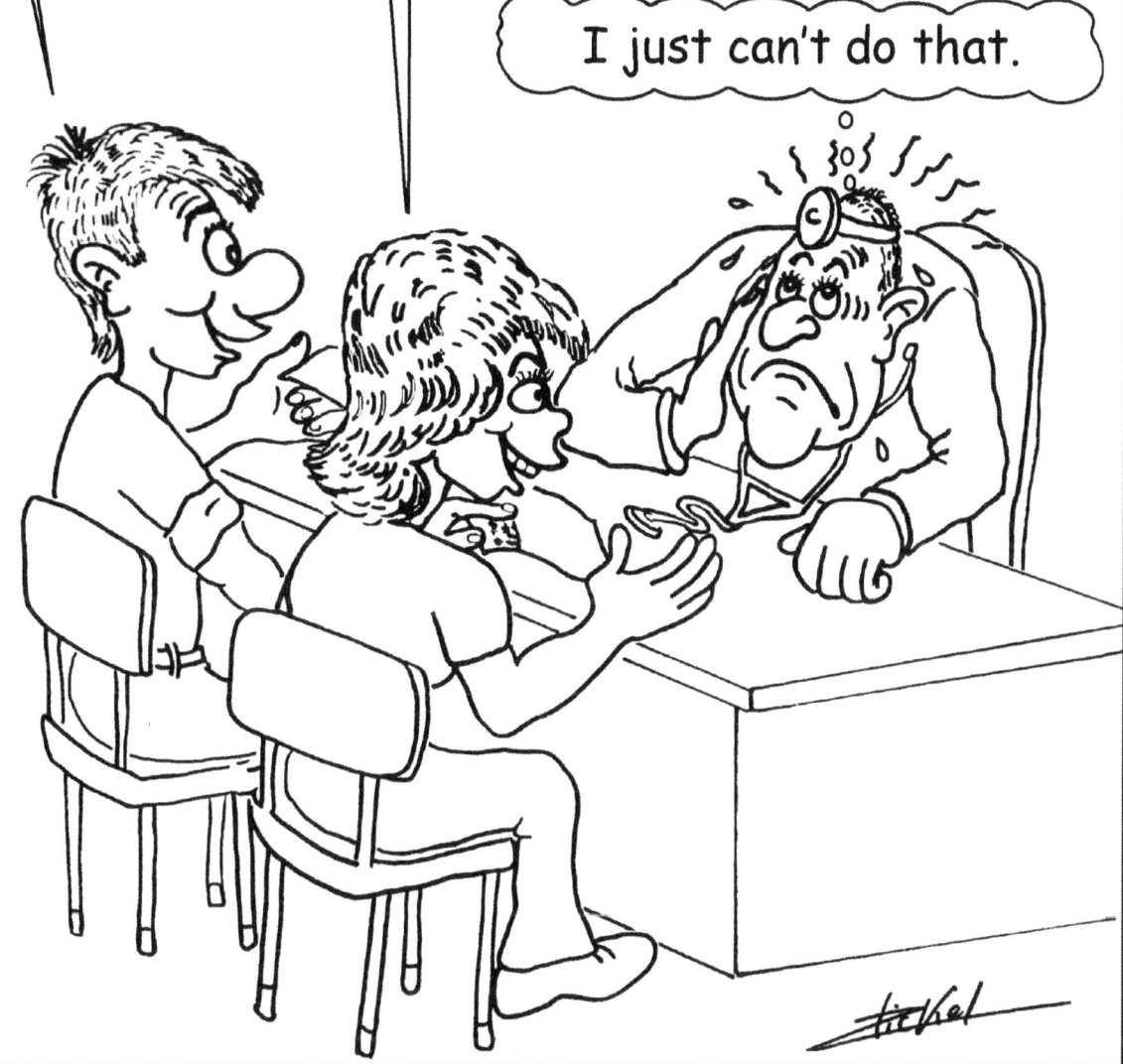

While the attitude and dictatorial claims of vaccination services are based on fanciful premises, our determination [against the vaccinal dogma] is conversely based **on current scientific knowledge.**

Dr. Jacques KALMAR

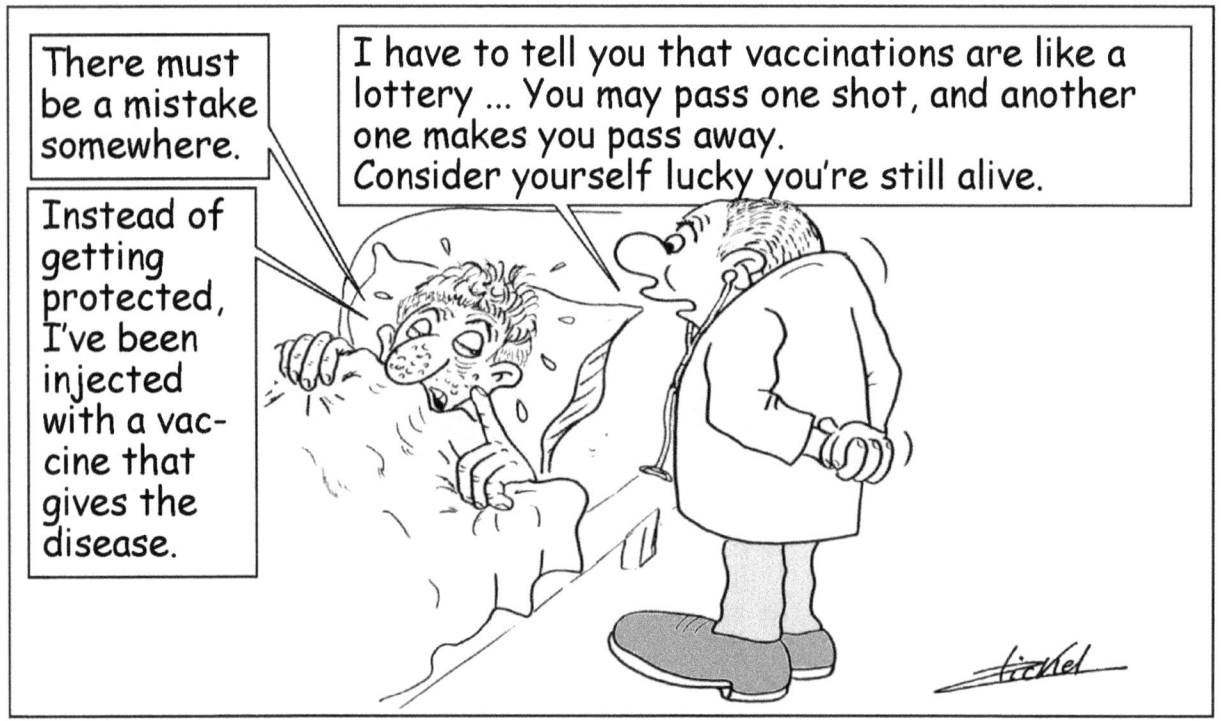

Vaccination is not a protection, but conversely a contamination.   **Dr. Jacques MICHAUD**
(For Another Medicine)

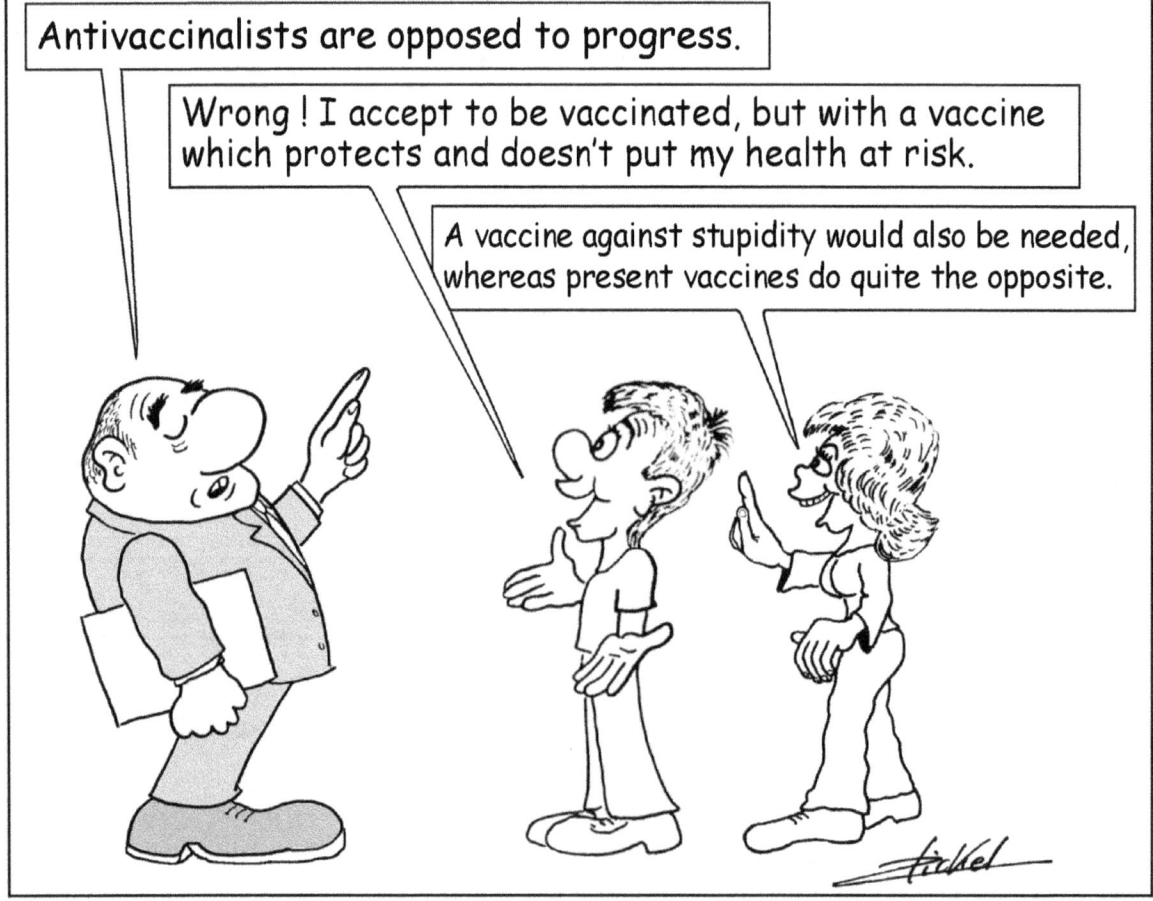

> *This is not a sensible medical practice to risk one's life by submitting to a probably ineffective intervention, in order to avoid a disease that will probably never arise.*
> Dr. Kris GAUBLOMME

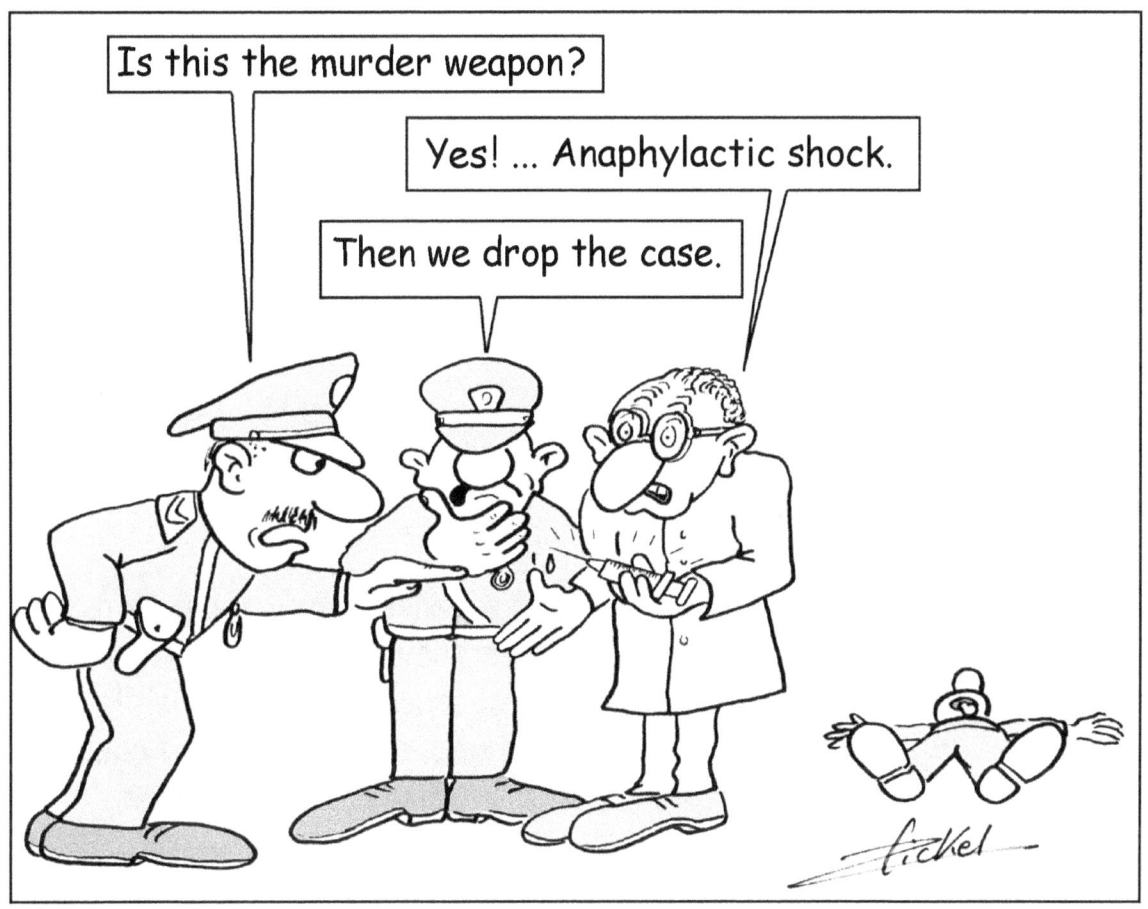

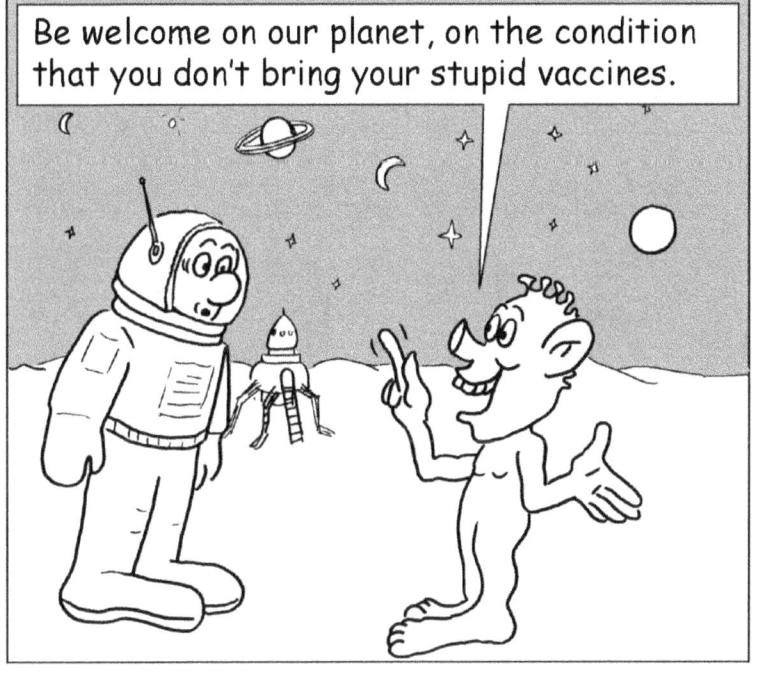

> *Human stupidity is the source of the worst disasters ...*
> Michel de Montaigne
>
> *... But also an inexhaustible gold mine for those who know how to exploit it.*
> Dr. Toulet

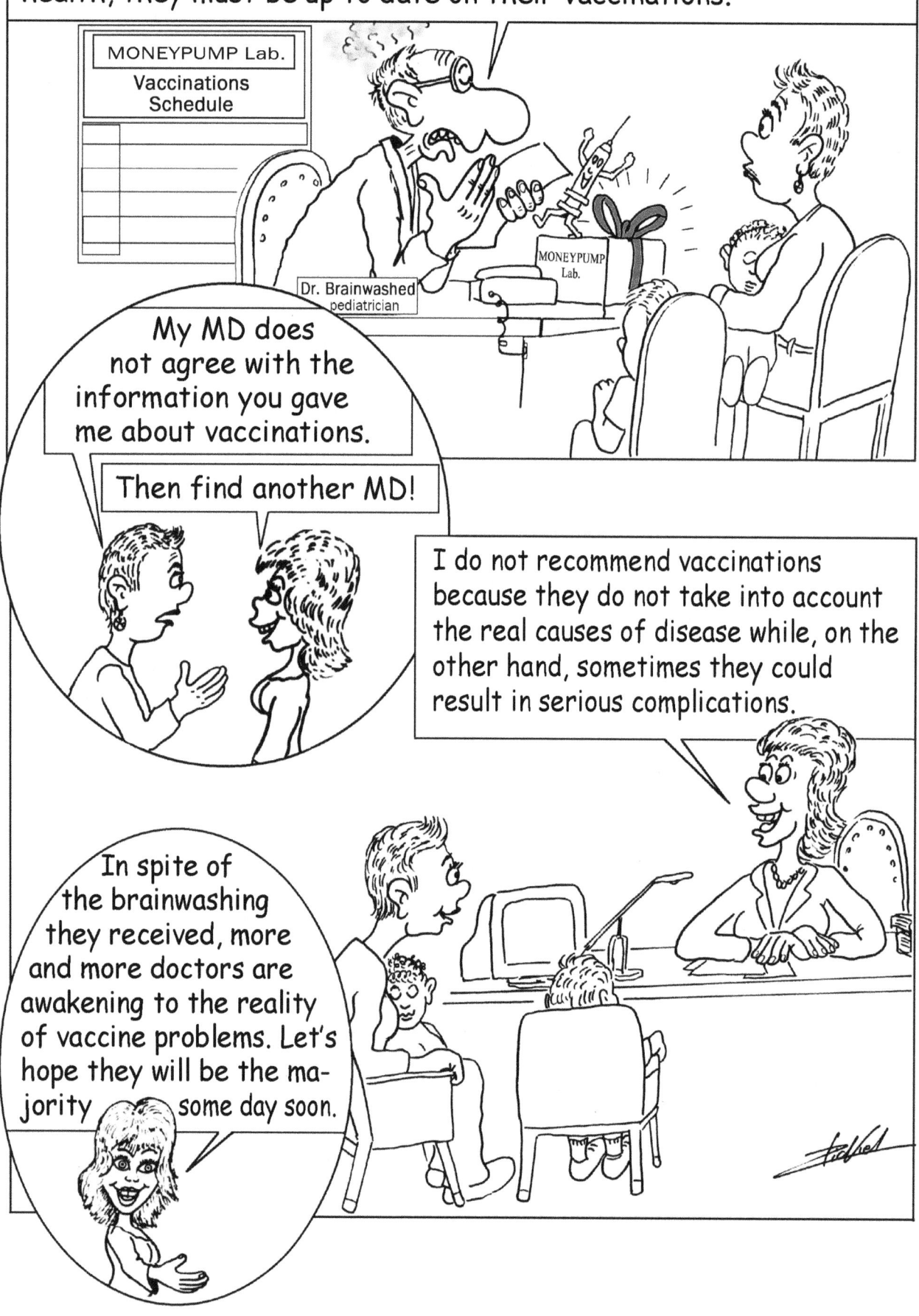

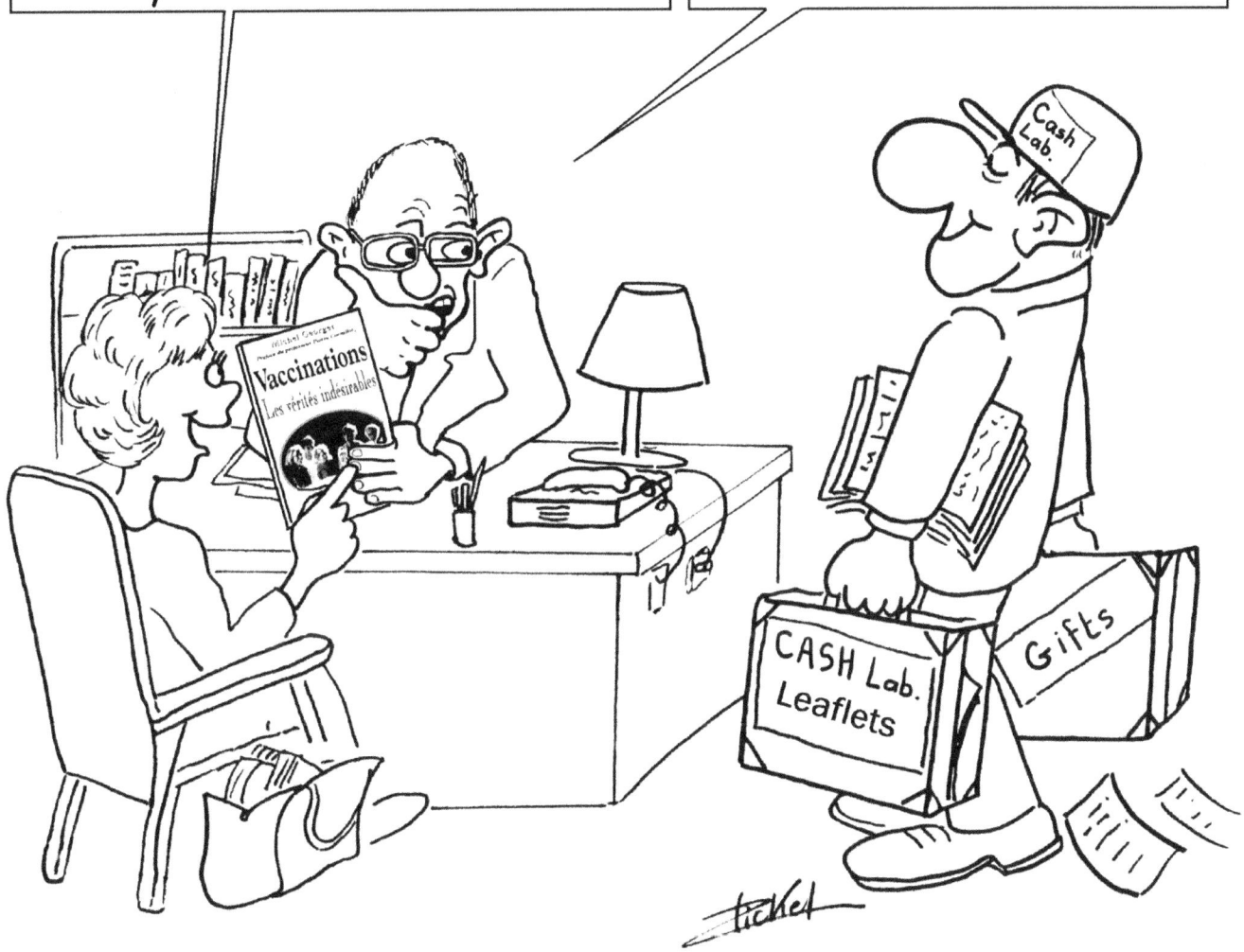

It is not indifferent either, as Jules ROMAINS pointed out in a famous play, that the reading of the pharmaceutical advertising is, in fact, the most usual mode of post-graduate education of the medical doctor.

Professor Henri PEQUIGNOT

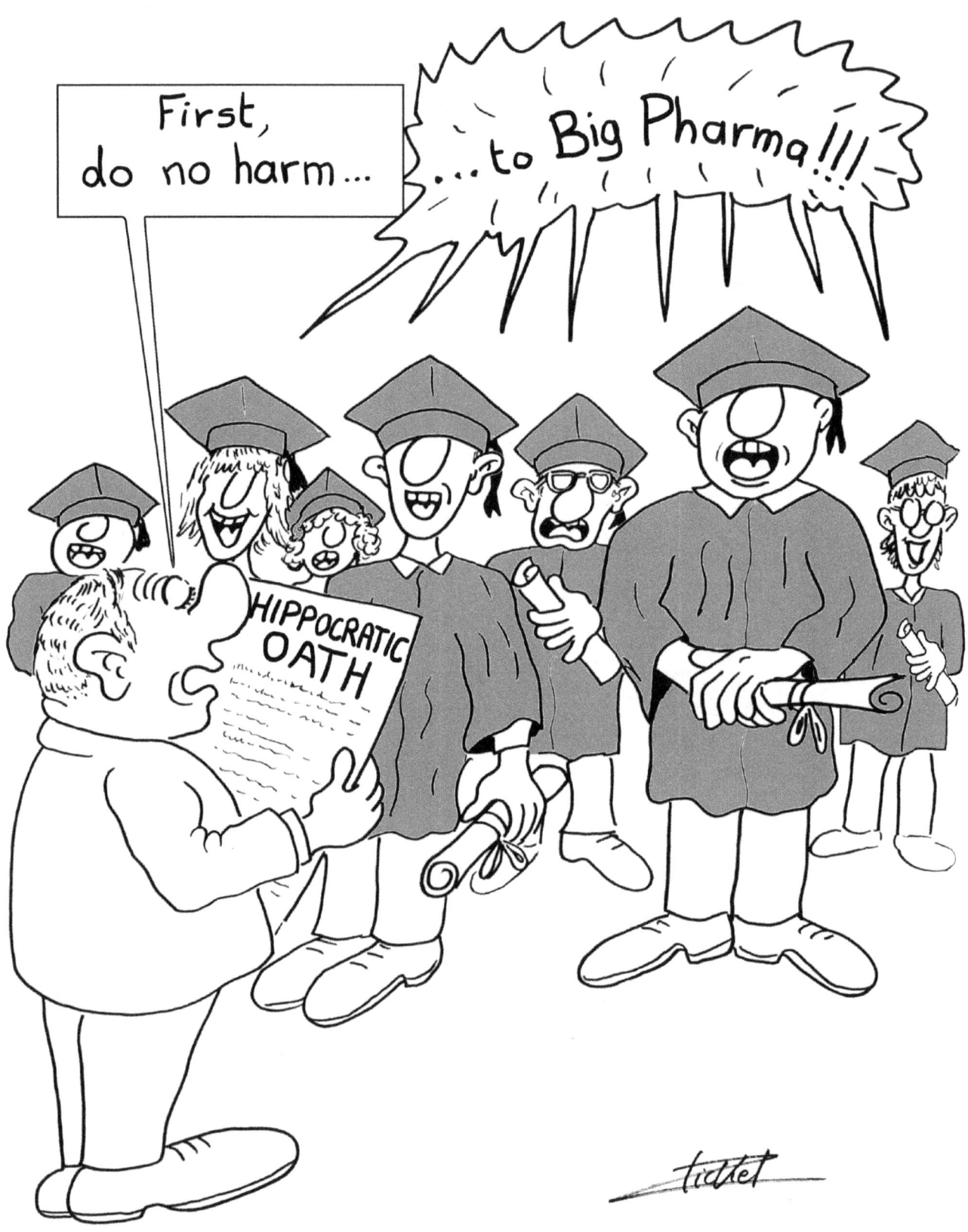

The industry of laboratories has become, by its excesses, a scourge for public health.

Dr. Paul CARTON

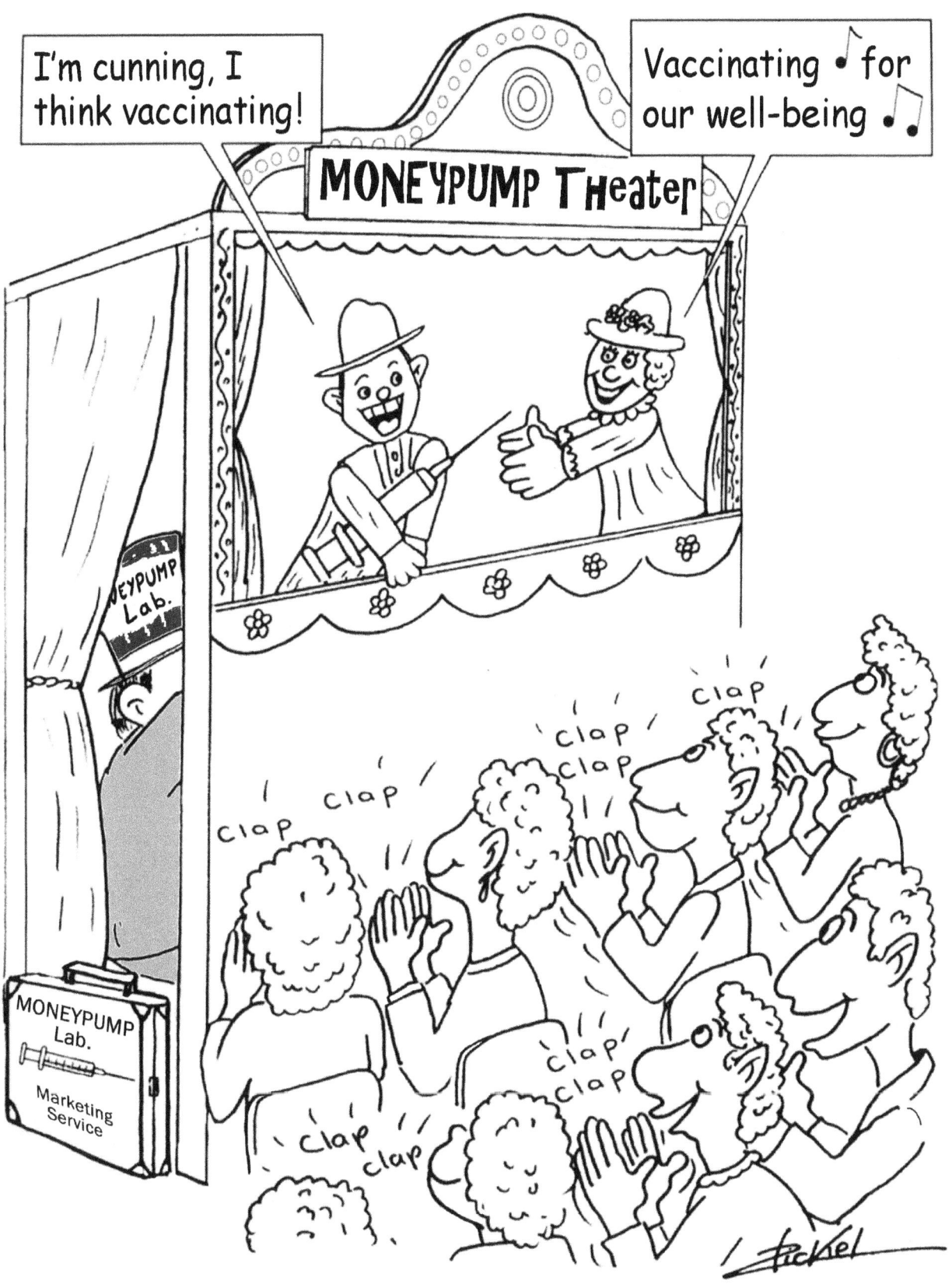

Supported by numerous advertising campaigns, the vaccine system has imposed its non-negotiable commandments.

Dr. Jacques KALMAR

Vaccines: The Great Illusion

> *Panic has the huge advantage to turn a compulsory coerced act into a medical act spontaneously claimed by the patient who, under the influence of an ageless fear, understood quite suddenly its value and interest. In order to "launch" this or that vaccine every now and then, the ministry of health would cunningly create a consensus of opinion, with the unconscious help of the popular press.*
>
> Concours Médical, 1955 (about the epidemic in Vannes - France)

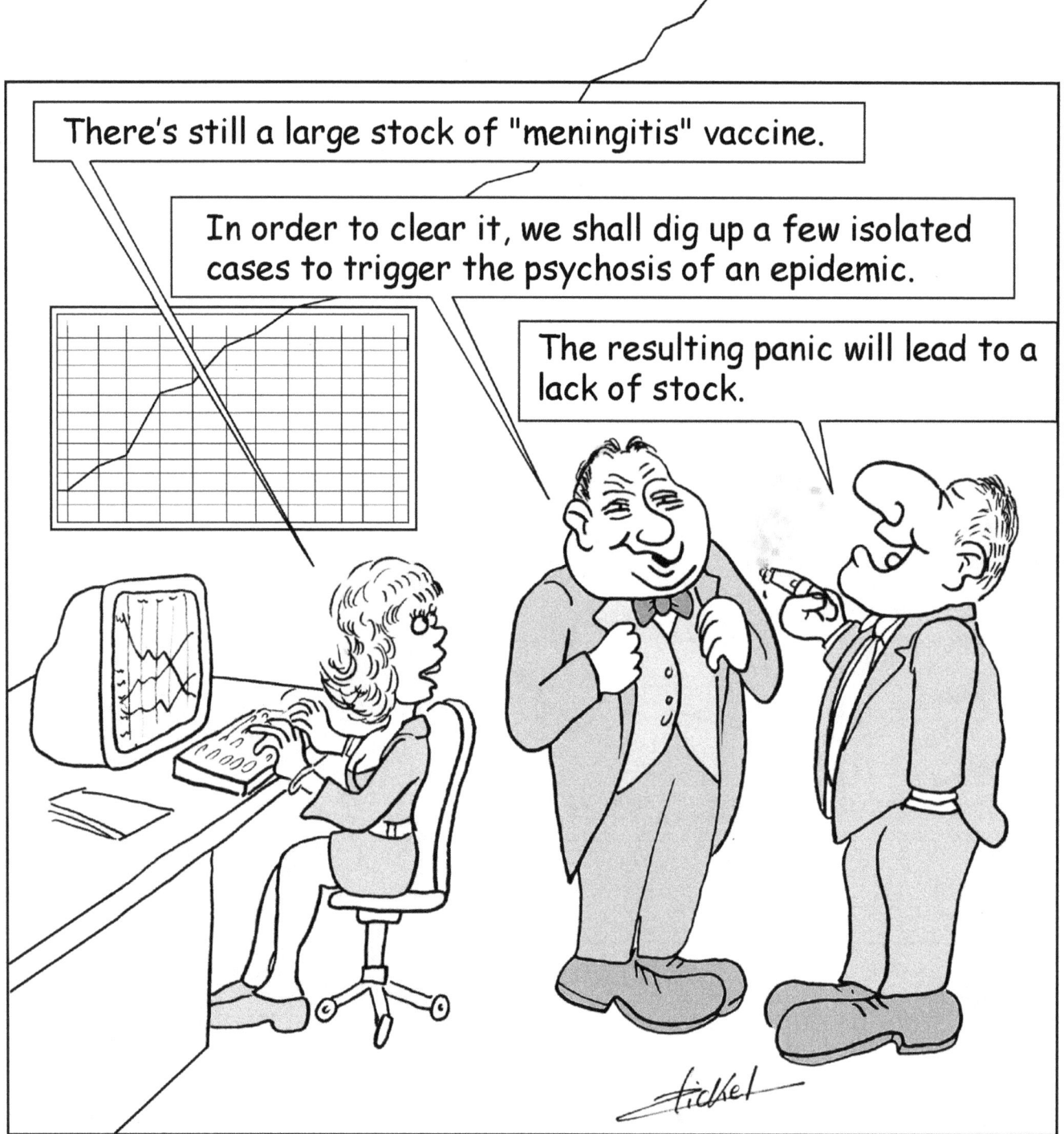

> The tragedy is that human beings are blind to the point of being receptive to error only. And hospitals, cemeteries are full of people who accepted, with satisfaction, to let themselves be stupidly assassinated, by the evil of the only force that they have cultivated with care: the strength of their IGNORANCE.
>
> Dr. Jacques KALMAR

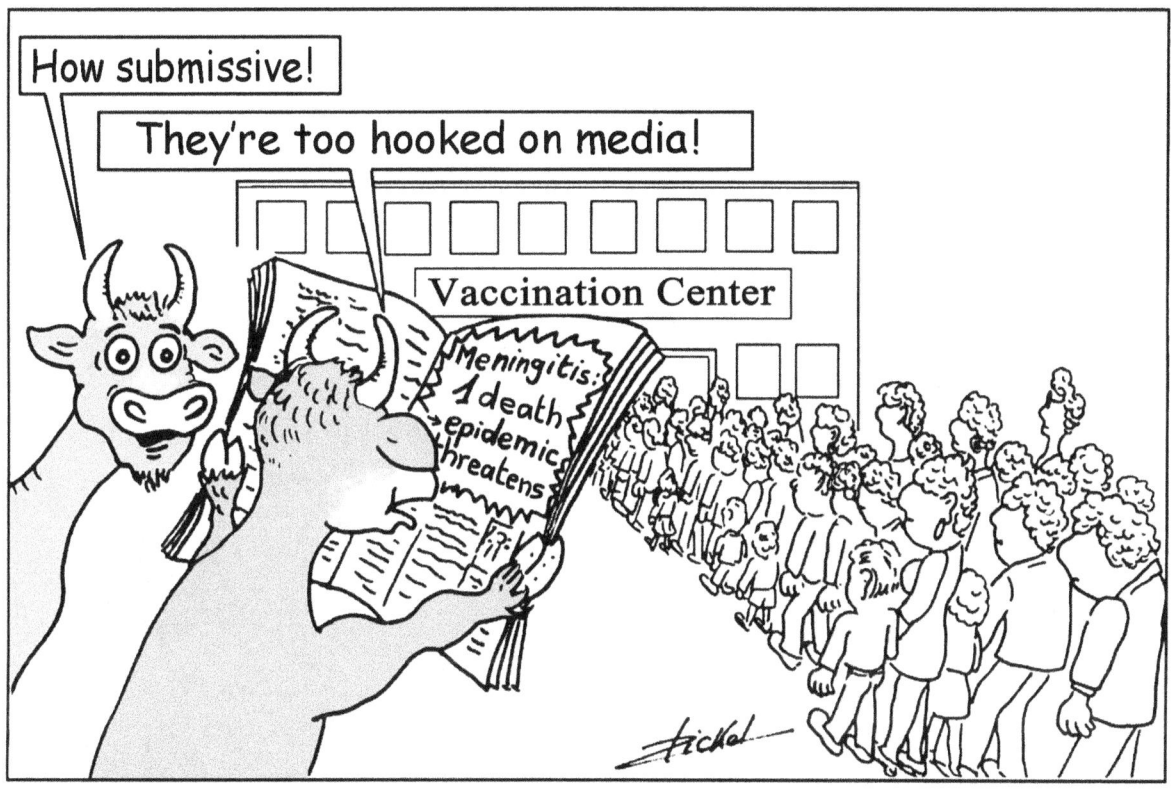

> It is awful to see how many huge portions of the human ocean have been programmed by invisible broadcast stations on a mental frequency which reduces human beings to the status of a parrot.
>
> Andrew THOMAS
> (On the shore of infinite worlds)

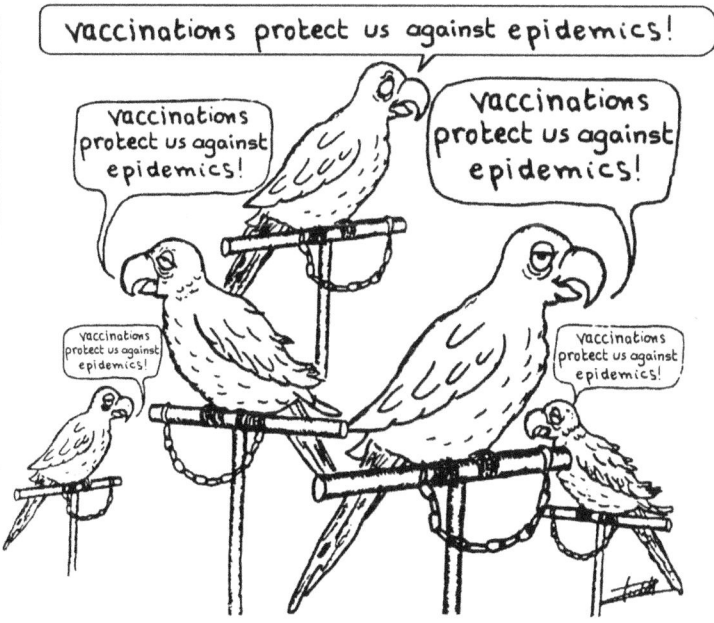

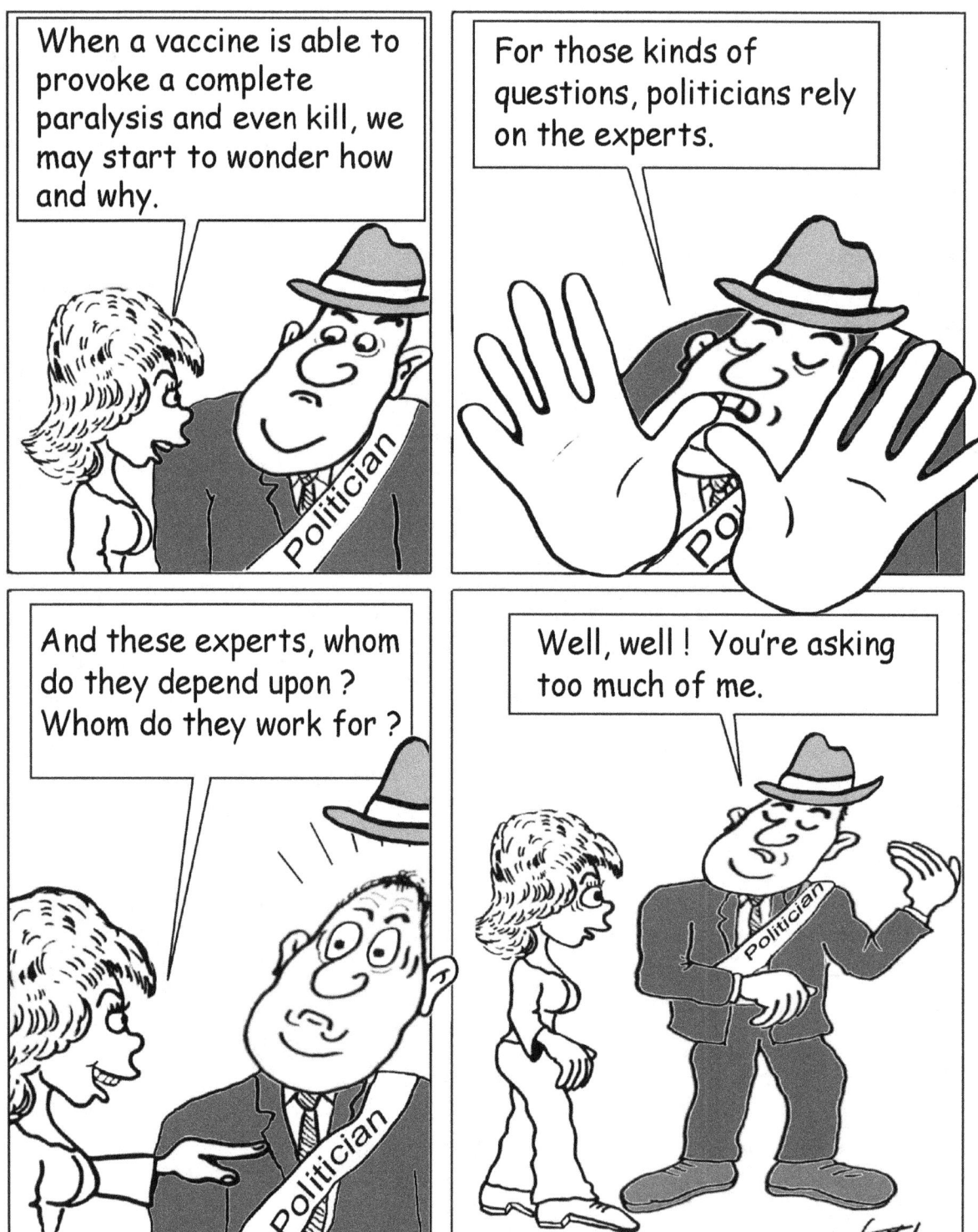

Politicians are therefore responsible and guilty now.
Their guilt is based upon the fact that they have in hand all information on the current system. They know perfectly well expertise works on a one-way basis. They know about the collusion between experts and sellers. They accept this state of affairs. Political leaders are accountable.

Dr. Jacques LACAZE

Vaccines: The Great Illusion

> « ... The launch of the BCG vaccine is a model of economic gangsterism, a gigantic and corrupt commercial operation. Nothing is missing in the scenario : a silly inventor, rigged lab experiments, a pseudo-scientific make-up, truncated statistics, a shameless advertising campaign, the remunerated support of the mandarins, and as a supreme trick, free access to the product... financed by the taxpayers !
> All this appears quite usuall. French public is accustomed to scandals. But what is new with the BCG, and reaches heights of smartness, is the ultimate and successful maneuver of devilish coercion imagined by its promoters, the Council of the Republic :
> BCG vaccination was made compulsory. »
>
> Dr. Jean ELMIGER (the Recovered Medicine)

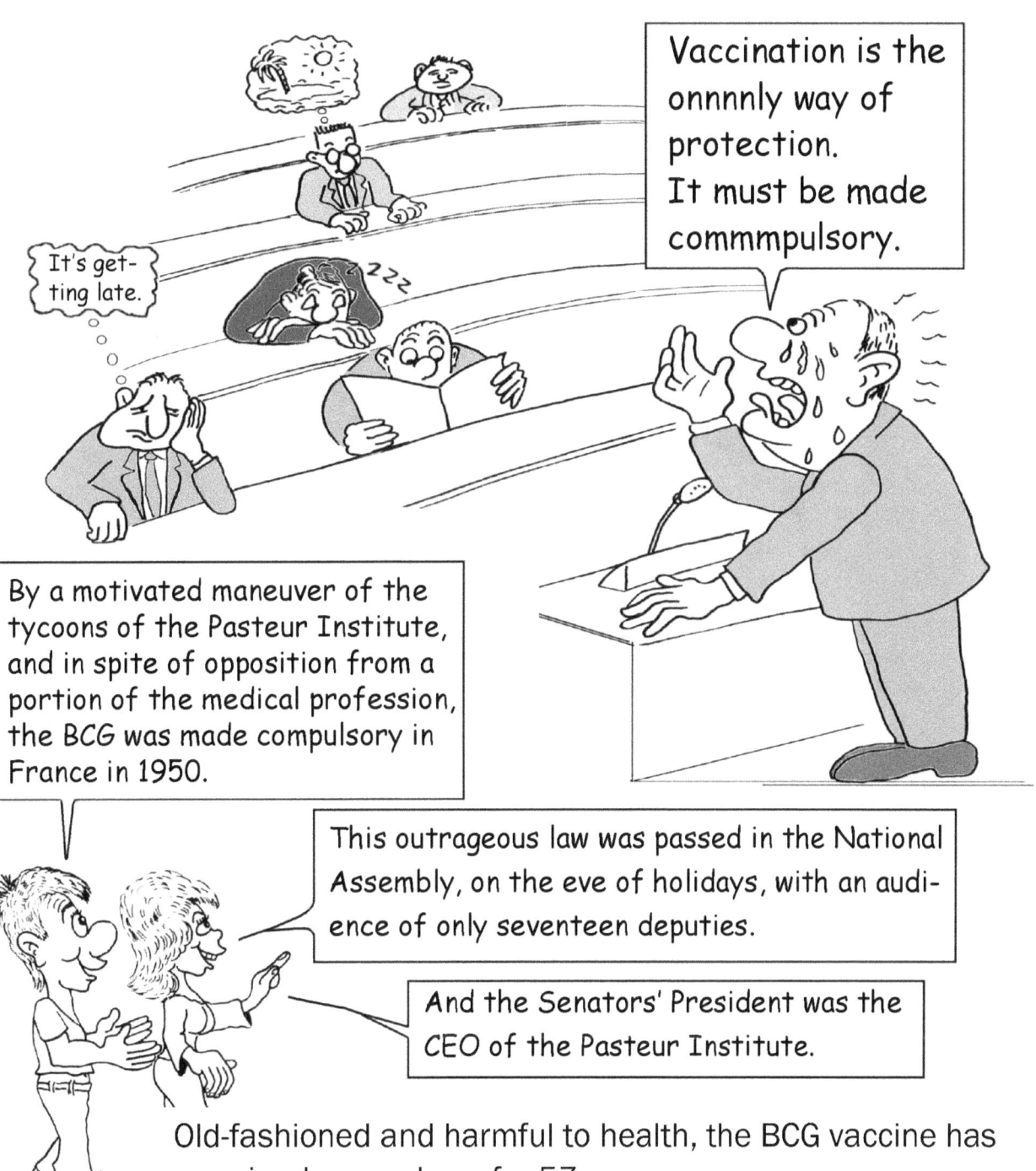

Old-fashioned and harmful to health, the BCG vaccine has remained compulsory for 57 years.

From mental rape to physical rape

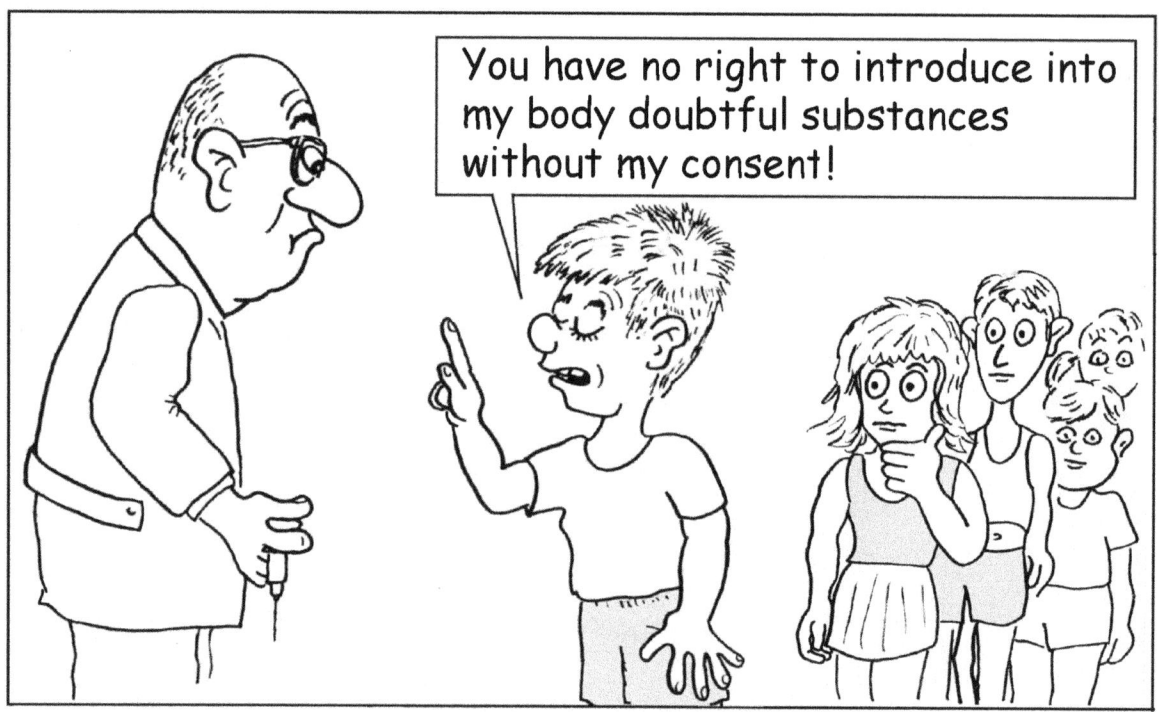

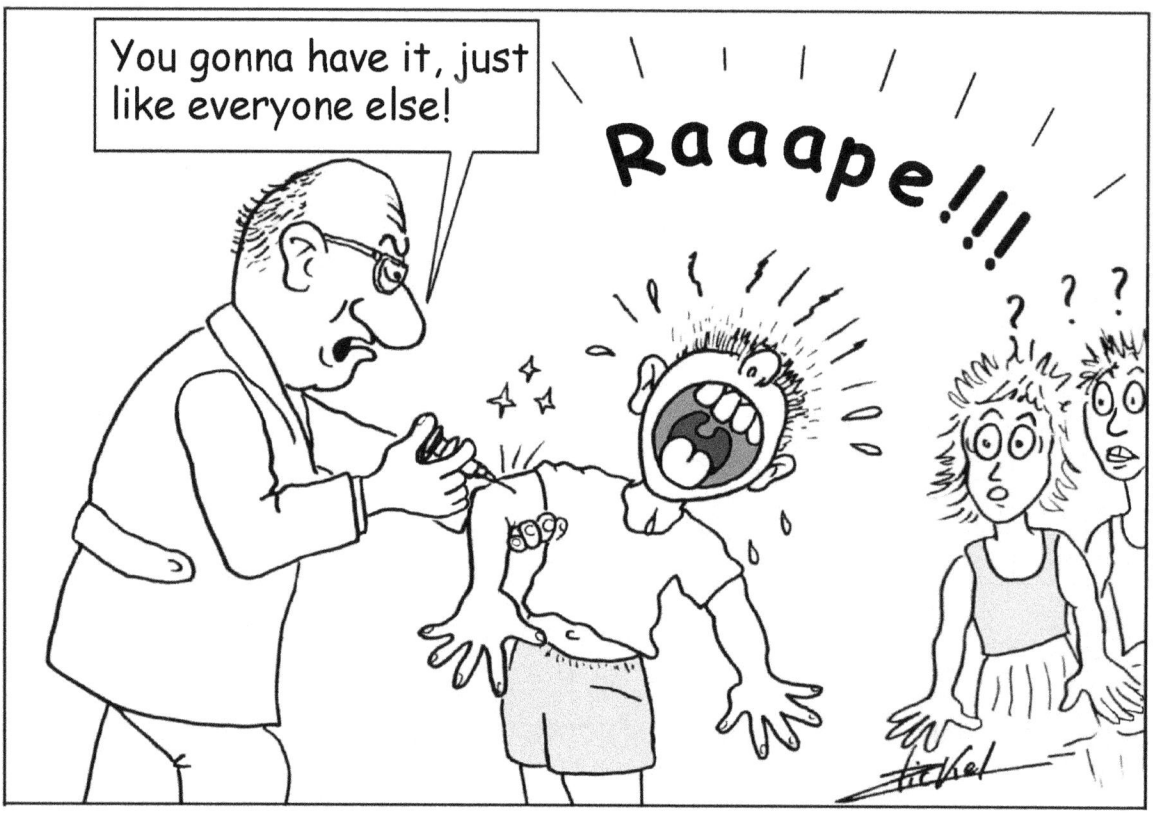

Whether the vaccination be mandatory or not mandatory, forced vaccination is a rape, and to cooperate with that is murderous.

Dr. Guylaine LANCTÔT (The Medical Mafia)

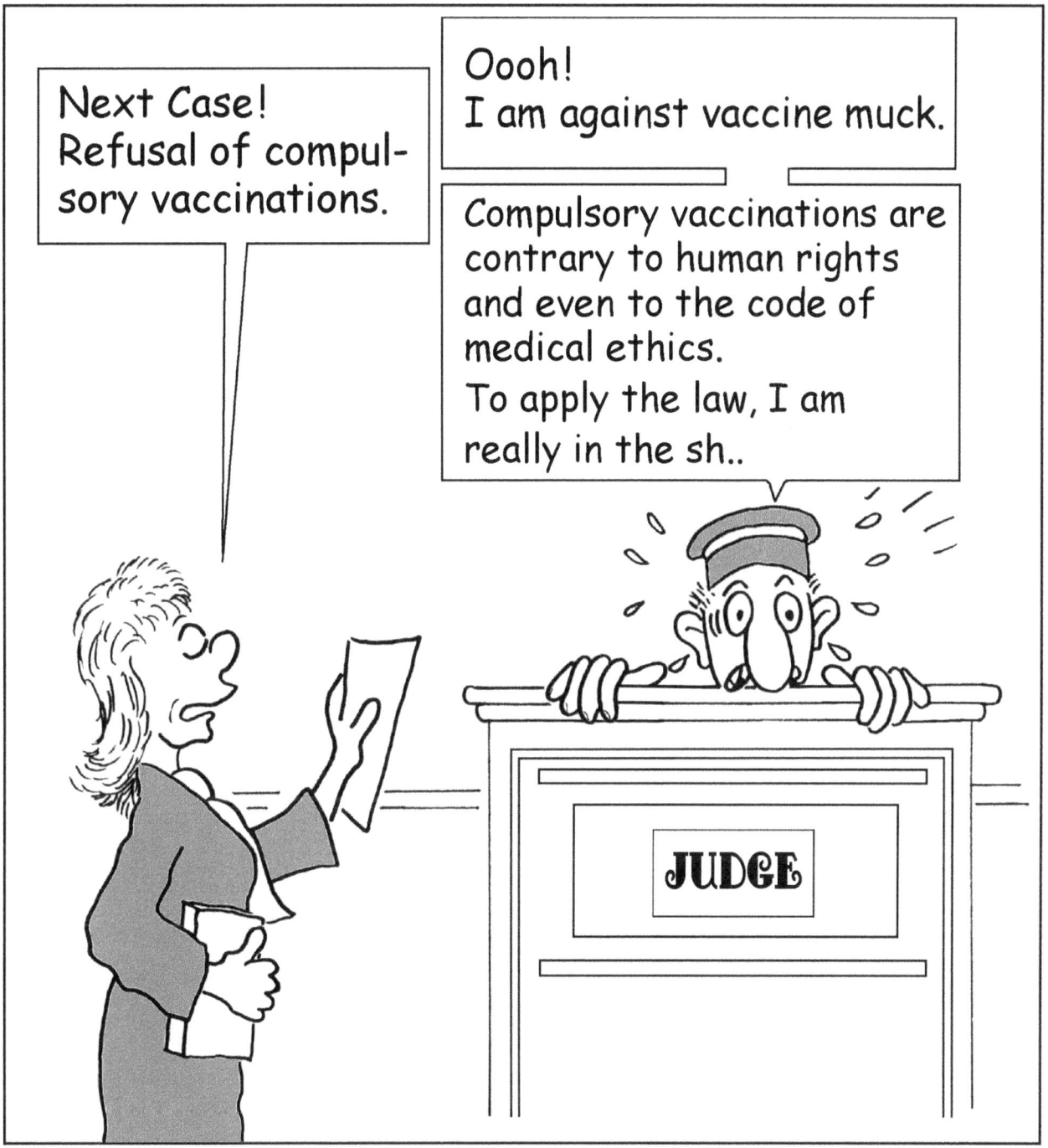

It is only by a constant struggle and by developing our solidarity that we may regain a freedom that has been confiscated from us with impunity, thanks to ignorance of the public, by a medical dictatorship that has no match elsewhere in the world.

Frederic HOFFET *(lawyer at the Bar of Strasbourg)*

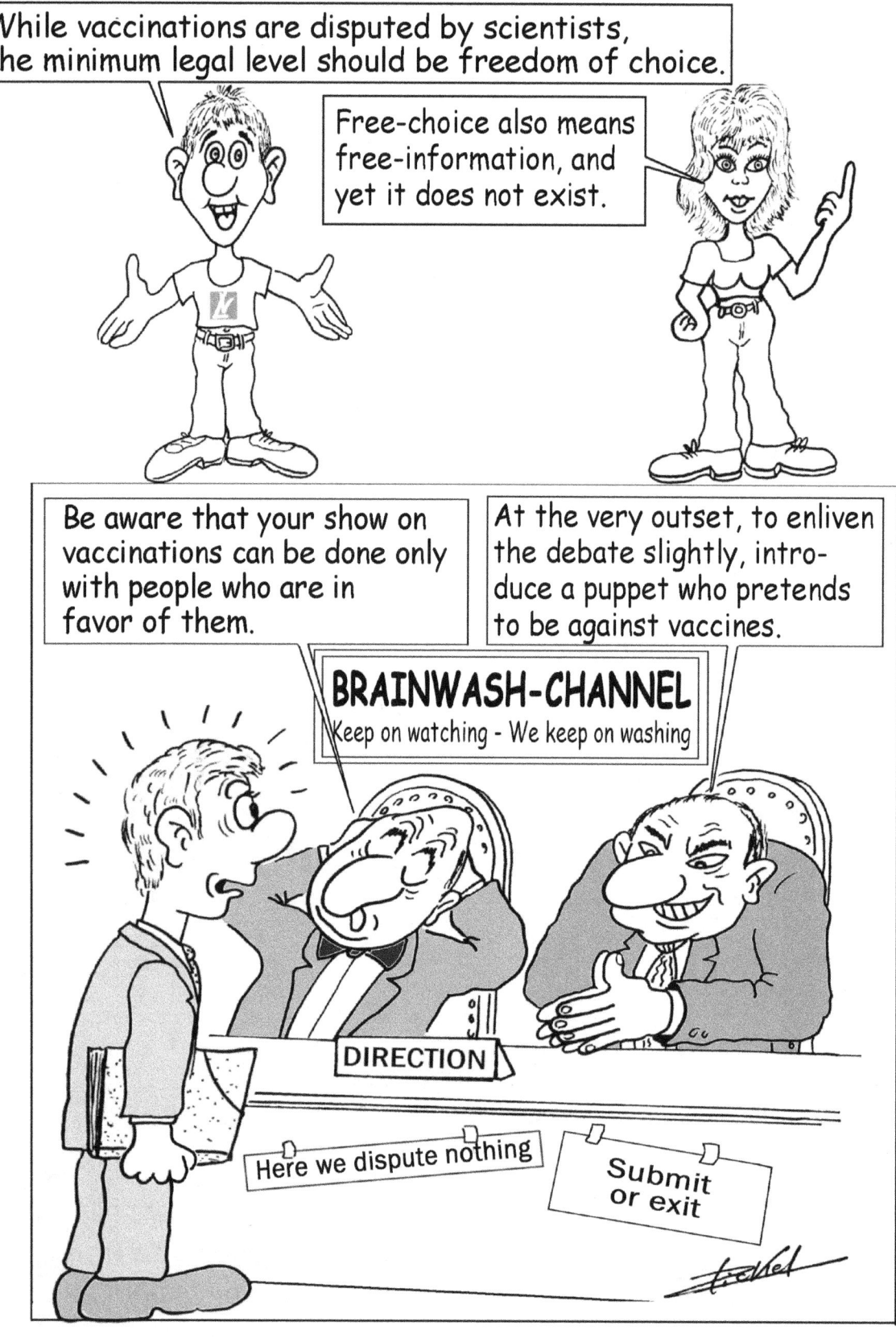

Vaccines: The Great Illusion

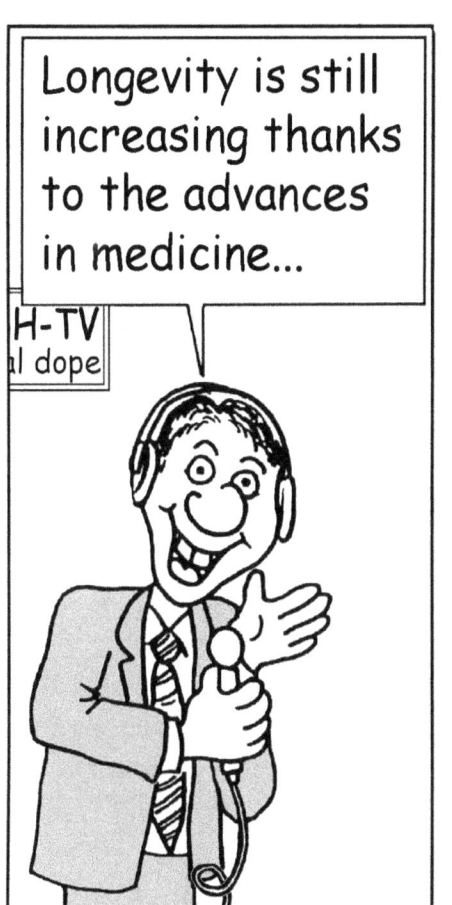
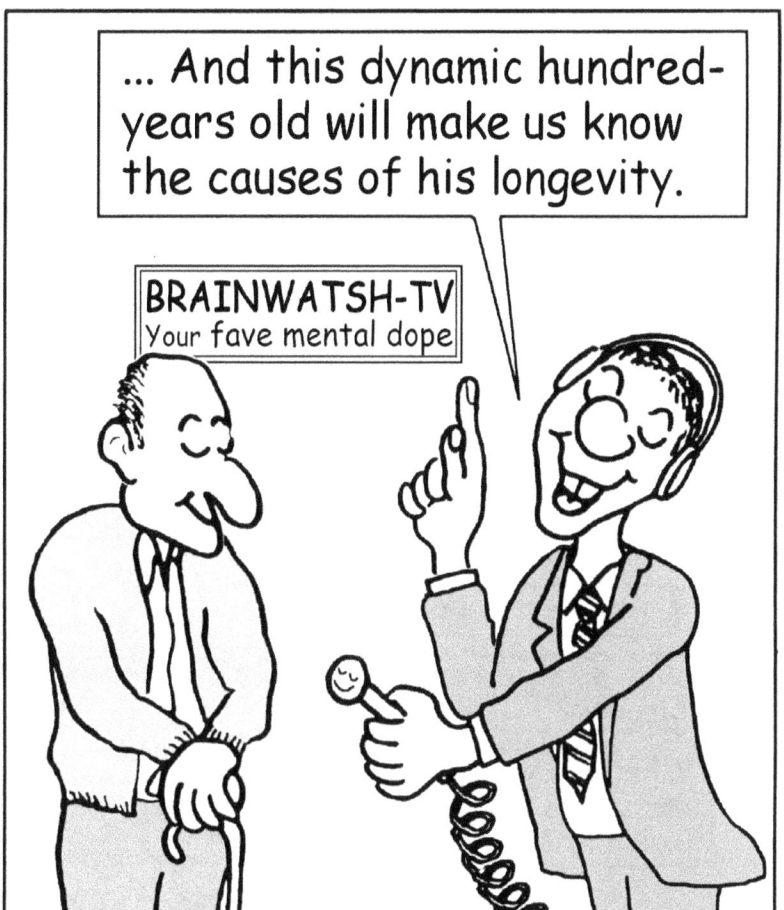
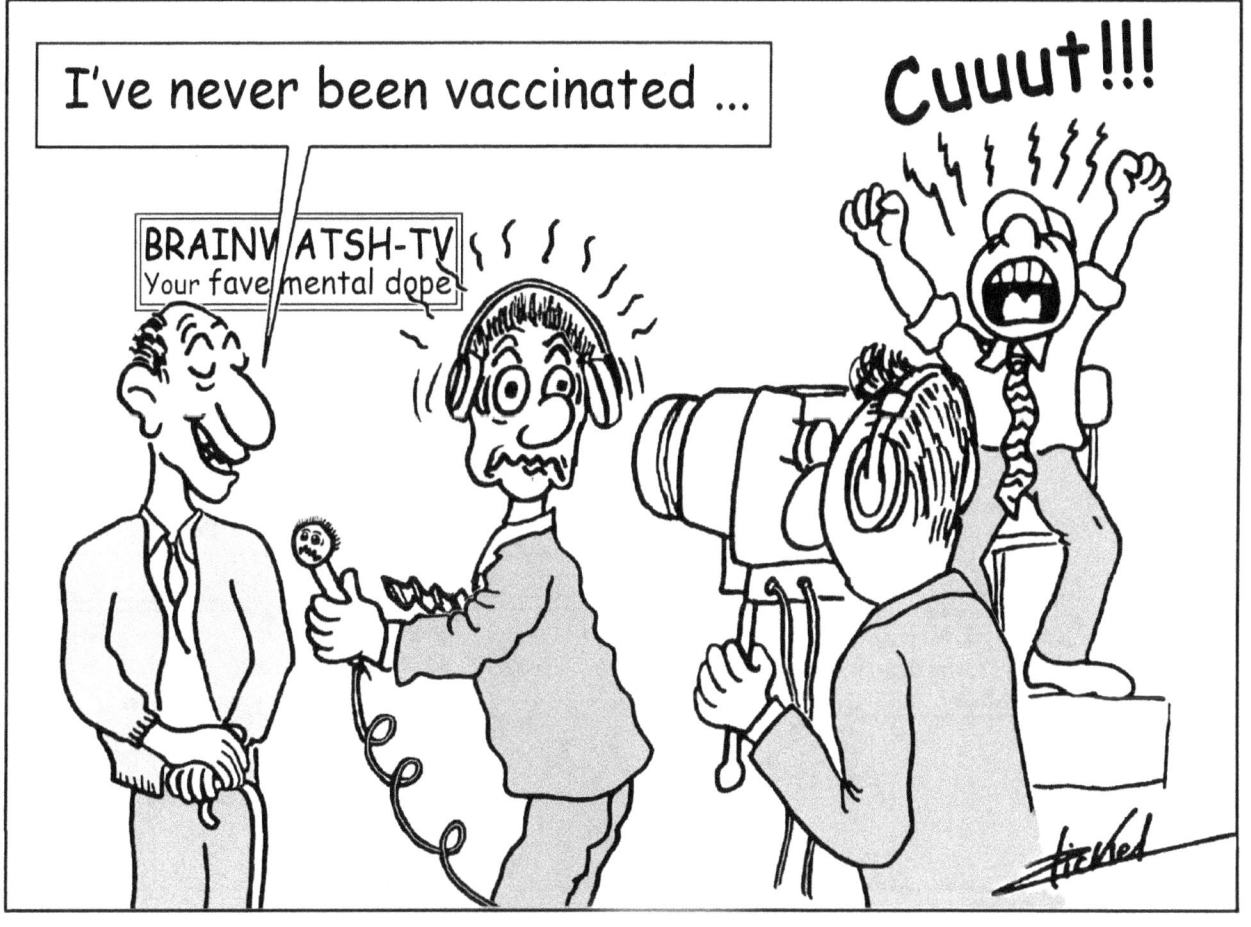

Vaccines: The Great Illusion

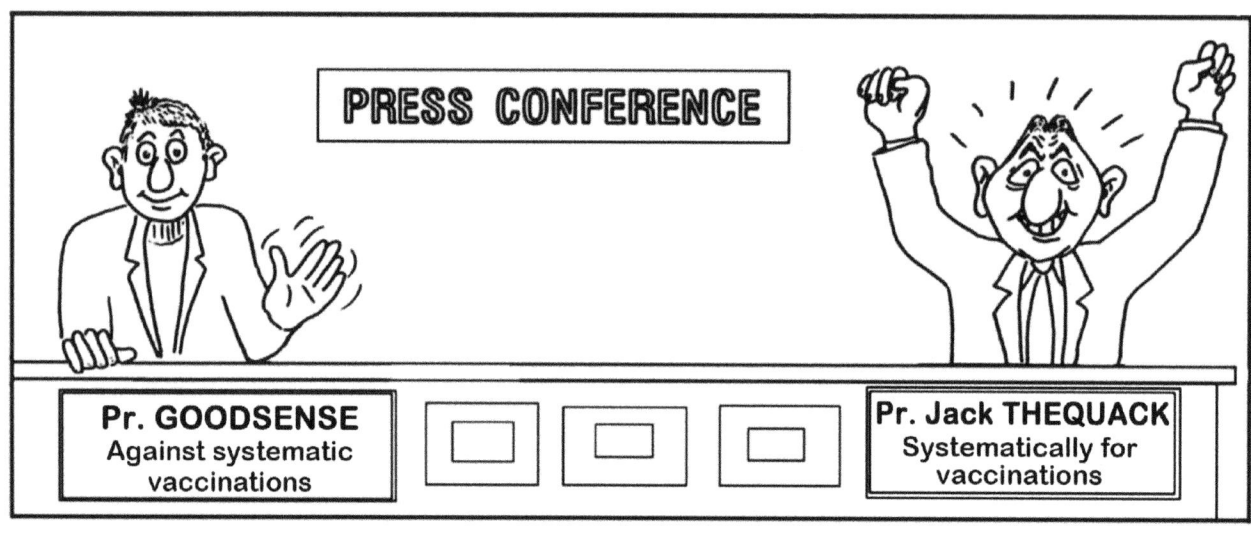
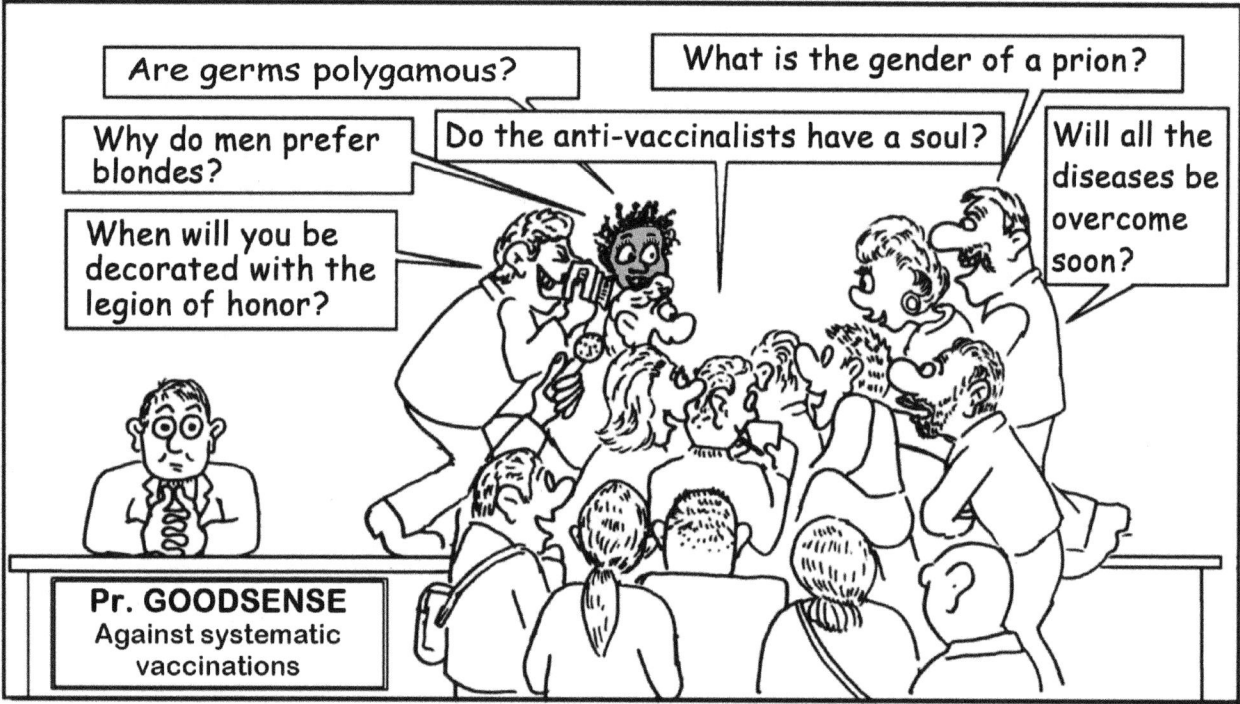
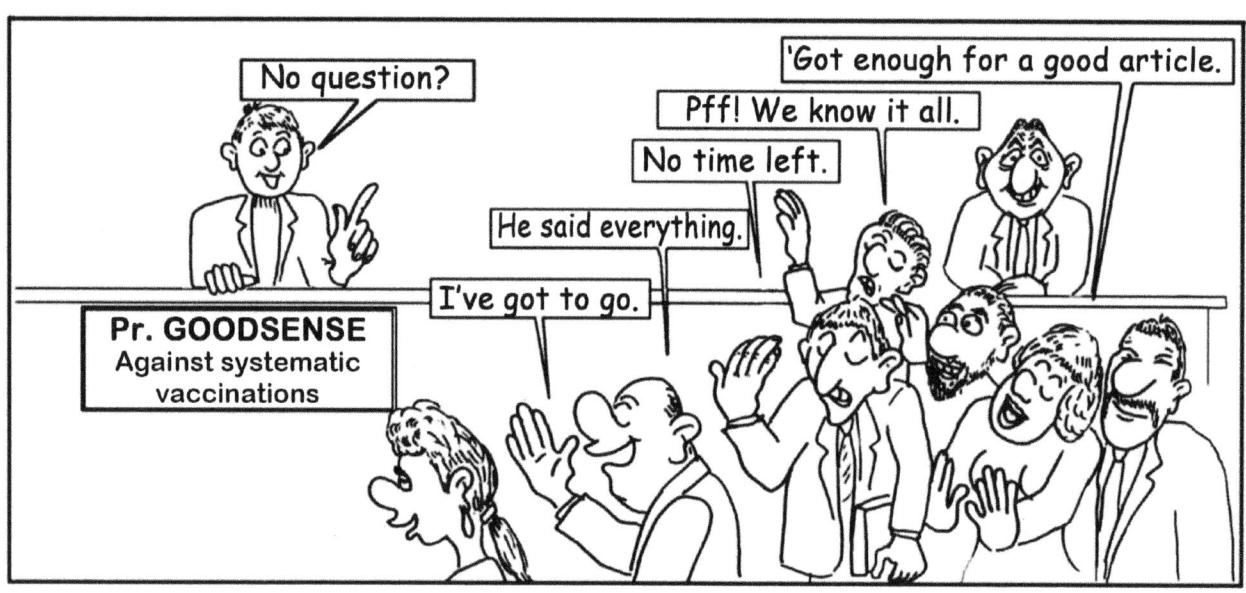

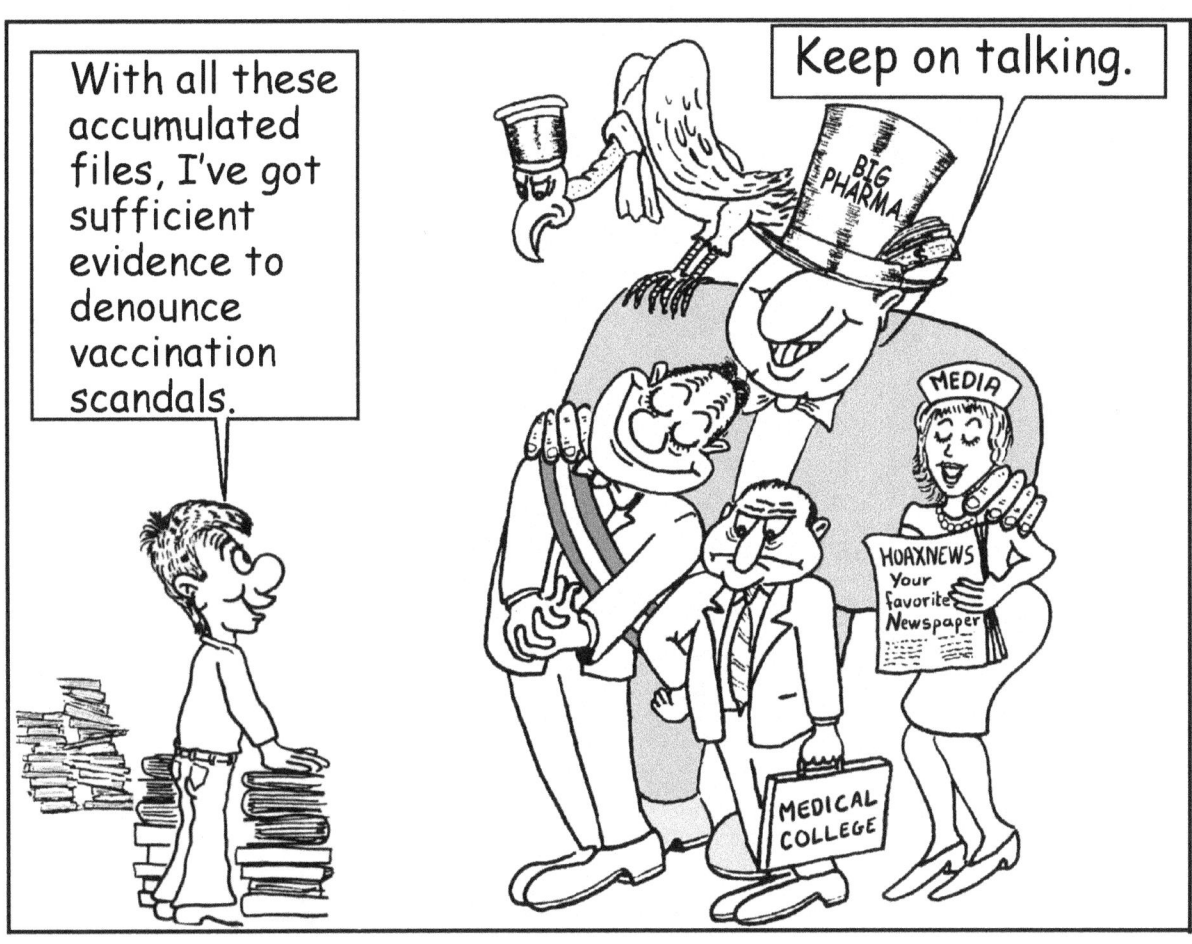
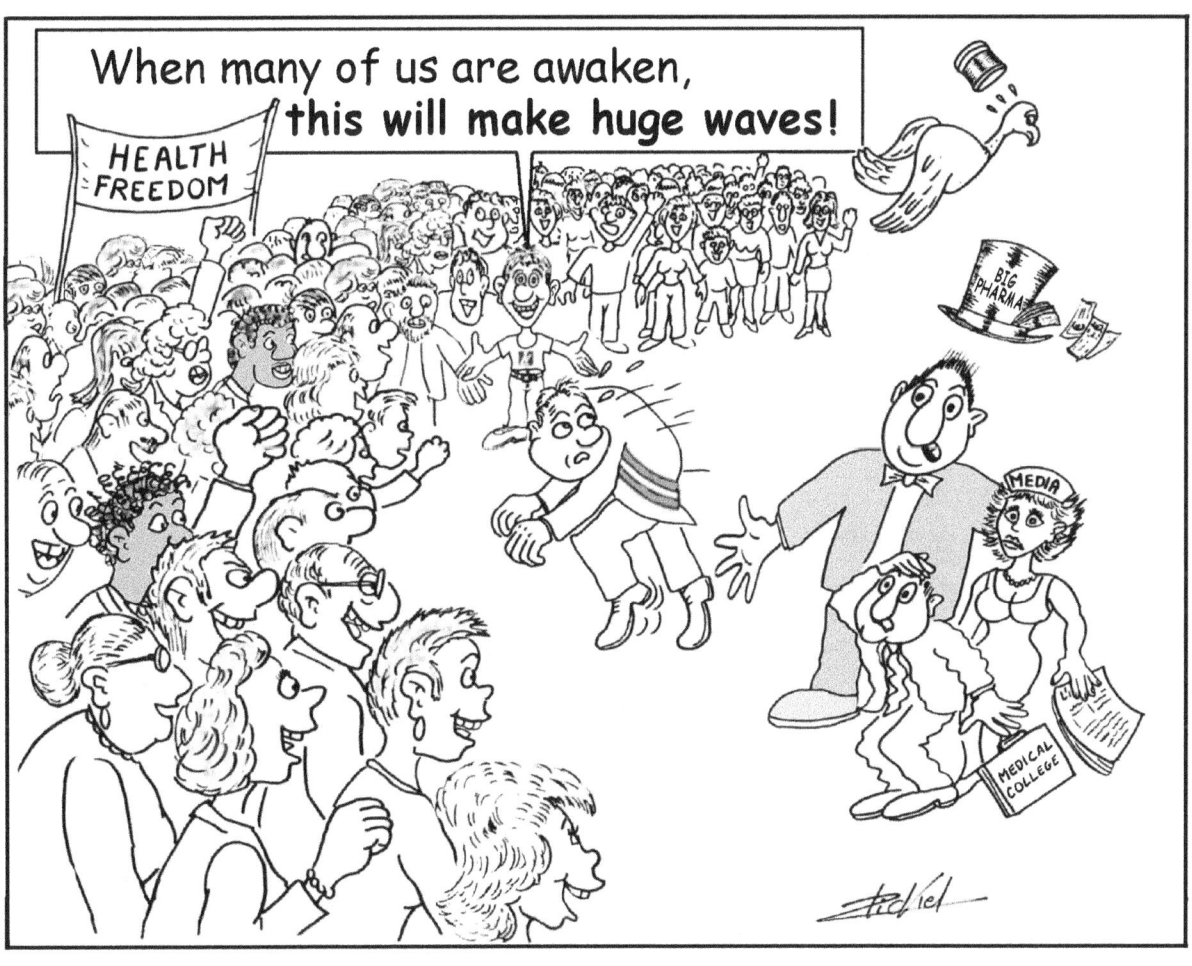

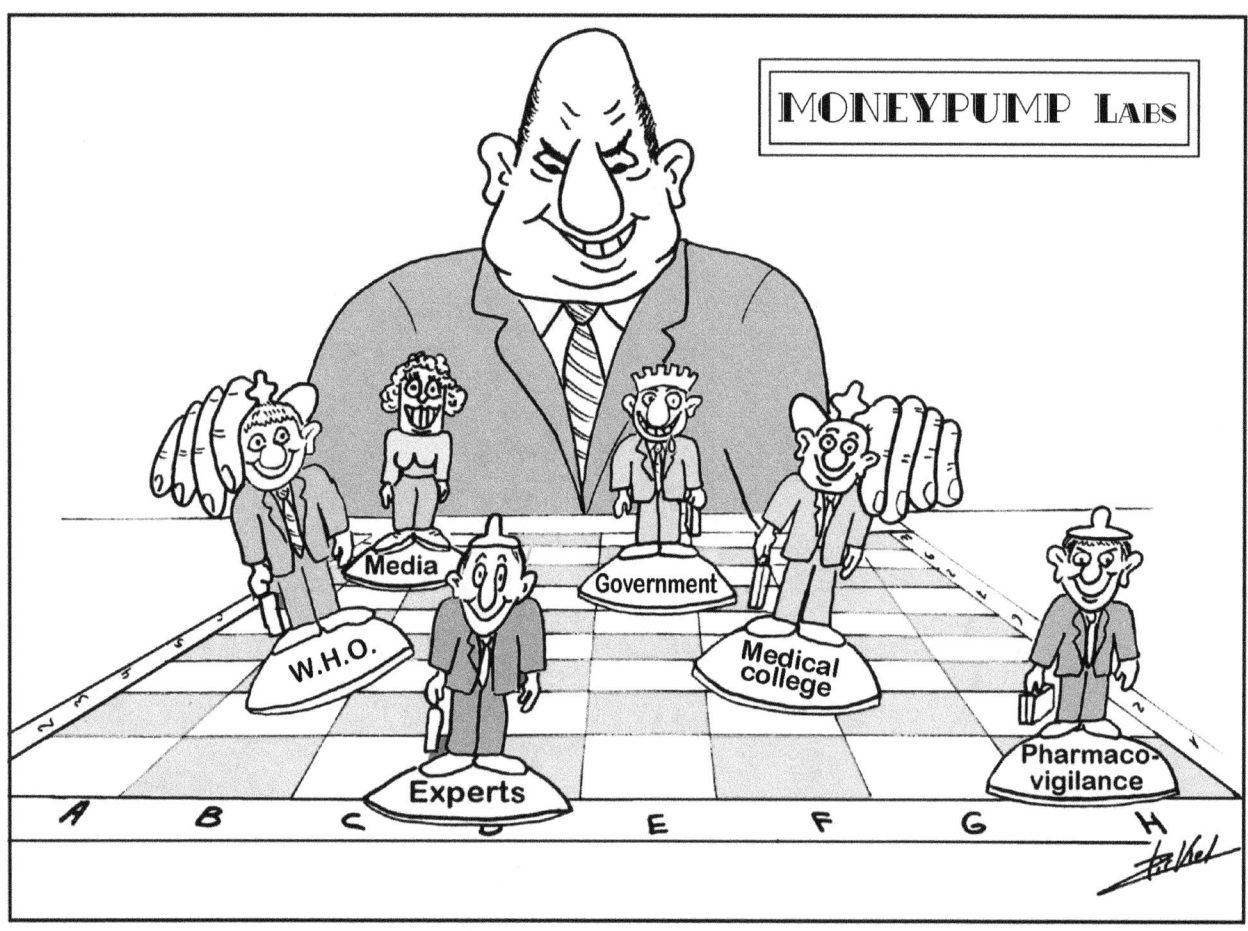

The experiment that humanity is undergoing nowadays is a "game" leading towards decay and death.

Consciences are awakening today, information flows on the fringes of the media. Those who pull the strings to make us dance in this macabre ballroom are powerful in appearance only.
Our life choices and the public pressure will make some of their puppets give in, and the rest will collapse like a house of cards.

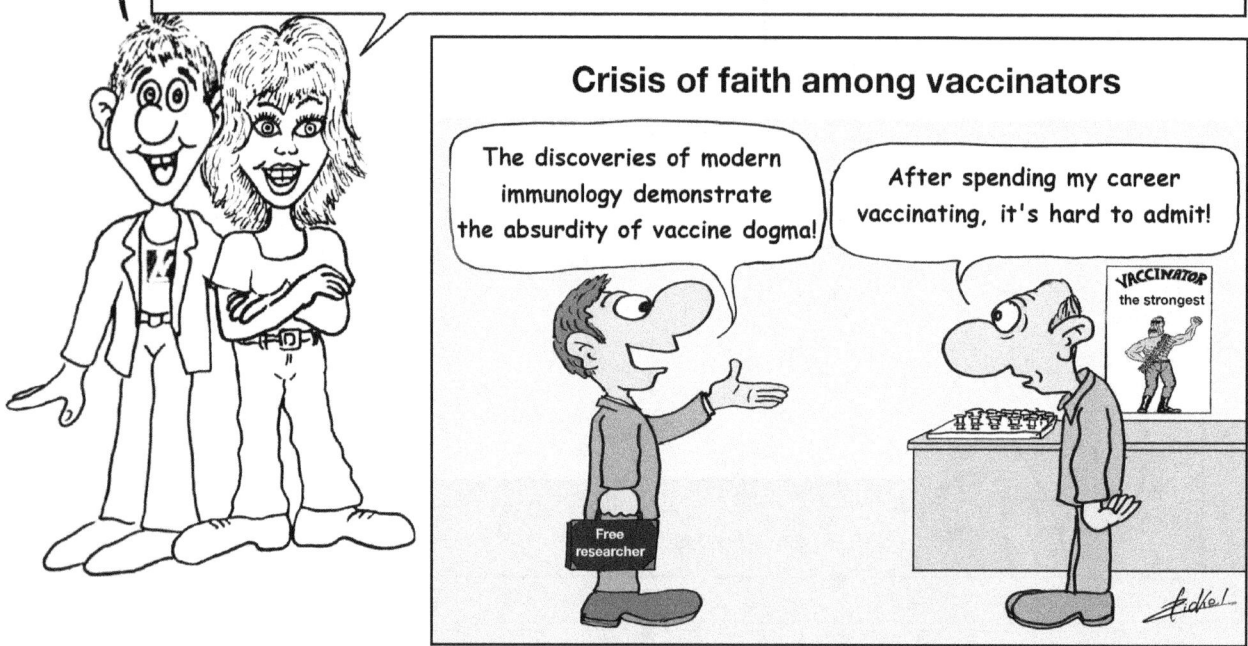

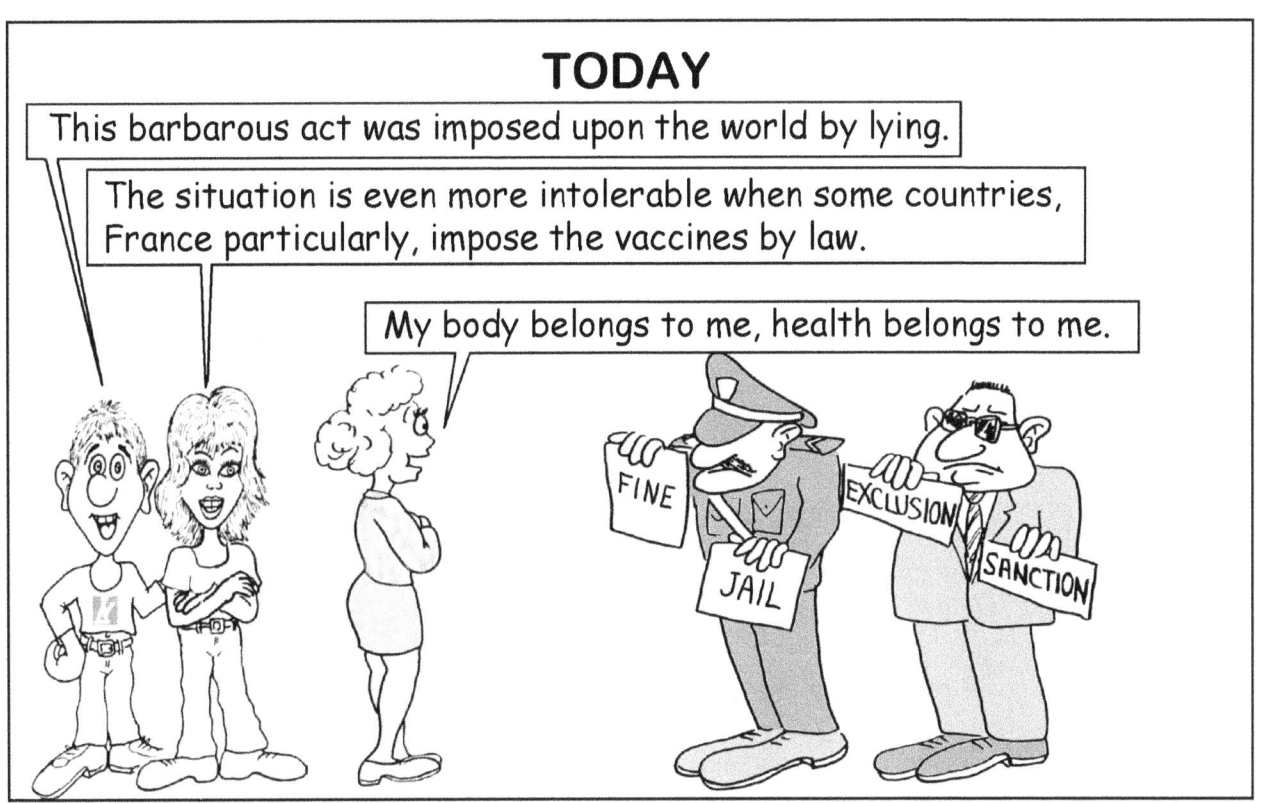

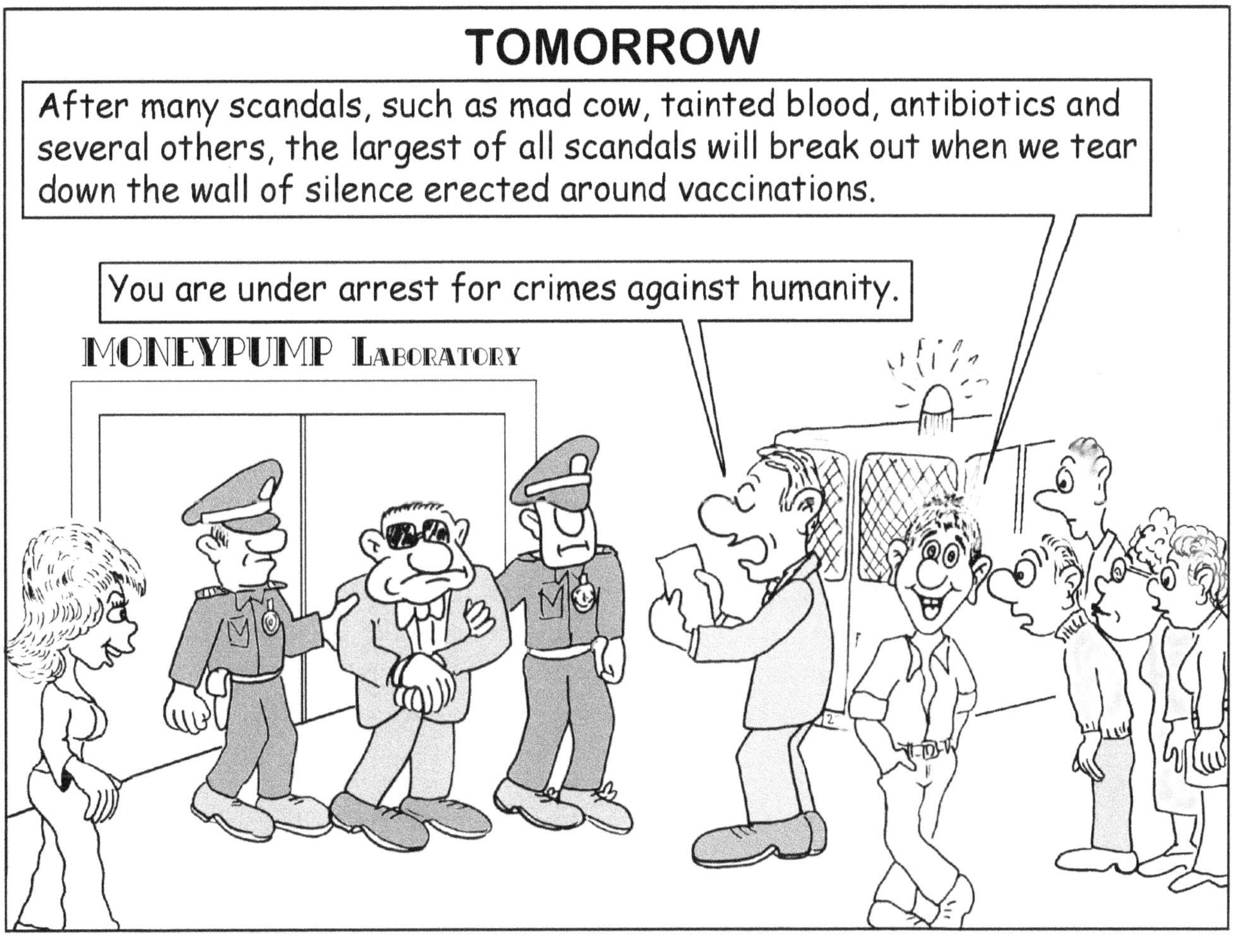

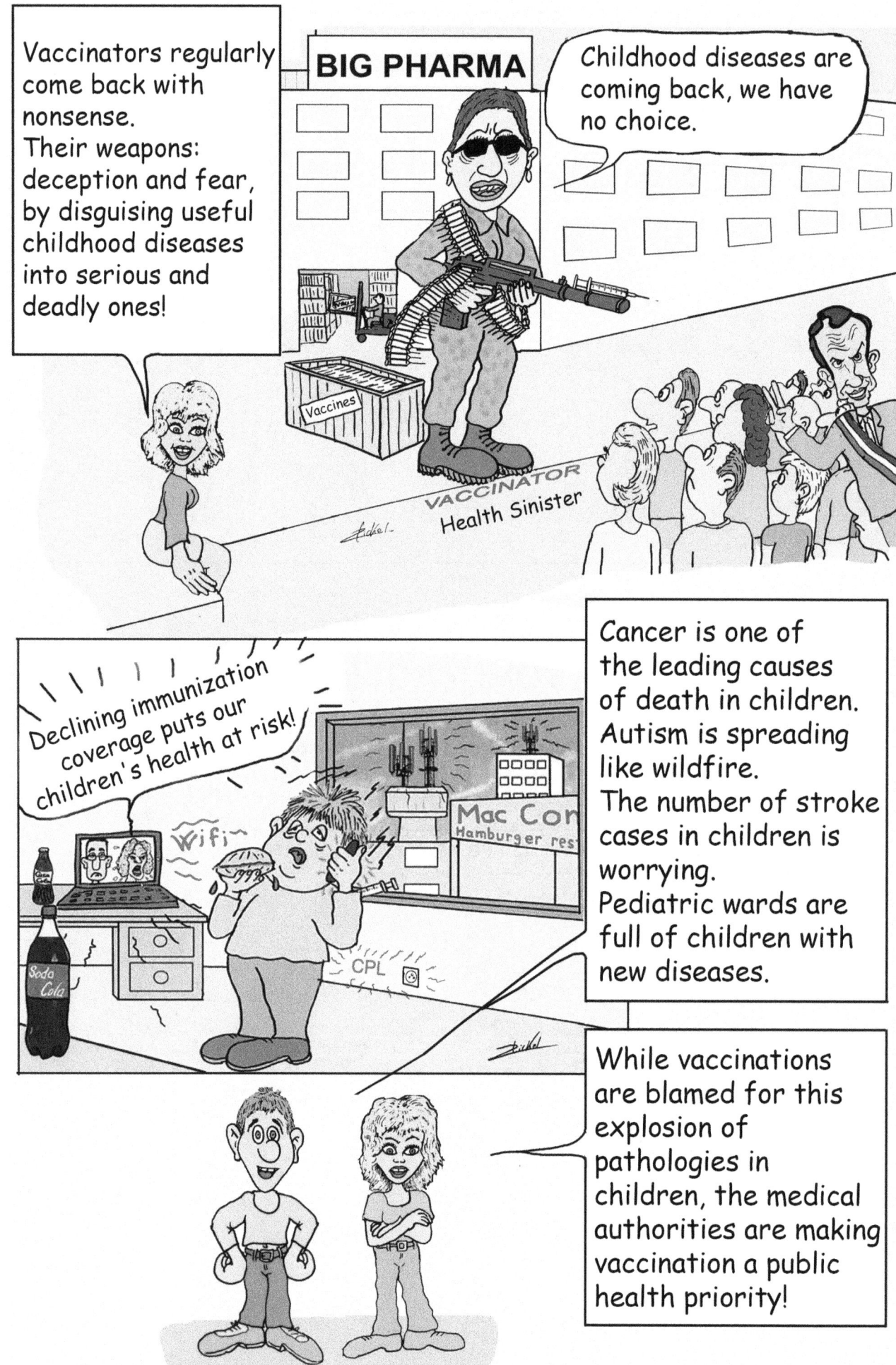

Vaccines: The Great Illusion

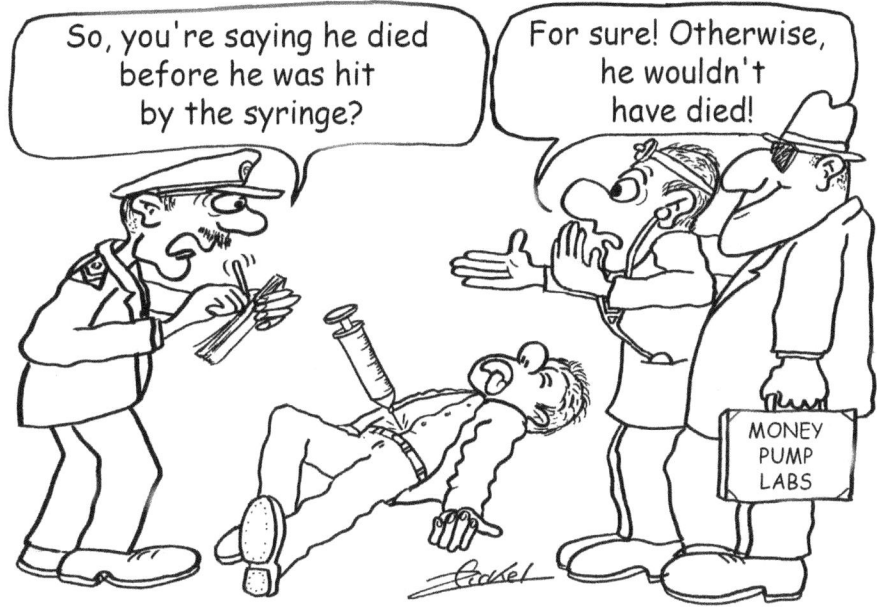

It's easier to fool people than to convince them that they have been fooled.

Attributed to Mark TWAIN

It is not disbelief that is dangerous to our society; it is belief.

George Bernard SHAW

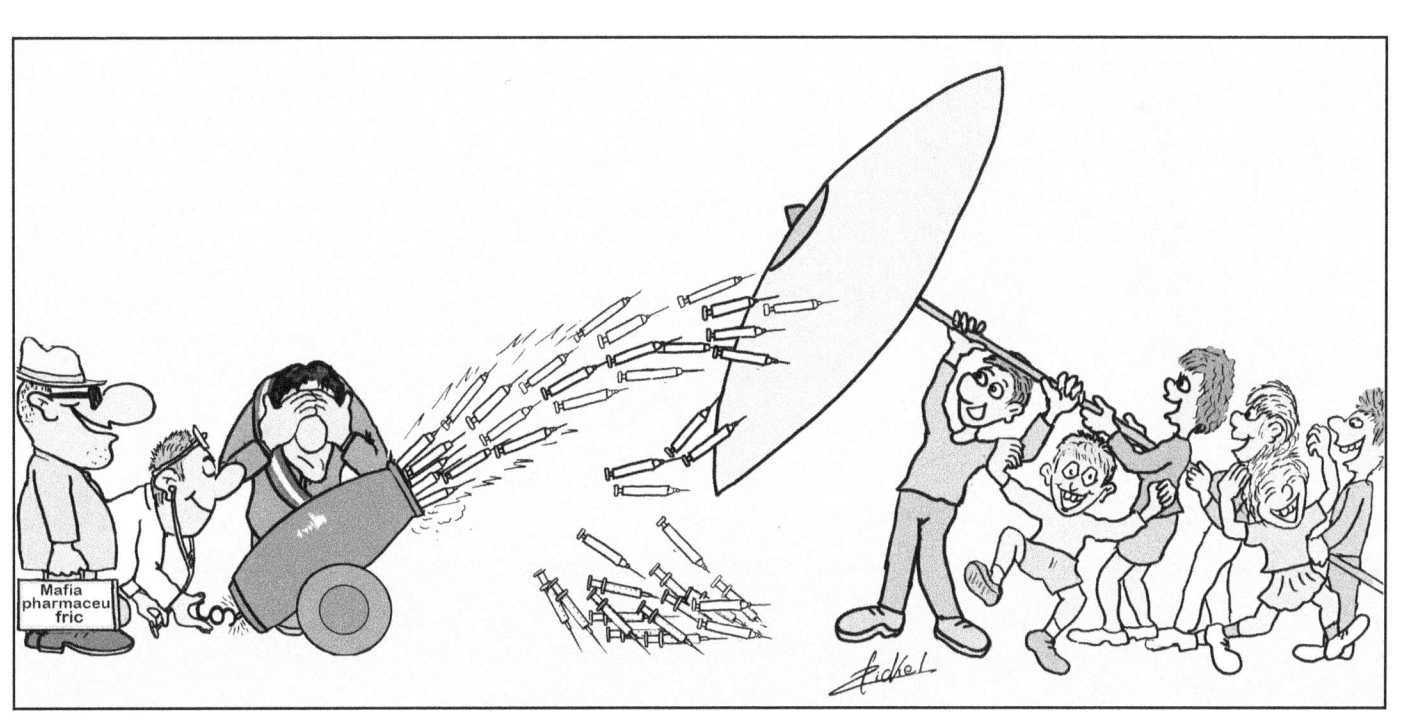

Vaccines: The Great Illusion

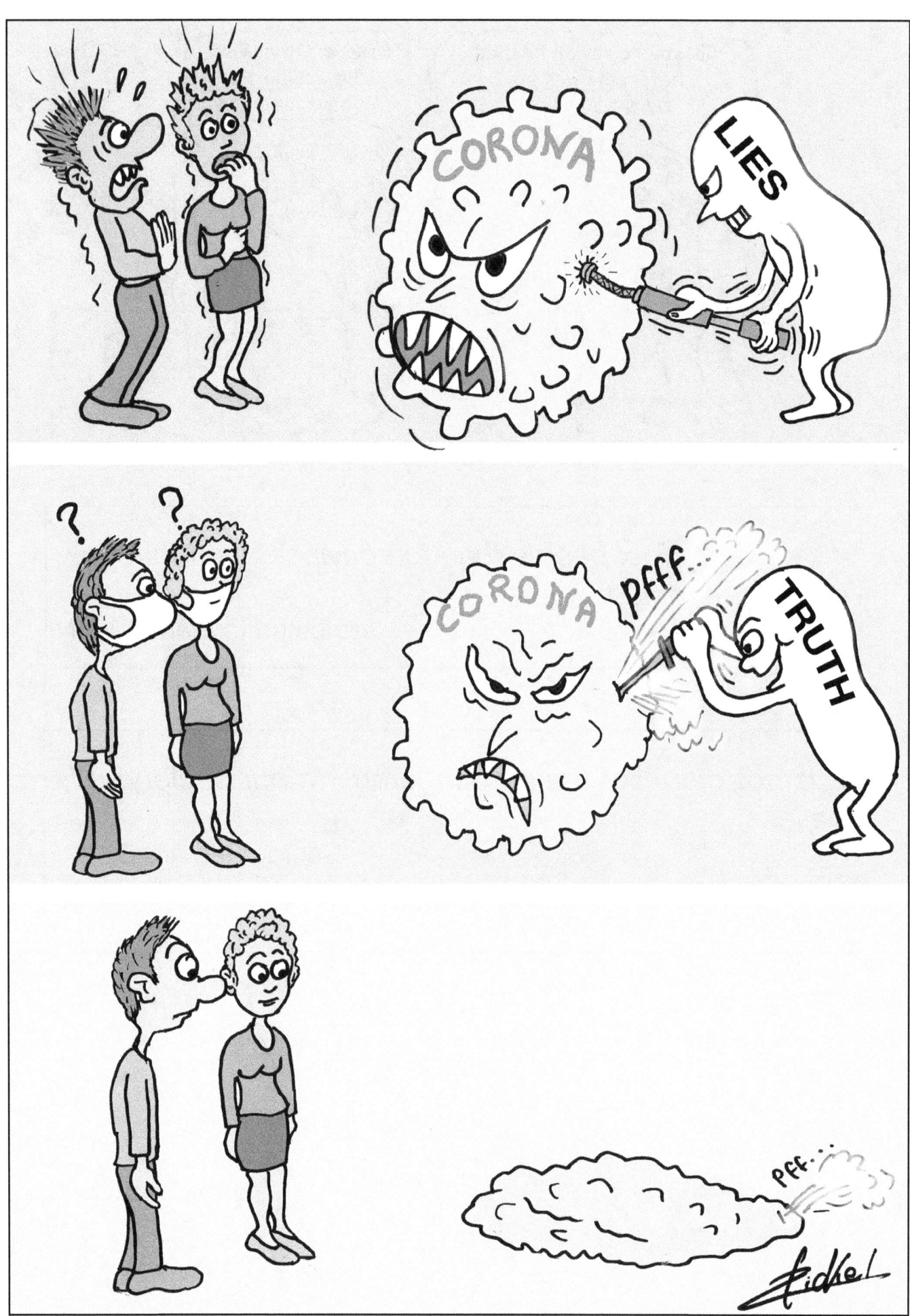

Vaccines: The Great Illusion

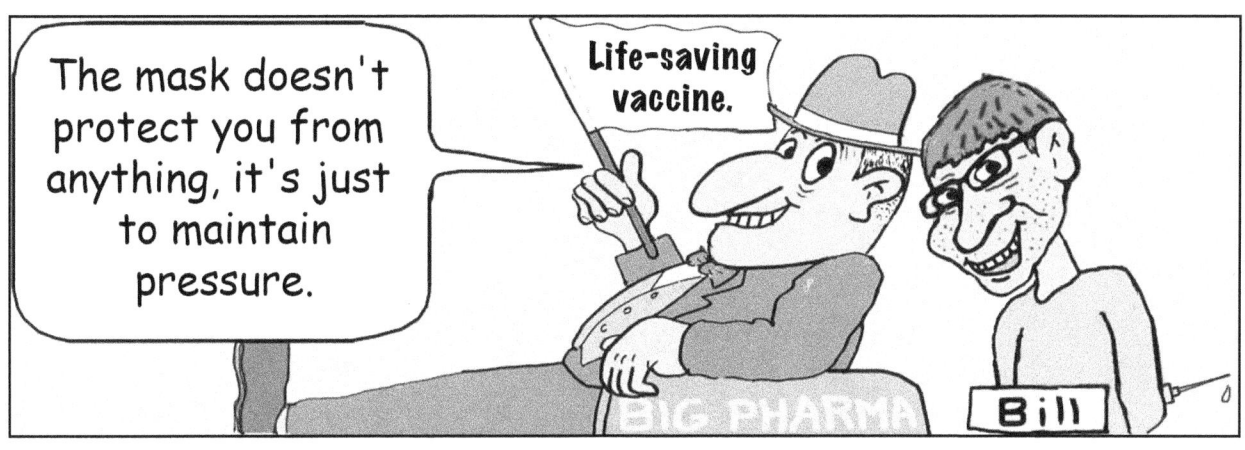

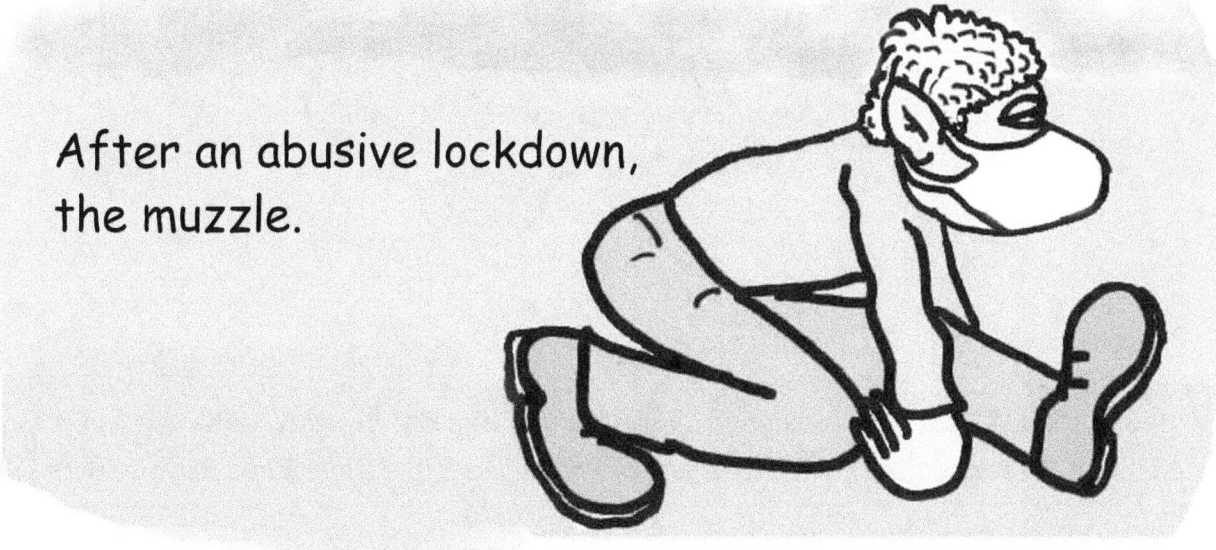

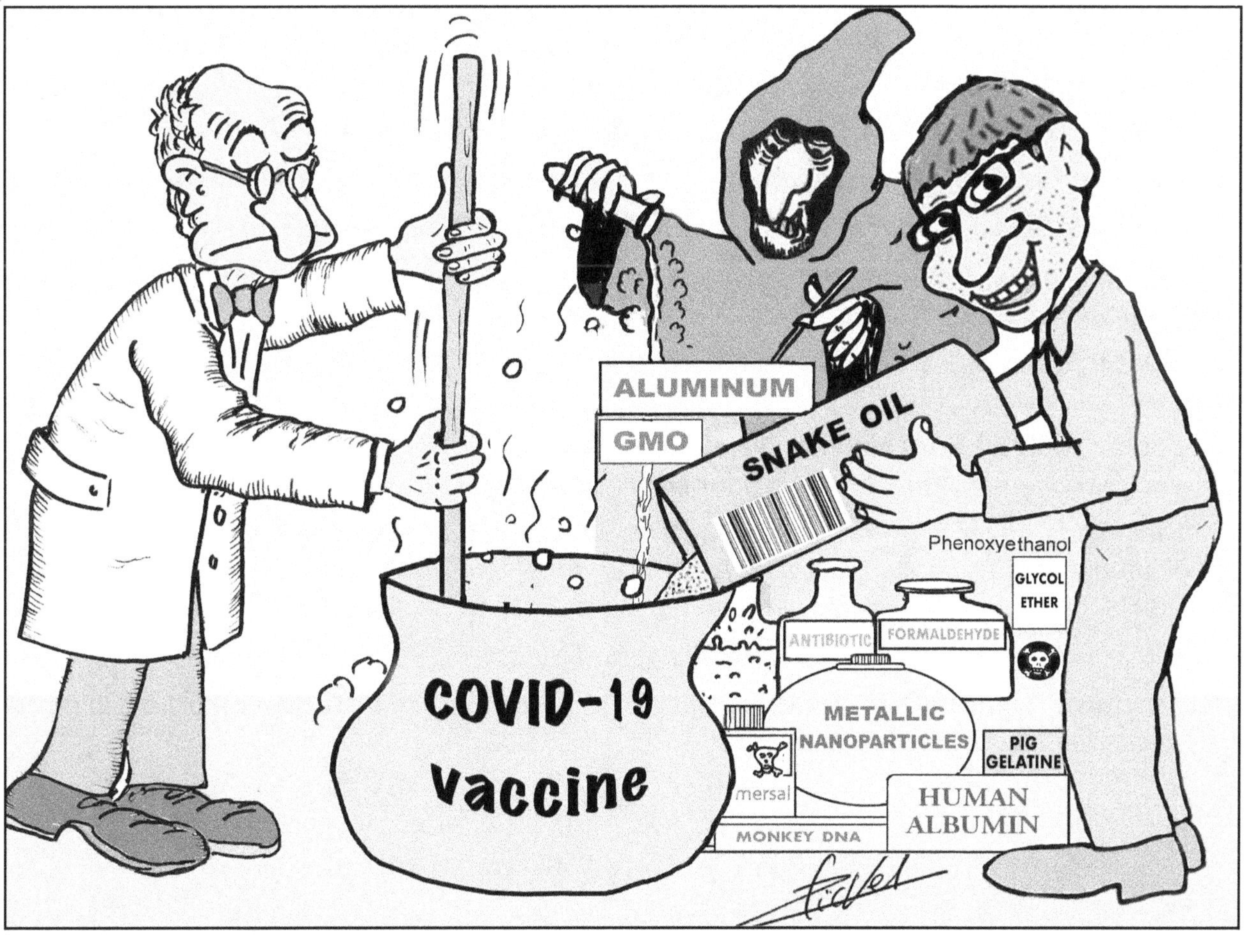

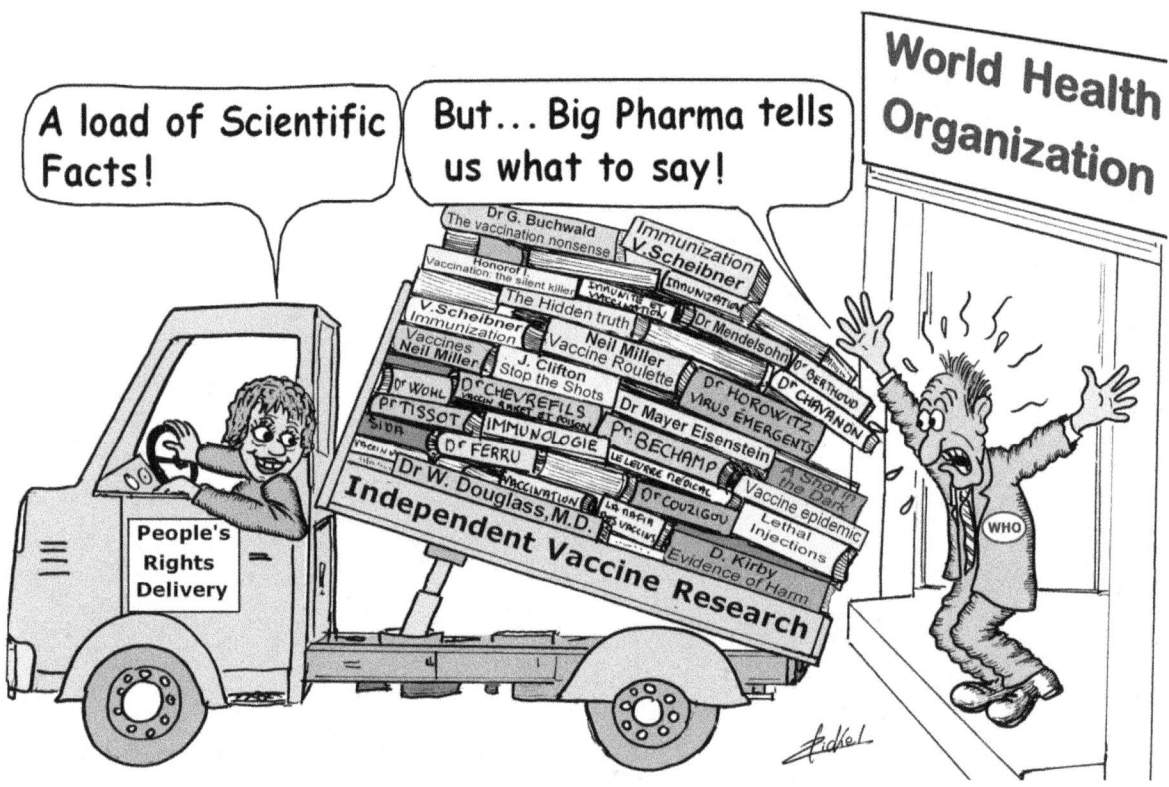

Bibliography

Hodge, John W, MD, *The Vaccination Superstition*, Harvard University 1902

Klenner, Frederick R, MD, *The Treatment of Poliomyelitis and Other Virus Diseases with Vitamin C*, 1949

Rimland, Bernard, PhD, *Infantile Autism: The Syndrome and Its Implications for a Neural Theory of Behavior*, 1964

Honorof, Ida and McBean, E, *Vaccination the Silent Killer, a clear and present danger*, 1977

Mendelsohn, Robert S, MD, *Confessions of a Medical Heretic*, 1979

Mendelsohn, Robert S, MD, *How To Raise a Healthy Child In Spite of Your Doctor*, 1987

Chaitow, Leon, ND DO, *Vaccination and Immunization: Dangers, Delusions and Alternatives*, 1987

James, Walene, Founder of vaclib.org, *Immunization - The Reality behind the myth*, 1988

Douglas Hume, Ethel, *Pasteur Exposed, Germs Genes Vaccines – the false foundations of modern medicine*, 1923-1989

Coulter, Harris L, PhD, *Vaccination, Social Violence and Criminality - the Medical Assault on the American Brain*, 1990

Coulter, Harris L, PhD and Loe Fisher, Barbara, *A shot in the dark - Why the P in the DPT vaccination may be hazardous to your child's health*, 1991

Bird, Christopher, *The Persecution and Trial of Gaston Naessens: The True Story of the Efforts to Suppress an Alternative Treatment for Cancer, AIDS, and Other Immunologically Based Diseases*, 1991

O'Mara, Peggy, Editor, *Vaccinations, The rest of the story*, 1992

Scheibner, Viera, PhD, *Vaccination: 100 years of orthodox research shows that vaccines represent an assault on the immune system*, 1993

Orient, Jane M, MD, *Your Doctor Is Not In*, 1994

Buchwald, Gerhard, MD, *Vaccination, A Business Based on Fear*, 1994

Buttram, Harold E, MD and Hoffman, John C, PhD, *The immune trio - vaccination and Immune Malfunction*, 1995

Lanctot, Guylaine, MD, *The Medical Mafia*, Bridge of Love 1995

Miller, Neil Z., Journalist, *Immunization Theory Vs. Reality: Expose on Vaccinations*, 1995

Duesberg, Peter H, Biologist, *Inventing the AIDS Virus*, 1996

Delong, Richard, Biologist, *Live Viral Vaccines: Biological Pollution*, 1996

Fried, Stephen, Journalist, *Bitter pills - Inside the hazardous world of legal drugs*, 1998

The Australian Vaccination Network, *Vaccination Roulette: Experiences, Risks and Alternatives*, 1998

Appleton, Nancy, PhD, *The Curse of Louis Pasteur*, 1999

Kalokerinos, Archie, MD, *Medical Pioneer of the 20th Century, an autobiography*, 2000

O'Shea, Tim, DC, *The sanctity of human blood - Vaccination is not immunization*, 2001

Rampton, Sheldon and Stauber, John, *Trust us we're experts - How Industry manipulate science and gambles with your future*, 2001

Regush, Nicholas, Journalist, *The Virus Within*, 2001

Whitlock, Chuck, *Mediscams, How to spot & avoid health care scams, medical fraud & quackery from the local physician to the major health care providers & drug manufacturers*, 2001

Cave, Stephanie with Mitchell, Deborah, *What your doctor may not tell you about children's vaccinations*, 2001

Boaz, Noel, *Evolving Health, the origin of sickness and how the modern world is making us sick*, 2002

Appleton, Nancy, PhD, *Rethinking Pasteur's Germ Theory: How to Maintain Your Optimal Health*, 2002

Tenpenny, Sherri J., DO, *Saying No to Vaccines: A Resource Guide for All Ages*, 2008

Elsner, Todd M, DC, *What The Pharmaceutical Companies Don't Want You To Know About VACCINES...*, 2009

Craig, Jennifer, PhD, BSN, MA, Dhom, *Jabs, Jenner and Juggernauts*, 2009

Elmiger, Jean, MD, *The Treatment of Auto-Immune Diseases*, 2010

Dunkelberger, Kathleen, RN BC CLNC, *No Vaccines for Me!*, 2010

Douglas Hume, Ethel, *Béchamp or Pasteur? A lost chapter in the history of Biology*, 1923-2010

Béchamp, Antoine, Professor of Biology, *The Blood and its Third Element*, 1912-2010

Buttram, Harold E, MD and England, Christina, *Shaken Baby Syndrome or Vaccine-Induced Encephalitis?*, 2011

Bachmair, Andreas, Homeopath, *Vaccine Free: 111 Stories of Unvaccinated Children*, 2012

James, Walene, Founder of vaclib.org, *The Vaccine Religion: Mass Mind & The Struggle For Human Freedom*, 2012

Frompovich, Catherine J., Health Researcher & Journalist, *Vaccination Voodoo: What YOU Don't Know About Vaccines*, 2013

www.ingramcontent.com/pod-product-compliance
Lightning Source LLC
LaVergne TN
LVHW080352070526
838199LV00058B/3801